MAKING IT BETTER

MAKING IT BETTER

Gender-Transformative Health Promotion

Edited by

LORRAINE GREAVES, ANN PEDERSON, AND NANCY POOLE

Canadian Scholars' Press
Women's Press
Toronto

Making It Better: Gender-Transformative Health Promotion
Edited by Lorraine Greaves, Ann Pederson, and Nancy Poole

First published in 2014 by
Canadian Scholars' Press Inc./Women's Press
425 Adelaide Street West, Suite 200
Toronto, Ontario
M5V 3C1

www.cspi.org/www.womenspress.ca

Canadian Scholars' Press Inc./Women's Press gratefully acknowledges financial support for our publishing activities from the Government of Canada through the Canada Book Fund (CBF).

Library and Archives Canada Cataloguing in Publication

Making it better : gender-transformative health promotion / edited by Lorraine Greaves, Ann Pederson, and Nancy Poole.

Includes bibliographical references and index. Issued in print and electronic formats.
ISBN 978-0-88961-519-9 (pbk.).—ISBN 978-0-88961-520-5 (pdf).— ISBN 978-0-88961-521-2 (epub)

1. Health promotion. 2. Women—Health and hygiene. I. Greaves, Lorraine, editor II. Pederson, Ann P., editor   III. Poole, Nancy, editor

RA427.8.M23 2014   613'.0424   C2014-904951-X   C2014-904952-8

Text design by Susan MacGregor
Cover design by Gord Robertson

Printed and bound in Canada by Marquis.

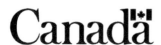

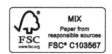

MIX
Paper from
responsible sources
FSC® C103567

Contents

PART 1

PART 2

Foreword

Marilyn Beaumont

In 2008 the Vancouver-based British Columbia Centre of Excellence for Women's Health (BCCEWH) approached Women's Health Victoria (WHV) to collaborate on developing a new approach and framework for health promotion for women. At the time I was the executive director of Women's Health Victoria. We quickly agreed to work together on this project. Six years later, this book is one of the results of that collaboration.

It was not our first collaboration. Our two organizations had worked together since the late 1990s. At the heart of this successful partnership are the different strengths of each organization—BCCEWH's research capacity and WHV's applied health promotion capacity. These strengths are evident in this book, *Making It Better: Gender-Transformative Health Promotion*.

I reflect on my own work over many years in health services and systems after reading this collection. Through my early nursing career I worked with homeless people, including the very young who were escaping difficult backgrounds to live on the streets of our cities. Over time I came to understand that I was providing only temporary solutions, and that individual-level interventions were insufficient. However, the relationships I developed with these girls, women, boys, and men were critically important and supported them as they connected with services to meet their other needs.

I was also involved in services working with women addicted to prescribed drugs. At the time, my curiosity about their access to the drugs led me to collect pharmaceutical industry advertisements from Australian medical journals and newsletters. I was particularly interested in Valium, a "minor" tranquilizer (the serious addictive potential of this drug was only later made clear). The purpose of this advertising—aimed at doctors' prescribing habits—was to increase the sale of Valium. The images in the ads—with the caption "When she can't cope"—were of women lying exhausted over the ironing board in the middle of a chaotic room with clothes and children's toys everywhere. At the time I knew this was wrong, but other than to say this to my colleagues, I had little capacity to raise questions that would change this situation. It seemed too big an issue to tackle, but the stereotyping of women and their poor health service outcomes were clearly linked.

As the secretary of the Australian Nursing Federation in South Australia, I attended the international health promotion conference held in Adelaide in 1988. All facets of my work and personal values came together at that moment. This book refers to this process as connecting "her or his personal and political identities." The Adelaide conference had followed the first International Conference on Health Promotion, which was held in Ottawa in November 1986. Both of these conferences continued the work to strengthen health promotion principles and practice, such as healthy public policy, supportive environments, building healthy alliances, and bridging the equity gap. These principles became the framework for all of my work since. Eventually, the global conversation about the determinants of health emerged, and that cemented this perspective for me.

While leading Women's Health Victoria, I became involved with many challenging health problems and issues for girls and women. As our mandate was focused on program and policy initiatives to better women's health promotion, we had to study the context of women's lives and bring life to a social model of health. Women's Health Victoria and, on the national level, the Australian Women's Health Network (AWHN) both clearly assert that health is created in the places we live and work, in our environment, and in our society.

Indeed, many health issues are socially determined by a mix of structures, systems, and cultural attitudes. Gender is a key and, some assert, a central determinant of health by virtue of the social expectations about what it means to be a woman or a man or a girl or a boy. As a result, the opportunities, role expectations, and subsequent consequences of gendered responsibilities make a huge difference to health.

The health system in most countries is funded predominately to respond to ill health, diseases, or chronic conditions, with only a small amount of funding going toward the prevention of illness, and even less toward health promotion. This is a conundrum for health systems worldwide as they face increasing and spiralling costs that burden national economies.

Globally—not only in Canada and Australia—if there is a desire to "promote health," there is a pressing need to move from a pathology-oriented perspective to one that seeks to explicate the social factors and gendered relational dynamics discussed so well in this book. While the case for working on girls' and women's health is strong, as health providers, program developers, and policy-makers, we must consistently advocate for a women-centred and gendered approach to health. This invariably has to rest on a social model of health, which means more than just paying lip service to the social determinants of health, and generating authentic partnerships with communities.

I was fortunate to lead an organization in the state of Victoria, Australia, that was mandated and funded for health promotion action at the population rather than individual level. Further, advocacy was deemed an essential and positive element of health promotion, unlike in some jurisdictions where advocacy is discouraged in publically funded organizations. This advocacy work is essential for making change in structures, systems, and cultural beliefs, and requires putting resources into key priority areas over a long period of time to achieve sustainable change in health outcomes. Upstream advocacy for change that is efficient, effective, and long lasting, along with innovative knowledge translation, are critical elements of a new gender-transformative health promotion.

This book emphasizes that in order to improve women's health, we must shift more health promotion resources away from a focus on individual behaviour change—which is the current tendency in much health promotion activity—and turn our attention toward critical structural inequities. By addressing these causes, change in women's health and in women's status will be possible. That change is the transformation of traditional gender roles, norms, and structures and will be key in the primary prevention of many girls' and women's health issues.

A central aim is to bring attitudinal and behavioural change at the cultural, institutional, and individual levels, with a particular focus on shifting negative gender norms and behaviours that affect girls and women in health-threatening ways. Addressing violence against women as a key women's health issue (not solely as a criminal or legal or cultural issue) is a good example of this. In Australia, as elsewhere, there has been some success in making this shift. It includes exposing and naming violence-supportive attitudes and behaviours, including those of bystanders. Women's health advocates around the world have worked hard over a sustained period to have mainstream health and well-being agencies, national and international governments, and non-governmental agencies acknowledge that violence against women and girls is a major health issue. Attaining a violence-free life implies equality and freedom from fear and opens up possibilities for girls and women.

Other manifestations of these types of changes include recognition that sexist and misogynistic attitudes are significant drivers of high and unacceptable rates of violence and discrimination toward women and girls. These sorts of attitudes cut off opportunities for women in political life and a range of occupations, and restrict women's freedom of movement and autonomy. Australia's National Plan to Address Violence against Women and Their Children is unprecedented in the way it focuses—across jurisdictions—on preventing violence by raising awareness and building respectful relationships in the next generation.

Advocating for women's equitable participation and engagement in decision-making processes in all spheres of public and private lives is another key manifestation of gender-transformative health promotion. The absence of women in leadership positions is now publicly acknowledged—including by the Australian Institute of Company Directors—as a problem that must be addressed and resolved. In Canada and the United Kingdom there are similar calls to take more aggressive steps to include women as directors. In 2012 the Australian Workplace Gender Equality Agency was established to oversee the establishment of a workplace program to remove the barriers to women entering and advancing in organizations, including in major listed companies and on government and industry boards. The correlation between increased gender equity and improved health with economic development is a key dimension of current thinking.

All of these efforts are continuing despite the violence in our national political discourse, particularly in Australia, which has resulted in international headlines and notoriety over the past few years. As the Australian Women's Health Network's 2012 Position Paper, *Women and Health and Well-Being*, states: "When women are demeaned at work, in their homes or in social situations, gendered social practices are operating to keep women in subordination. Efforts to change these social practices are frequently met with resistance and ridicule which, in turn, produce and reproduce conditions that create unequal conditions or working relationships for women."

Many of us, including myself, have experienced the silencing that happens to us when expressing ideas about gender equity, feminism, or advocating for women's rights. This is also a possibility as we push forward with gender-transformative health promotion work. It is critically important that we do not become discouraged or pressured to choose the "easy" option of focusing on individual behaviours when doing health promotion work, or be satisfied with gender-exploitative or gender-accommodating health promotion. It is also important to consider how men may contribute to gender-transformative health promotion and indeed may also benefit from changing negative and limiting gender norms.

Gender-transformative health promotion aims to redefine harmful gender norms, challenge gender stereotypes, and develop and strengthen equitable gender roles and relationships. Implementing the framework is in the hands of policy-makers, health care practitioners, researchers, communities, and women. This won't happen simply because the evidence for it is overwhelming. As Lorraine Greaves states in Chapter 15, it will happen only through "strategy, imagination, creativity, courage and passion" and, most of all, persistence. This book is a courageous and timely contribution to the evidence base available to us in making this aim a reality.

Marilyn Beaumont is the chairperson of the Australian Women's Health Network and formerly the executive director of Women's Health Victoria, an Australian women's health promotion and advocacy service. Trained as a registered general and mental health nurse, she held several leadership positions in the Australian Nursing Federation and served on the boards of several national health organizations, including the Health Employees Superannuation Trust Australia, the Health Insurance Commission, and the Melbourne Health Board.

Preface

This book is about gender and improving women's health through more effect-ive health promotion. While health promotion is a well-established field of practice, research, and policy, it has lagged in aggressively addressing gender and integrating evidence of sex- and gender-related factors and considerations into its development. Even though the social determinants of health are well recognized as critically important to shaping the opportunity for and access to health, and gender is consistently understood to be one of the social determinants, there has been a critical blind spot in fully considering the implications of sex and gender in a systematic and relevant manner in the practice of health promotion.

This book, aimed at rectifying this oversight, is the culmination of six years of study intended to improve health promotion for women by a two-country, multi-sec-toral, and interdisciplinary team. More effective health promotion for women, if achieved, will have positive effects on health care and health policy, potentially changing their purposes, activities, and scope. More effective health promotion for women and girls will lessen the need for acute women's health care and may high-light and support the need for inter-sectoral policies to enhance health. In addition, achieving improved health for women will also generate individual and social capital, improve child and family health, and improve the level of community health.

In 2008 we established a team of researchers, policy-makers, and practitioners in Canada and Australia to address how health promotion might be made more effect-ive for women and girls. We had a blank slate, but were informed by our collective experiences of how women's health promotion seemed unidimensional and stuck on changing women and their behaviours, as opposed to aiming to change the wider social and economic forces that affect health in ways specific to women and girls.

We were also struck by the lack of gender considerations in health promotion, even though local and international agencies had identified gender as an established and widely identified social determinant of health. But, in practice, we noted that gender, if recognized at all, was often simply acknowledged as one of several determinants of health, often conflated with sex in practice, and rarely conceptually developed and measured with any precision. And perhaps more significantly, critical reflections on the role of gender in health promotion remain, unfortunately, rare. When sex or gender has been considered in health promotion, often it is superficial or, worse, exploitative or reinforces damaging stereotypes.

These concerns led our team to begin with a critique of generic health promotion and its typical gender-blind treatment of women's health. We then progressed to developing a framework and tool for practitioners and policy-makers to use in addressing health promotion for women from a more specific, deeper, and enlightened perspective.

Along the way, we reviewed many approaches to understanding gender, a critical factor in understanding health. We also reviewed how sex and gender are operationalized (or not) in current health promotion and health research. We examined health promotion practices in the form of campaigns, messages, and programs aimed at women and girls, and brought a critical lens to those activities and initiatives. We also engaged with gender theory and the few typologies for understanding gender that have been tendered in the past few years. We engaged with research practices in health promotion, as well as examining health policy and its effects on health promotion for women. We also consulted widely with experts in these areas, along with women in a range of settings, and with decision-makers and health care providers.

We quickly realized that simply doing more to integrate gender into health promotion would not be sufficient to change and improve women's and girls' health. Rather, we realized that to really change women's health and to engage with the gendered effects of the social determinants of health, we had to be explicit about a dual goal. We creatively critiqued a range of health promotion approaches with a view to improving the status of women and girls while simultaneously improving women's health. Throughout, we tried to work out how we could combine these dual goals in both policy and practice. And we tried to work out how to conceptualize this approach in a framework and a planning tool, so that others might more easily take up this dual challenge as well.

As we worked through these processes among our team, and with a widening circle of informants and discussants and women, we turned to numerous cases of health promotion practice to examine and test our ideas. We considered issues such as tobacco control, obesity, physical inactivity, mental health, heart health, alcohol use and misuse, sexual and reproductive health, and violence against women, among others, to determine how health promotion was often conducted and experienced, and how more effective women's health promotion might be different. We also considered how different populations of women and girls differentially experience health and health promotion, and how different settings offer opportunities for improving women's health.

We also encountered health promotion campaigns designed to improve women's health by focusing on men, such as those that engage men in taking responsibility for violence against women. And, as our work progressed, we recognized that gender-transformative approaches to health promotion not only hold promise for women and girls, but also for men and boys. Addressing dual goals in all health promotion activities, not just those that were designed with women in mind, will ultimately advance health for all.

A serious transformation in health promotion practice is long overdue. Similarly, reducing gender inequity in the wider health and social and economic arenas remains a pressing worldwide issue. In our view, these two issues can—and must—be tackled together. The forces that create and perpetuate gender inequities are reflected in women's access to health and health status and then often reflected again in health promotion practices aimed at women. These forces manifest in sexist approaches, gendered assumptions about roles, and disempowering practices. But their roots run deeper in assumptions about male power, privilege, roles, and decision making, and about lesser values and opportunities ascribed to the lives and health of girls and women. In these areas, it is sometimes necessary and relevant to address men and boys about how gendered assumptions may be hindering or helping them achieve health as well. And it goes without saying that if gendered male norms that negatively view or impact women and girls are shifted, then all will benefit: women, men, girls, and boys. There are varied approaches to challenging such norms and values and their related practices. One way is through health promotion.

Lorraine Greaves, Ann Pederson, and Nancy Poole
January 2014

Acknowledgements

This book is one of the results of a program of activity investigating gender and health promotion, with a particular eye to improving women's health. It reflects the work and thinking of a large team of researchers, advisers, and community partners in two countries. As a team comprised of researchers, practitioners, and policy-makers, we took up the challenge of changing the gender blindness of current health promotion discourse, theory, and practice. Funding from the Canadian Institutes of Health Research's Institute of Gender and Health made the creation of our team possible and supported our work for five years under an Emerging Team Grant.

Our activities drew together researchers and community partners from across Canada and beyond. Our key partnership with Women's Health Victoria in Melbourne, Australia, assisted us in garnering the views and participation of many Australian colleagues. Key informants from the United Kingdom also shared their wisdom on health promotion and gender and commented on our framework and planning tool as they emerged.

Our original research team included Lorraine Greaves, Ann Pederson, Nancy Poole, Jan Christilaw, Wendy Frisby, Karin Humphries, Beth Jackson, and Lynne Young. Our trainees included Sue Mills, Pam Ponic, Brenda Kent, and Sirad Deria. Our Advisory Committee included Irv Rootman, Liz Whynot, Joan Geber, Paola Ardiles, Rose Durey, and Petra Begnell. Over the years many staff members and contractors—including Lauren Bialystok, Marie Dussault, Mei Lan Fang, Karen Gelb, Julia Gerbrandt, Natalie Hemsing, Mona Izadnegahdar, Phoebe Long, Rehana Nanjijuma, and Wendy Rice—have greatly assisted in developing our work.

Many thanks to our publisher, Canadian Scholars' Press Inc., especially Nancy Reilly for her help in the early stages of book development, and Daniella Balabuk and Caley Clements for their patience and skill in producing this book. We appreciate their important feedback and enthusiasm for sharing our ideas through this publication.

We thank all of these individuals and agencies, as well as the anonymous key informants, survey respondents, and reviewers of our work as it developed for their insight, interest, and contributions. Many of these colleagues shared with us the desire to improve the way health promotion integrates gender, and welcomed the opportunities to offer suggestions and critiques of existing and future improvements. Our interest in women's health has been sustained over the years through strong partnerships among the Centres of Excellence for Women's Health Program, previously supported by Health Canada, and with women's health advocates, researchers, and policy-makers in Australia. This book was vastly enriched by these relationships.

INTRODUCTION

Raising the Bar
on Women's Health Promotion

Lorraine Greaves

This book is about shifting health promotion practice, policy, and research. It issues a call for not only including gender in health promotion, which in itself would be progress, but also to include gender in thoughtful and transformative ways, so that gendered norms are changed for the better and health is improved for both women and men.

This book is also about improving women's health, status, and empowerment. Women's health has been an expanding field of research, practice, and policy for over two decades and is continuing to grow, inviting an increasingly critical lens. The basic arguments for distinguishing women's health practice, policy, and research from generic or mainstream health practice, policy, or research rest on increasing evidence of the pertinence of sex and gender in determining human health (Oliffe & Greaves, 2011; Wizemann & Pardue, 2001).

Both sex and gender affect health. Over the past decade and a half, sex (the biological aspects of health and bodies) and gender (the social, economic, and cultural aspects of being female or male) have emerged as critically important factors affecting trajectories of disease, access to health care, responses to health and social policy, the design and interpretation of research, and women's overall opportunities for health. Clearly, sex and gender also affect men's and boys' health, but addressing girls' and women's health is critically important for the health and well-being of individuals, families, children, and communities, and has become a priority for global development, both economic and social (see, for example, Action for Global Health, n.d.).

In real life, gender is complicated: it is always in motion, culturally specific and temporal, always developing, difficult to measure, and cross-cuts other determinants and factors that affect health (Johnson, Greaves, & Repta, 2009). Gender is a

1

challenged and challenging construct. These factors undoubtedly make it difficult to include gender in research, practice, or policy developments affecting women's health. But even recognition of gender's complexities was, and is, mostly missing from health promotion practice, research, and related policy. This has been a serious omission from the literature and practice, perpetuated despite rapid developments in the past 10 years in sex and gender theory, measurement, and conceptualization, with many applied resources made available to the public, researchers, practitioners, and policy-makers intended to assist in integrating gender in health promotion and health more generally (Clow, Pederson, Haworth-Brockman, & Bernier, 2009; Johnston, Greaves, & Repta, 2007; Oliffe & Greaves, 2011; Pederson, Hankivsky, Morrow, & Greaves, 2003). But the field of health promotion, with a few exceptions, has been slow to engage with these developments and ideas (Gelb, Pederson, & Greaves, 2012).

As one of the social determinants of health, gender cross-cuts all of the other biological and social determinants that construct human health. Gender influences education, income, reproductive roles, and caring responsibilities, among other determinants, all areas where, globally, women and girls often experience inequities or specific biological processes that directly affect their health. Moreover, ongoing serious gender inequities that persist around the world and victimize women disproportionately, such as interpersonal violence and sexual assault, highlight the critical need for blending the design of health promotion with clear and conscious goals of empowerment and gender transformation.

Much of what passes for gender considerations in health promotion is often only lip service to sex-based demographic categories or the reflection of uniform notions of women (or men) based on fixed attitudes or beliefs. While these mistakes may be excused as reflecting prevailing evidence and practice, these assumptions also often inform research, creating loops of evidence to practice that are misinformed or based on prevailing fixed assumptions about what gender means when it comes to women's health. For example, the assumption that women and girls are concerned about and motivated by their appearance has informed many a health promotion campaign, from obesity control to physical activity to alcohol and tobacco use. And this assumption creates more campaigns based on the same assumption, reinforcing girls' and women's views of their appearance as motivation and feeding the evidence wheel by setting up research questions to examine these links.

It is hard to break these cycles of thinking, but in this book we try to do that by examining how to address gender as a component affecting women's and girls' health from a different viewpoint. In creating the framework for this book, we asked ourselves a series of questions, including how to measure and take note of gendered assumptions, how we in health promotion might be perpetuating some gendered assumptions, and how we might channel the use of gender analyses to create new pathways to health for women and new approaches to health promotion for practitioners. These are difficult questions as they force us to turn many assumptions about women, girls, and health promotion on their heads, and to generate a collective understanding of the meaning of typical health promotion and its impact on the dual goals of improving women's status as well as women's health.

A range of experts in various countries have recently addressed the needs in women's health. For example, Garcia et al. (2010) reviewed the progress and priorities in girls' and women's health in the United States, reflecting on two decades of activity. An expert interdisciplinary panel representing 48 Centers of Excellence in Women's Health was assembled and concluded that individual-level interventions were insufficient, and endorsed a preventive health promotion approach that addressed the social determinants of health. In particular, increased empowerment of women and measures of health education, interpersonal violence, and access to health care were identified as the most important indicators of change.

In 2009, Armstrong and Deadman edited a book on the state of women's health research, policy, and practice in Canada (Armstrong & Deadman, 2009). They stressed the importance of carrying out gender-based analyses of every health issue, policy, or initiative, as well as analyzing the gendered nature of the health care workforce, concluding that much remains to be done to advance women's health practices. In that book I noted (Greaves, 2009) that the definitions of women's health in Canada emerged via a strong women's health movement that began in the 1970s, initially in reaction against forces such as medicalization, paternalism, lack of health information, consent, and inclusion, as well as general sexism in social norms and values that expressed themselves in health care, research, and policy.

A similar history of women's activism arising in reaction to a lack of information and poor health care led the way to significant changes in women's health in Australia. Gwen Gray Jamieson (2012) charted the detailed history of the effects of the movement on public policy in Australia, culminating in the first National Women's Health Policy in 1989. The National Policy incorporated several advances, notably a social model of health, women's participation in decision making, less focus on reproduction, and improved research. Among the highlighted priorities were, significantly, issues such as violence against women and the effects of sex-role stereotyping. These shifts resulted in changes in practice such as separate women's health services and mainstreaming of better practices on issues such as rape crisis. The National Women's Health Policy was renewed in 2012, with a new focus on health inequity, health issues among different groups of women, and prevention.

In a cogent summary of ethnographic themes that have emerged in women's health in a range of countries, most with incomes lower than those in the United States, Canada, and Australia, Marcia Inhorn (2006) points to the health issues that women themselves have identified as important. Central to these is the power to define one's own health as a woman, nodding to the persistence of lists of women's health issues that reflect medical, disease, or body-related issues while ignoring the social context of women's lives. The essentializing of women's reproductive capacities and the ignoring of men's roles in reproduction, along with the ongoing cultural definitions of women's bodies, are all critically important (and ignored) critiques of how women's health is currently defined. But the effects of the hegemony of biomedicine and the widespread negative health effects of patriarchy further define and limit the definition of women's health. Inhorn calls for more input from women in "defining" women's health, and more ethnography with women to uncover this input.

Overarching these country-based efforts and ethnographic forays are global and international documents that specifically guide the field of women's health, sometimes through a "gender" lens, such as those of the World Health Organization (WHO). For example, the WHO Gender Policy (World Health Organization, 2002) identifies the right to health for all and the factors determining health and illness between women and men, including the impact of resource allocation, decision making, and access to care. It further reflects on unequal gender relations and their interactions with social and economic variables, which contribute to increased risks to health.

A set of global documents also frame and inform the field of health promotion, such as the Ottawa and Bangkok charters (World Health Organization, 1986, 2005), among others. These charters outline grand perspectives on health promotion, bringing forward the importance of the field, as well as the notions of linkages with other structures that produce the opportunity for health. The Ottawa Charter, developed in 1986, promised considerable reorientation of health promotion efforts by pledging to create positive action in five areas: healthy public policy, supportive environments, community actions, personal skills, and health services. Significantly, the Ottawa Charter makes the explicit point that "those involved should take as a guiding principle that, in each phase of planning, implementation and evaluation of health promotion activities, women and men should become equal partners." The Ottawa Charter was intended to instigate action to achieve "Health for All" by the year 2000 and beyond, and was widely influential in promoting health promotion and integrating it into public health practice. A critical dimension of the Ottawa Charter was that it "emphasizes the relationship between an individual and their broader social context, as well as the notion of health equity" (Gelb et al., 2012), concepts that highlight the importance of structural factors on health, and implicitly engage with the effects of gender.

The Bangkok Charter took a different approach, noting that "the global context for health promotion has changed markedly since the development of the Ottawa Charter" and focusing on the effects of globalization on health. As Gelb et al. (2012) note, "The Bangkok Charter departs from the Ottawa Charter dramatically in that it introduces the private sector into the conversation, suggesting that building partnerships and alliances with the private sector is a required strategy for health promotion in a globalized world" (p. 450). Porter applied a critical discourse analysis to both of these important documents and concluded that the Ottawa Charter exhibited a "new social movements" discourse, compared to the "new capitalism" discourse of "law and economics in Bangkok" (Porter, 2007, p. 75). This change is illustrated by a shift from themes of "democratization, equity and diversity" in the Ottawa Charter, to a more economic and rational approach in the Bangkok Charter (Porter, 2007). The implications of this shift, according to Porter, is that the progressive, community-building, equity-oriented formulations underpinning the Ottawa Charter were lost in favour of regulation and legislation, thereby reinforcing, rather than changing, the structures affecting health (p. 78).

Early in our work, we reviewed these two charters and three other key health promotion documents released between 1974 and 2010 to assess their consideration and treatment of gender (Gelb et al., 2012). To our dismay, we discovered that these main tropes in health promotion were paying only lip service, at best, to gender and its integration into health promotion practice and research. Specifically, gender was generally excluded in health promotion frameworks, creating a blind spot, given that gender is one of the key social determinants of health affecting numerous aspects of health promotion, such as access to and control over resources, information, and education.

When gender was considered, its complexity typically went unaddressed and remained only superficially understood. For example, sex and gender were considered most often in reproductive health and sexual health and HIV/AIDS, where a more direct link between sex, gender, and health can easily be drawn. However, limiting the integration and consideration of gender to such issues is insufficient. We concluded that health promotion that "does not acknowledge the specific needs of women and men will not ultimately be able to provide health for all" (Gelb et al., 2012, p. 446), particularly when the complexities of gender were not considered as foundational concepts or variables. In fact, in these key documents, gender was never identified as critical to successful health promotion, contrary to significant scholarship and practice on the myriad effects of gender, gender relations, institutional gender, and gender roles on health (see, for example, Johnson et al., 2007; Keleher, 2004).

The WHO Commission on Social Determinants of Health was carried out between 2005 and 2008, constituting an all-important stage setting for the integration of the social determinants into health promotion, health care, and health reform (Commission on Social Determinants of Health, 2008). This commission, led by Sir Michael Marmot, raised the profile of the impact of social determinants on health and has had a direct and positive effect on the content of the global conversation about health inequities. The commission called for an end to health inequity in a generation, and highlighted the unequal distribution of power and resources as an issue. Within this category, the commission recommended that gender equity be promoted through enforceable legislation.

In order to delve into the impact of gender more thoroughly, the WHO Commission included a Women and Gender Equity Knowledge Network, which submitted a final report in 2007 (Sen & Östlin, 2007). This report boldly states that "gender inequality damages the health of millions of girls and women across the globe" (p. xii). Sen and Östlin go on to say that "taking action to improve gender equity in health and to address women's rights to health is one of the most direct and potent ways to reduce health inequities and ensure effective use of health resources" (p. xii). Sen and Östlin zero in on gender relations as the pivot on which inequality balances as they shape everyday experiences of health and access to health care, and reflect power distributions in society.

Our team approached our critique of women's health promotion in this context of 40 years of health promotion, global leadership on social determinants, and a key report on gender as a social determinant of health. We reflected on emergent understandings of women's health, gender as a key cross-cutting social determinant of health, and how gender manifests and affects everyday life. We critique current health promotion practices and related policy and research, and propose transformative changes that not only include gender, but do so in progressive and innovative ways, paving the way for a dual transformation. We created a conceptual framework to guide future health promotion by focusing on both improving women's health as well as women's status by specifically interrogating gender and pointedly focusing on diminishing the effects of negative gender norms. We hope that our proposal for gender-transformative health promotion points the way to a refreshed goal of health promotion for women. Ultimately, we hope our vision for gender-transformative health promotion sees action in the field.

This transformative vision has several elements. We are focused on shifting the gaze in health promotion from the individual—from exhorting women to change their behaviours or to adopt particular lifestyle changes in order to be healthy—to generating a shared social responsibility for women's health. We are interested in generating an understanding of the impact of structural factors affecting women's health—those factors that remain out of an individual's control, yet profoundly affect health—and to figure out how to shift attention to changing them. We are drawing attention to the inequities of both structures and experiences that are aligned with gender in all of its manifestations.

We are also consistently explicit about the dual goals of improving women's status along with women's health, and suggesting concrete steps and mechanisms for planning and translating these notions into action in health promotion. All of these elements inspired us to create a new framework and a planning tool to systematically address these concerns, and to inspire others to do the same. At root is the explicit and integrated aim of not only changing health outcomes for women and girls, but also changing negative gender norms and practices that contribute to women's and girls' inequity. This is the essence of gender-transformative health promotion.

In 2014, there are still serious and ongoing gender inequities in the economic, social, and health status of girls and women when compared to men and boys, despite progress toward global gender equity in many areas. The links between women's health and economic and social development are still being studied and drawn, but there is an increasing focus on the impact of gender equity and girls' and women's empowerment on health and economic well-being as a critical factor in development. And, as Sen and Östlin (2007) indicate, not only is gendered health inequity unfair and unequal, it is also inefficient and a poor use of health care resources.

This correlation of increased gender equity and improved health with economic development is a key dimension of current thinking. Countries that have intervened to generate empowerment for women in decision making have reported improved health among children, and better disease control and sanitation (CARE International, 2012). CARE International carried out a program in Bangladesh to increase women's empowerment on three levels: individual, structural, and interpersonal. Everyday experiences were challenged and changed by direct interventions on issues such as access to schools and private sanitation for girls and women; discussing domestic violence and confronting street harassment; gaining access to money and the marketplace; and challenging laws and cultural pressures that encourage child marriage, curtail freedom of movement, and limit decision-making powers. CARE International (2012) reports empirical evidence linking these interventions to increased nutrition in women, reduced childhood malnutrition, and healthier newborns. Most important, though, is that women's leadership opportunities had a direct influence on their health by generating more self- and community respect for their roles in the family and community.

It is now generally understood that "in poor countries … the under-utilization of women stunts economic growth" and that educating girls "is probably the single best investment that can be made in the developing world" ("Women and the World Economy," 2006). But even in higher income countries there is increasing attention to women's economic equality and economic progress as key indicators of national development. The World Economic Forum measures these linkages in its annual Global Gender Gap reports (Hausmann, Tyson, & Zahidi, 2012), which index progress in all countries on four main pillars, one of which is "health and survival." The index measures health and survival using two measures: sex ratios at birth and life expectancy. In 2012, it again reported a strong correlation between global competitiveness and a country's gender gap.

These examples illustrate that there are payoffs to societies that embrace women's talents by increasing the value placed on women's and girls' lives, increasing opportunities for education and employment for females, and generating cultural shifts in gender norms and practices governing issues such as independence, violence, harassment, and freedom of movement. These initiatives offer hope for both women's status and women's health and point to the importance of pursuing improvements in both at once. They also illustrate the profound shifts required in politics, culture, society, and the economy to achieve improvements in gender equity and women's health.

It is clear that it is not enough to aspire to the goal of simply integrating gender into health promotion by slipping awareness and increased quality processes into program and policy development, or by improving research methods and designs in health promotion research. While these improvements are necessary, they are not sufficient for achieving the dual goals of improving women's health and status concurrently. Rather, the integration of gender must be purposeful and transformative, aimed at changing negative gender norms by questioning and challenging them as an integral goal and aspect of health promotion practice, policy, and intervention.

Although gender-based inequities and problems may appear more stark in some societies than others, similar mechanisms function around the globe to keep women and girls in particular positions so that they are confined to specified roles, enjoy less power as a group, and often have limited aspirations when compared to men and boys. For example, gendered assumptions are supported by socialization that ascribes more caretaking and housekeeping roles to girls and women and encourages women (and men) to internalize gendered assumptions that further define and demarcate social roles, thus complicating efforts to transform gender and health promotion. Further to our example about exploiting women's aspirations of external beauty to motivate changes in their health behaviour, it may well be that such efforts "succeed" as they fall on willing and ready ears, sensitized by gender role socialization.

To explore these issues more fully, this book is divided into three sections. Part 1 introduces in detail the issues of gender, women's health, and health promotion.

The inadequacies of current health promotion and the specific needs of women and girls for a different health promotion approach are articulated along with the process and content of the development of our gender-transformative health promotion framework. Gender theories are reviewed and accessed to bring a wider and deeper understanding to an improved health promotion for women, and a range of options in incorporating gender into health promotion are assessed.

We document how we engaged with many partners and stakeholders to develop the framework for gender-transformative health promotion, and what methods and media we used in doing so. We complete this section with a consideration of two key elements of women's health promotion. First, the intersectional nature(s) of health and gender with factors and characteristics such as ethnicity, age, culture, class, and disability, recognizing the intricacies of multiple and cross-cutting pressures and opportunities for women to achieve health and access health care and promotion. Second, we delve into theories of power, recognizing that within this arena are some of the key issues and potential solutions to generating not just better health promotion for women, but also improved status and ultimately gender transformation.

In Part 2 we examine a range of health issues and more deeply illustrate the state of health promotion in examples affecting the health of, and health promotion with, women. Each of the cases considered in this section presents a different scenario: different assumptions, norms and values, and histories and external factors surrounding the case or issue, different populations of women, or different settings. The many different and multiple locations occupied by women reflecting complex and multifaceted lives are investigated, but the essential threads of sex and gender woven throughout the cases are recognized as defining and pivotal themes.

A number of points of contrast and comparison surface in these cases: differing levels of assignation of women's responsibility for their condition and their responsibility for change; differing stigmatizing forces from society at large; differing assumptions about women's roles in each of these; and differing levels of knowledge regarding the influence of sex and gender. These cases also show how gender, or some understanding of gender, has been used historically to either encourage or discourage practices and behaviours among women and girls, whether health promoting or not. These cases also illustrate how gender-transformative health promotion might assist in improving women's health, in different ways and using different approaches, depending on the case and context. In this section we examine issues such as tobacco and alcohol use, preconception and maternity care, physical activity, and mental health promotion.

Part 3 addresses the many complex issues in going forward. What knowledge translation challenges might be either obstacles or opportunities for generating support and understanding for gender-transformative health promotion? How can knowledge translation itself be gender-transformative? What key ingredients and qualities should it have? And how should men be engaged in gender-transformative health promotion?

There are growing calls for men's involvement in issues affecting women's health. We present one such project where men in their workplace were directly engaged in reducing violence against women. Engaging men raises some key questions, however. How do men figure into improvements in women's health promotion, and is it the responsibility of the women's health movement to integrate and create opportunities for men to engage? Should scarce resources for women be expended on initiatives to engage men? These questions are critically important and arise with some frequency, highlighting interesting and provocative arguments. We also consider how health promotion and gender have been considered in the hospital setting by presenting reflections from a former leader of a women's hospital. These chapters raise numerous issues about institutional and organizational cultures and how they may provide opportunities or create barriers to introducing considerations of gender and gender-transformative health promotion.

We conclude with a review of potential options for pursuing changes in gender and health promotion in the wider spheres—the community, state, province, nation, or worlds—and what influences might be shaping ongoing pressures and new opportunities for generating more gender-transformative health promotion. There is no doubt that generating a clear understanding of gender-transformative health promotion, and making that case simply and realistically, is the first and most basic challenge. Further to that, collecting useful data to inform health promotion practice, intervention development, and research is essential in building the case for a more effective, refined, and complex view of gender and its place in health promotion. Specifically, developing more nuanced indicators of both gender and transformative processes such as empowerment and freedom of movement so that changes can be more accurately measured is a critical challenge.

Our call is for new thinking in health promotion (Pederson et al., 2010). First, the inclusion of a sex, gender, and diversity analysis is essential to fully understand the complexities and cross-cutting effects of gender and other social factors. Second, key to a progressive and critical health promotion is serious engagement with the debate about the balance and/or impact of women's agency respecting health and health behaviours versus the structural factors affecting women's health that often lie beyond an individual's control. Third, a significant broadening of "what counts as evidence" in generating knowledge about gender and health promotion is long overdue, as Inhorn (2006) and Armstrong and Deadman (2009), among many others, have long argued. Women themselves have considerable knowledge about their health and how to improve it, but such knowledge is rarely tapped or respected.

Finally, innovative knowledge exchange that calls for true engagement with and among women, researchers, and practitioners in a spirit of co-developing more inspired gender-transformative health promotion is critical to the ongoing project of improving women's health. This is a creative as well as a scientific challenge. There is no doubt that the shift we envisage in creating gender-transformative health promotion is progressive, but it is a shift that will in key ways harken back to the social and equity goals embedded in early health promotion documents and the engagement processes first developed in the women's movements of the 1970s, yet with more sophisticated understandings and measures of gender woven in.

A focus on including gender in health promotion for women is long overdue. In particular, reducing gender inequity in health and social and economic arenas is a worldwide issue requiring immediate action. Women especially will benefit from successful gender-transformative health promotion. Gender inequity thrives on exploitation, power imbalances, history, and culture, and operates through limits on decision making and access to resources such as money, land, or positions of authority, all of which affect health and well-being. There are varied approaches to challenging such norms and values and their associated practices. One way is through health promotion.

REFERENCES

Action for Global Health. (n.d.). Engendering global health. Retrieved from www.action-forglobalhealth.eu/uploads/media/Engendering_Global_Health.pdf

Armstrong, P., & Deadman, J. (Eds.). (2009). *Women's health: Intersections of policy, research, and practice.* Toronto: Women's Press.

CARE International. (2012). Reaching new heights: The case for measuring women's empowerment. Retrieved from www.care.org/getinvolved/iwd/images/CARE_IWD_2012.pdf

Clow, B., Pederson, A., Haworth-Brockman, M., & Bernier, J. (2009). *Rising to the challenge: Sex and gender-based analysis for health planning, policy, and research in Canada.* Halifax: Atlantic Centre of Excellence for Women's Health.

Commission on Social Determinants of Health. (2008). *Closing the gap in a generation: Health equity through action on the social determinants of health.* Final report of the Commission on Social Determinants of Health. Geneva: World Health Organization.

Garcia, F., Freund, K. M., Berlin, M., Digre, K., Dudley, D., Fife, R. S., & … White, H. (2010). Progress and priorities in the health of women and girls: A decade of advances and challenges. *Journal of Women's Health, 19*(4), 671–680.

Gelb, K., Pederson, A., & Greaves, L. (2012). How have health promotion frameworks considered gender? *Health Promotion International, 27*(4), 445–452. doi:10.1093/heapro/dar08

Gray Jamieson, G. (2012). *Reaching for health: The Australian women's health movement and public policy.* Canberra: Australian National University Press.

Greaves, L. (2009). Women, gender, and health research. In P. Armstrong & J. Deadman (Eds.), *Women's health: Intersections of policy, research, and practice* (pp. 3–20). Toronto: Women's Press.

Hausmann, R., Tyson, L., & Zahidi, S. (2012). *The global gender gap report 2012.* Cologny/Geneva: World Economic Forum.

Inhorn, M. (2006). Defining women's health: A dozen messages from more than 150 ethnographies. *Medical Anthropology Quarterly, 20*(3), 345–378.

Johnson, J. L., Greaves, L., & Repta, R. (2007). *Better science with sex and gender: A primer for health research.* Vancouver: Women's Health Research Network.

Johnson, J. L., Greaves, L., & Repta, R. (2009). Better science with sex and gender: Facilitating the use of a sex- and gender-based analysis in health research. *International Journal for Equity in Health, 8*(14). doi:10:486/1475-9276-8-14

Keleher, H. (2004). Why build a health promotion evidence base about gender? *Health Promotion International, 19*(3), 277–279.

Oliffe, J. L., & Greaves, L. (Eds.). (2011). *Designing and conducting gender, sex, and health research.* Thousand Oaks, CA: Sage Publications.

Pederson, A., Hankivsky, O., Morrow, M., & Greaves, L. (2003). *Exploring concepts of gender and health.* Ottawa: Women's Health Bureau, Health Canada.

Pederson, A., Ponic, P. L., Greaves, L., Mills, S., Christilaw, J. E., Frisby, W., … Young, L. (2010). Igniting an agenda for health promotion for women: Critical perspectives, evidence-based practice, and innovative knowledge translation. *Canadian Journal of Public Health, 101*(3), 259–262.

Porter, C. (2007). Ottawa to Bangkok: Changing health promotion discourse. *Health Promotion International, 22*(1), 72–79.

Sen, G., & Östlin, P. (2007). Unequal, unfair, ineffective, and inefficient. Gender inequity in health: Why it exists and how we can change it. Final report to the WHO Commission on Social Determinants of Health, Women and Gender Equity Knowledge Network. Geneva: World Health Organization.

Wizemann, T. M., & Pardue, M.-L. (Eds.). (2001). *Exploring the biological contributions to human health: Does sex matter?* Washington, DC: National Academy of Sciences.

Women and the world economy: A guide to womenomics. (April 12, 2006). Retrieved from www.economist.com/node/6802551

World Health Organization. (1986). Ottawa Charter for health promotion. *Canadian Journal of Public Health, 77*(6), 425–430.

World Health Organization. (2002). WHO gender policy: Integrating gender perspectives in the work of WHO. Geneva: World Health Organization.

World Health Organization. (2005). The Bangkok Charter for health promotion in a globalized world [Editorial]. *Health Promotion Journal of Australia, 16*(3), 168–171.

PART 1

1 Envisioning Gender-Transformative Health Promotion

Ann Pederson, Nancy Poole, Lorraine Greaves,
Julieta Gerbrandt, and Mei Lan Fang[1]

In 2000, Geeta Rao Gupta challenged the audience at the 13th International AIDS Conference in Durban, South Africa, to consider the ways that gender norms, roles, and relations contributed to furthering the HIV/AIDS epidemic. Building on work she had done examining HIV interventions (Gupta & Weiss, 1993), Gupta argued that those offering prevention, diagnostic, and treatment programs for HIV/AIDS needed to understand how their efforts may exploit, accommodate, or transform the gender norms, roles, and relations that put men and women at risk for contracting HIV, infecting others, and/or seeking diagnostic or treatment services: "To effectively address the intersection between HIV/AIDS and gender and sexuality requires that interventions should, at the very least, not reinforce damaging gender and sexual stereotypes" (Gupta, 2000, p. 8). This challenge—that health promotion services and programs should, at the very least, "do no harm" with respect to gender—inspires us to argue for a vision of health promotion that seeks to transform harmful and negative gender norms, roles, relations, and structures within health promotion research, policy, and practice.

As discussed in the Introduction, health promotion needs to embrace gender considerations. But not only should gender be "considered" and possibly "integrated" into health promotion activities, changing gender roles, relations, and practices to reduce discriminatory assumptions, language, and practices should become one of the explicit goals of health promotion activity because these social practices and structures are routine, pervasive, and changeable determinants of health. Combining the empowering core of health promotion (see Chapter 2) with a commitment to transforming limiting gender norms, roles, relations, and institutions will not only improve women's and men's health, but also change their social and economic status.

To these ends, we have developed a framework designed to encourage gender transformation as an explicit aim of health promotion practice, policy-making, and research. This approach means addressing what Sir Michael Marmot (2007) and others have called the "causes of the causes," recognizing sex and gender as fundamental determinants of health, and interrogating the links between sex, gender, and other determinants such as income, education, occupation, and the social and built environments: "The differential status of men and women in almost every society is perhaps the most pervasive and entrenched inequity. As such, the relation between the sexes represents as pressing a societal issue for health as the social gradient itself" (Marmot, 2007, p. 1155). Only with this full recognition of the significance of sex and gender as determinants of health can health promotion contribute to more than minor changes in health and social outcomes; indeed, it may even exacerbate health inequities (World Health Organization, 2010).

In this chapter, we describe our framework for gender-transformative health promotion and the thinking behind it. We also explain some of the processes involved in creating the framework, particularly an extensive stakeholder consultation process that involved over 150 people in several countries. We illustrate the core of the framework with examples from cardiovascular disease prevention for women. We conclude with suggestions of what we see as some of the promise of gender-transformative health promotion for improving health, strengthening community action, and fostering gender equity. Though the framework was originally derived from work with women, there is evidence to suggest these approaches are also relevant to, and indeed essential for, promoting the health of men.

Developing a Framework for Gender-Transformative Health Promotion

Working with an expert advisory group of researchers, practitioners, and policy-makers, we generated this framework for gender-transformative health promotion over several years through an iterative process of literature reviews, case studies, and dialogue. We began with meetings and brainstorming sessions within the research team itself and with our advisory group members. As our ideas gelled, we entered into a broad consultation process comprised of interviews (n = 4) with health promotion and gender experts from Canada and Scotland, focus groups (n = 36 participants) in Canada and Australia, and an international online survey (n = 100). Consistent with the Ottawa Charter (World Health Organization, 1986) principles of health promotion, this consultation strategy—as a method—embodied the tenets and assumptions of inclusion and empowerment in the opportunity for dialogue created among a wide range of individuals, including women, students, academics, community researchers, policy-makers, and health practitioners. Qualitative data were transcribed, coded, and analyzed using NVivo8 software (Bazeley, 2007) for common themes and suggestions, while quantitative data describing the characteristics of their respondents and their involvement in health promotion were analyzed using SPSS software. Our choice of methods was informed by our need for detailed feedback on the framework as well as the opportunity that group discussions present for generating critical feedback (Kitzinger, 1994).

Overall, consultation participants—who included self-identified academic researchers, policy-makers, health promotion practitioners, students, and health care providers—thought a framework would be useful for increasing awareness about gender transformation as a health promotion approach and guiding action. The majority of the respondents (85 percent) had experience working in the health promotion field, and many were familiar with women's health. In their feedback, respondents encouraged us to articulate the framework's theoretical foundations and to make clear how we understood gender as a determinant of health. For example, one respondent said,

> If you get that the economic influences intersect with gender to keep the problem in place, then you're going to be able to easily see the logic of the fact that, you know, simply putting up another women's shelter is not going to be—not going to be a long-term solution to ending violence against women.

Respondents also urged us to explicitly link the framework to the determinants of health, address the feasibility of its application, and consider how the framework could build capacity for gender-transformative practice. One respondent linked these issues to the larger discussion of addressing health equity within health promotion:

> Health promotion practitioners are finding that they need an equity lens of some sort to figure out how to address the needs of diverse populations and not increase disparities between populations. It should help people look at the structures and barriers that women and girls face and develop health promotion plans that reduce or address those barriers and structures.

This quotation was a response to an open-ended question in an online survey conducted in the summer of 2012 to review an early draft of the framework. The respondent clearly articulated the need for analytic and practical tools for health promotion to address issues of equity and diversity, and to support the development of interventions for girls and women. We hope that the framework, outlined next, offers some direction for how health promotion can contribute to gender transformation to enhance both health and gender equity.

A Framework for Gender-Transformative Health Promotion

The framework for gender-transformative health promotion (see Figure 1.1) is a conceptual tool designed to illustrate the ways in which health promotion interacts with multiple factors to either improve health and social outcomes for women or, through a feedback loop, maintain health systems and social structures that are based on and foster biased and discriminatory norms and practices.

In our figure, each section is understood to affect the one(s) to its right. On the left is a representation of gendered structures and systems, which affect everything from relationship roles and economic opportunities to power structures and personal choices. Gendered health determinants are created through the interactions of numerous gender facets of the social, cultural, political, and economic context and the environmental and biological conditions (which have important sex-based influences). Gendered social structures and systems, as Sen and Östlin (2010) have outlined, are reflected in discriminatory values, norms, and practices that advantage some and disadvantage others. These are intimately connected to differential power dynamics and influence how women and men, girls and boys experience different vulnerabilities and exposures to health-enhancing or health-diminishing environments, conditions, and actions. This complex set of gendered social structures and systems include the "health" system—that is, the infrastructure of health policy, research, and practice—as well as individual social and biological determinants. All these determinants contribute to direct health outcomes for women as well as socio-political outcomes such as the distribution of power and resources, which ultimately contribute to both health status (and health inequities) as well as gender equity (or inequities).

Health promotion, understood to be a diverse set of information, education, organization, community, and political practices that operate at multiple levels (see Chapter 2), is diagrammatically depicted as a continuum cutting across all these contexts and effects. Depending on the specific approach taken, health promotion interventions are understood to either reinforce existing gender norms, structures, and relations or challenge them. If health promotion activities are gender-transformative, they produce health and social outcomes that contribute to gender equity. If not, they reinforce existing gendered social structures, as signalled through a feedback loop.

Gupta's provocative question of whether health promotion and disease-prevention efforts sustain or challenge aspects of cultural and social norms, as expressed through gender and gender relations, underpins the core of our framework for gender-transformative health promotion. We have illustrated this vision in a continuum (see Figure 1.2), building on concepts outlined in Gupta's work as well as a number of publications of the World Health Organization (see, for example, World Health Organization, 2009, 2010). The continuum permits us to envision the various

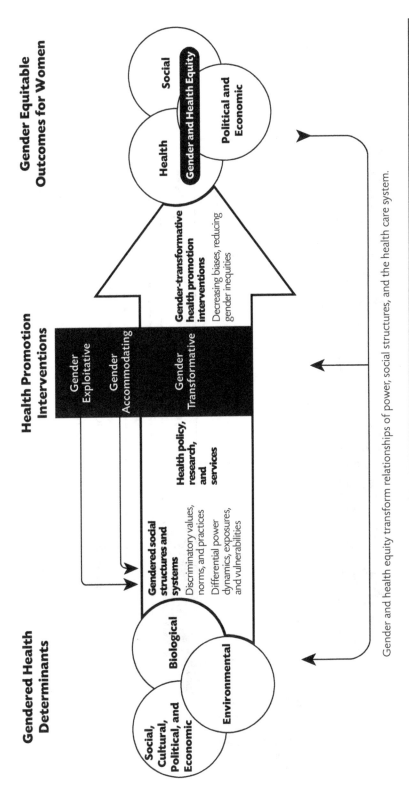

FIGURE 1.1:   A Framework for Gender-Transformative Health Promotion for Women

Source: Authors

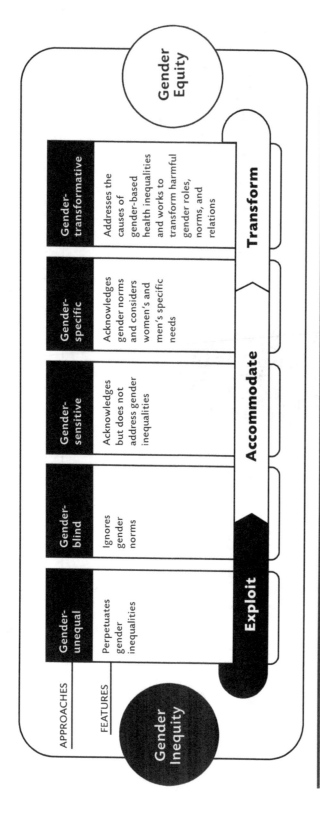

FIGURE 1.2: A Continuum of Approaches to Action on Gender and Health

Note: Inspired by remarks by Geeta Rao Gupta, Ph.D, Director, International Center for Research on Women (ICRW) during her plenary address at the 13th International Aids Conference, Durban, South Africa, July 12, 2000: "To effectively address the intersection between HIV/AIDS and gender and sexuality requires that interactions should, at the very least, not reinforce damaging gender and sexual stereotypes."

Source: Authors

characteristics of interventions in relation to whether they contribute to gender inequity or gender equity by virtue of the extent to which they perpetuate, ignore, acknowledge, consider, or address the causes of gender-based health inequities.

Approaches may be explicitly gender unequal, as when images are used in social marketing and health education campaigns that privilege men over women or women over men. Gupta (2000) referred in her Durban speech, for example, to the prevalence in early HIV/AIDS activities of imagery and campaigns that fostered "a predatory, violent, irresponsible image of male sexuality and portrayed women as powerless victims or as repositories of infection" (p. 8), both of which represent sexist and limited stereotypes that deny women and men the capacity for agency, mutually respectful relations, and positive, responsible expressions of their sexuality.

Gender-blind interventions tend to be the dominant approach in health promotion (Gelb, Pederson, & Greaves, 2012). Gender-blind interventions typically use vague terms to describe the population of interest, such as "people" or "health care system users" or "the urban poor" rather than "low-income women" or "women who experience violence and abuse," thus obscuring a clear understanding of who is affected by a problem or who is being studied, and failing to make distinctions based on gender in the design and reporting of programs (World Health Organization, 2010). In so doing, many interventions may inadvertently reinforce privilege such that those individuals or social groups with existing knowledge and skills or access to technology, among other things, are more likely to benefit from the intervention, policy, or resource. For example, the WHO (2010) has identified how out-of-pocket payments for health services widen gender inequities because of women's disproportionate need for such health expenditures and their lack of economic resources.

A Planning Tool for Gender-Transformative Health Promotion

From the beginning of our consultations about the framework, colleagues urged us to consider its practical application. In particular, participants in a consultation workshop in Melbourne, Australia, in April 2012 encouraged us to think about how researchers, policy-makers, and health promotion program developers would apply the framework in practice. This feedback led to the creation of a separate planning tool that is informed by the principles of gender transformation, engagement, and empowerment (discussed in detail in Chapter 11). The planning framework follows a traditional project planning cycle but incorporates critical reflective practices; encourages the engagement of key stakeholders; and challenges users to identify the known or potential sex, gender, diversity, and equity effects of a program, policy, or research project. This planning tool incorporates a number of principles of action, discussed in further detail in Chapter 11. The most significant of these is that health promotion interventions must be evidence-based. Given the limited work on gender-transformative practice to date, there is a critical need for more research to support this work (but see, for example, World Health Organization, 2011, as a promising direction).

In the balance of this chapter, we describe the foundations of the framework, illustrate the continuum of action on gender and health through the example of heart health promotion for women, and outline the principles for action that we believe should inform interventions—whether individual or collective, local or global—that are consistent with this framework.

Framework Foundations

Overcoming a History of Gender-Blindness in Health Promotion

The starting point for our work on gender equity and health promotion was the Ottawa Charter for Health Promotion (World Health Organization, 1986), which defines health promotion as the process of enabling people to increase control over and improve their health. Despite the call within the Ottawa Charter for programs and policies "to respond to the health gap within and between societies, and to tackle the inequities in health produced by the rules and practices of these societies" (p. 1), a close look reveals that health promotion has generally failed to consider gender and its implications for opportunities for health (Gelb et al., 2012).

A number of critics have argued that the field's failure to clearly embrace gender considerations has reduced the effectiveness of health promotion while contributing to or exacerbating health inequities (Cohen, 1998; Daykin & Naidoo, 1995; Doyal, 1995; Keleher, 2004; Reid, Pederson, & Dupéré, 2007). For health promotion to increase women's control over and improve their health, it needs to pay explicit attention to the determinants of health—which include sex and gender (though some lists of determinants, such as the framework developed by Robert Wood Johnson Foundation, 2010, fail to name them)—and acknowledge that issues of power, engagement, and access to resources form vital challenges within health promotion practice (see Chapter 2).

Daykin and Naidoo (1995) argued almost 20 years ago that health promotion programs often hold women responsible for the health behaviours of children, male partners, and other family members while failing to recognize women's complex social positioning, including the gendered and racialized power imbalances and differential access to material resources that shape their ability to influence the health of others. More recently, the reports of the Women and Gender Equity Knowledge Network (Sen & Östlin, 2007) and the WHO Commission on Social Determinants of Health (Commission on Social Determinants of Health, 2008) have argued for more intense discussions of gender as a determinant of health. Yet the translation of these frameworks and discourses into practice has been hampered by the lack of models, program evaluations, critical evidence bases, and experience in gender-responsive programming (Benoit & Shumka, 2009).

Early discussions of gender-responsive programming in health promotion and disease prevention appeared within the fields of HIV/AIDS prevention (e.g., see World Health Organization, 2009) and reproductive and maternal health (Rottach, Schuler, & Hardee, 2009). Possibly the obvious associations between intimate relationships and these health issues facilitated these links; presumably, this approach was also a response to the scale and nature of the problems that HIV/AIDS and reproductive health pose for girls and women globally and the need for effective, efficient programs. Regardless, a decade of work in some of these areas has produced some important findings that can be used to inform gender-responsive—ideally gender-transformative—health promotion more broadly. Our work extends the use of this approach into other topic areas beyond sexual and reproductive health, including women's tobacco use (see Chapter 4), housing among women who experience violence in their relationships (see Chapter 8), and cardiovascular disease prevention (Chapter 7).

Theoretical Origins

The framework draws on theories in various disciplines, including feminist theory, philosophy, and cultural theory (Barker, Hulme, & Iversen, 1994; Hankivsky et al., 2010; Kelly, 2008; Ridgeway, 2009; Risman, 2004), which provide a rationale and strategy for gender-transformative health promotion. The framework is also contextualized in the long history of health promotion theory itself as expressed in major texts, various charters, and frameworks (e.g., Rootman, Dupéré, Pederson, & O'Neill, 2012) and recognizes the major tensions in the field. These tensions include questioning the appropriate site of intervention (individual versus structural) and debates on how the neo-liberal focus on individual responsibility for health reinforces a form of health promotion aimed at changing individual knowledge and behaviours rather than addressing the social, cultural, and economic conditions that shape the opportunities for women's health (Pederson, Haworth-Brockman, Clow, Isfeld, & Liwander, 2013).

Though discourse on social responsibility clearly contends that health is shaped by social conditions (Ponic & Frisby, 2010), the field of health promotion has long confronted these tensions regarding where to locate responsibility for health, whether on the individual or on society (Petersen & Lupton, 1996). Although health promotion has debated how structure and agency affect health behaviour, health promotion interventions have largely targeted health behaviours and the related individual characteristics of those most at risk of diminished health (Ponic & Frisby, 2010; Raphael, 2004). These are often poor and underserved women and men. When considering gender and women's health, it is therefore crucial that health promotion addresses women's agency and acknowledges how gender norms, roles, relations, and expectations uphold social structures that influence women's health behaviours and affect women's health outcomes. To address this gap in current health promotion practice, the framework development process considered gendered structural constraints, such as the different environments in which girls and women spend their time (i.e., home, work, clinic, school, etc.) and how these intersect with women's identities (i.e., mother, caregiver, daughter, sister, wife, etc.). These constraints are ultimately shaped by societal norms and expectations of women. While elements of these debates remain vital within the field of health promotion as a whole, as well as within the sphere of women's health, our focus is fundamentally on how gender identities, norms, roles, relations, institutions, and structures can be health-damaging or health-promoting. To that end, Chapters 2 and 3 in Part 1 develop two specific and highly relevant aspects of theory in greater depth, namely, power and intersectionality.

Briefly, analysts of health promotion have called for a theory of power to complement health promotion's explicit attention to "empowerment" as the core mechanism for change. Power can be understood as a mechanism to prevent some groups from participating in decision-making processes through social stratification (Gaventa, 1980; Sadan, 1997; Saunders, 1990). Hierarchical structures, systems, and norms are dictated by individuals who hold the power, typically those who possess socially desirable traits such as heterosexual white men. There needs to be an acknowledgement of the unequal and unjust power dynamics that exist as a function of gender relations (Reid et al., 2007). Dominant health promotion discourse, which tends to depict gender as "difference," contributes to the trivialization of challenges experienced by women as a result of gendered social structures and systems. On the other hand, empowerment discourse within health promotion holds promise for improving women's health. Empowerment can be understood as a collection of social processes that aim to increase control and transition power back to those who have less power or who are powerless (Sadan, 1997). Even so, as Ponic et al. discuss in Chapter 2, we must be wary of our ability to empower others as opposed to entering into a process of mutual change that entails acknowledging and engaging with one another's relative power and limitations in any given instance. Empowerment requires the integration of micro-, meso-, and macro-level relations between the individual, community, and society to achieve a structural system that allows for equitable participation and engagement in decision-making processes (Sadan, 1997).

Gender as a Determinant of Health

Every step in the framework emphasizes the role of gender in producing health outcomes and is intended to orient the user toward those particular effects in the type of health issue or health promotion strategy at hand. The pervasiveness of gender as a determinant of health grounds the need for health promotion strategies that are gender-informed and that specifically consider the needs and experiences of women (Keleher, 2004). Moreover, it is necessary to understand gender in the context of other social determinants of health (such as socio-economic status, age, ethnocultural identity, location, etc.) in order to develop health promotion strategies that will be meaningful for diverse groups of women (Reid, Pederson, & Dupéré, 2012).

In considering how to articulate our perspective on gender as a determinant of health, we drew on Sen and Östlin's framework in their book, *Gender Equity in Health: The Shifting Frontiers of Evidence and Action* (Sen & Östlin, 2010), among others, because it identifies social determinants as both processes and systems of social stratification that vary with gender. Gendered health determinants produce a set of discriminatory values, norms, practices, and behaviours and lead women and men to have different types of vulnerabilities to diseases, injuries, and disabilities, and to experience different levels and types of exposures to health risks and conditions. These are affected by biases within the health system and health research—but also contribute to producing those biases. Through complex interactions, these factors produce two sets of outcomes: health outcomes (e.g., life expectancy, health status, mental health) and social and economic consequences (e.g., level of education and income, relationship status, place of residence, membership in valued social networks, and so on). Both women and men, as well as intersexed and transgendered people, are affected by gendered structural determinants, but with different outcomes.

With respect to women, Sen and Östlin (2010) note that some girls are fed less and educated less, and are more physically restricted than boys in their families or communities, and women often have lower-paid, less secure, and more informal employment.

> Girls and women are often viewed as less capable or able, and in some regions are seen as repositories of male or family honor [*sic*] and the self-respect of communities.... Restrictions on their physical mobility, sexuality, and reproductive capacity are perceived to be natural; and in many instances, accepted codes of social conduct and legal systems condone, and even reward, violence against them. (p. 5)

Gender connects biological and psychological differences with social and relational experiences (Keleher, 2004). This relationship predicts women's health and social out-comes as it drives and delineates pathways of inequity, especially in "socioeconomic circumstances that manifest in women's lower levels of income across the lifespan and in relatively subordinate positions of power and lower levels of decision making, whether in political arenas, workplaces or within families" (Keleher, 2004, p. 278).

Both gender and sex matter in understanding health, and both are continuous and fluid variables, open to redefinition in various temporal and cultural settings (Johnson, Greaves, & Repta, 2007; Krieger, 2003). Assuming gender is a dichot-omous, categorical variable can lead to the further assumption that all women are different from all men, while women themselves are a homogeneous group. One danger of this assumption is that it can lead to conceptualizing women's needs and interests as those of the dominant group in any given context. By not examining within-population differences, some groups of women may be marginalized. It is critical that health promotion therefore identifies and is sensitive to the fact that while most women experience some level of gendered inequality and inequity, women may experience those inequalities differently from one another, depending on their unique social positioning (Reid et al., 2007).

Women's health and social identities are defined by other elements of social inequities such as race/ethnicity, age, sexuality, disability, culture, and religion (Crenshaw, 1989; Daykin & Naidoo, 1995). The interplay between these dimensions places some women in more vulnerable positions than others (Hankivsky et al., 2010). An intersectional analysis, by focusing on social relationships of power instead of on differences in resources, encourages researchers and program developers to examine social experiences and how they intersect at multiple forms of oppression (McCall, 2005) in their work.

Intersectional theory posits that gender is distinct from but interacts with other social features like social class or race/ethnicity such that their effects are mutually constitutive rather than separate. Intersectional theory focuses on the ways that power shapes, sustains, and transforms social identities, sexualities, and social relations. It arose among black feminist scholars as an explanatory framework to understand the multiple rather than singular dimensions of social inequities, including gender, race/ethnicity, class, sexual orientation, age, disability, and so on (e.g., Collins, 1989). With its focus on how power aligns with privilege, intersectional theory is particularly useful for identifying the expression of complex lived experiences and the ways that overlapping systems of discrimination shape health and other social experiences.

Challenging the Evidence
We regard evidence as the foundation for gender-transformative health promotion.

As a multidisciplinary team, we have observed that in all substantive topic areas—whether alcohol or tobacco use, mental health, physical activity, occupational health, preconception care, or housing—there is an intellectual tradition, a set of methodological practices, and practice or policy approaches that are largely gender-blind or gender-neutral. In each of our fields, we have therefore been active in generating new evidence, revisiting theory, and identifying new methods that incorporate sex and gender and engage with their intersection with other forms of social stratification, marginalization, and oppression (see, for example, Johnson et al., 2007). Though not depicted in our framework per se, we see continued research and program evaluations in all areas of health promotion action as essential to either confirm or challenge the evidence base for health promotion interventions.

Translating the Framework into Practice

Kurt Lewin, a twentieth-century social psychologist, is famous for having said "There is nothing so practical as a good theory" (Lewin, 1951, p. 169), and "If you want truly to understand something, try to change it" (in Tolman, Cherry, van Hezewijk, & Lubke, 1996, p. 31). In that vein, we recognize that the strength of our framework will ultimately be in its usefulness to practitioners, policy-makers, and researchers. To support the model of planning depicted in Figure 1.3, we have generated a set of guiding principles to inform action. We have also identified several examples of health promotion interventions that are gender-exploitative, gender-accommodating, or gender-transformative respectively.

Principles of Action

Through literature reviews, our own experiences in health promotion, and discussions with practitioners, researchers, and policy-makers throughout the framework consultation process, we derived a set of principles to inform gender-transformative actions in health promotion. These principles are both background values that inform the use of the framework and criteria for checking that the outcomes generated by the framework are likely to be gender-transformative and positive for women. Drawn from promising practices in health promotion and women's health, they are intended to ensure that health promotion outcomes are meaningful for women of diverse backgrounds and that the outcomes promote positive encounters with the health system. We have identified eight principles of gender-transformative health promotion interventions:

1. Evidence-based
2. Equity-oriented

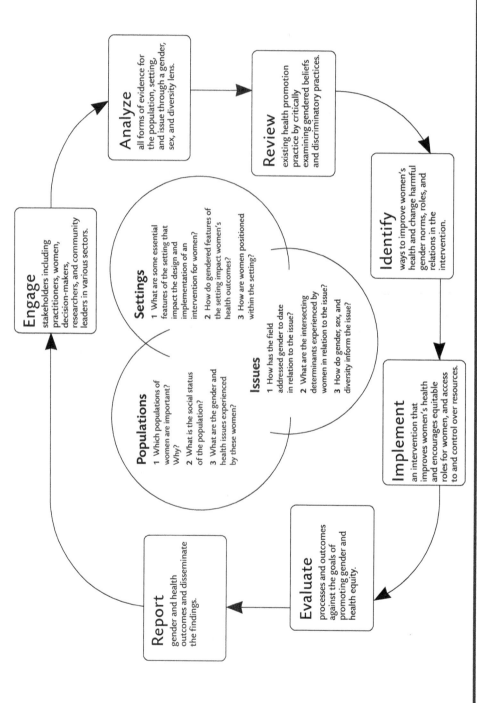

FIGURE 1.3: Creating Gender-Transformative Health Promotion Interventions for Women

Source: Authors

3. Action-oriented
4. Women-centred
5. Culturally safe
6. Trauma-informed
7. Harm reduction–oriented
8. Strengths-based

Summary of Key Principles

Evidence-Based

Health promotion interventions must be based upon research evidence of all kinds, including knowledge derived from clinical, policy, and program work, as well as from women's experience and traditional indigenous ways of knowing. Inclusive and collaborative approaches to research are essential to generate evidence and information for program and policy design, and to support the synthesis of these forms of knowledge to create effective, women-centred interventions (see, for example, Greaves & Ballem, 2001; Moya, 2002; Poole, 2008; Rycroft-Malone et al., 2004).

Equity-Oriented

Health promotion approaches with an equity orientation recognize how social, cultural, and economic conditions can affect access to resources and power and therefore health. They seek to reduce disparities in health that are a result of systemic, avoidable, and unjust social and economic policies and practices that create barriers to opportunity. Sometimes this means that tailored approaches are required in health promotion to achieve the reduction of inequities in health (see, for example, Browne et al., 2012).

Action-Oriented

Linking and translating such multi-faceted evidence into change at any level (from local to global) are central to the women's movement and women-centred research. Action is a central principle of women's health, evidenced at multiple levels and issues in consciousness-raising groups in the 1970s, to Action Agendas during the UN Decade for Women, to current efforts to challenge the negative impacts of economic globalization, end violence against women, and resist the erosion of women's rights (see, for example, Greaves, 2004; Kirby, Greaves, & Reid, 2006; Miles, 2013; Reid, Tom, & Frisby, 2006).

Women-Centred

Women-centred health promotion approaches recognize that women's health is important in and of itself, in addition to being linked to fetal, child, family, and community health. Women-centred health promotion and care involve women as informed participants in their own health care and improve women's overall health and safety. Women-centred care acknowledges women's rights to control their own reproductive health, avoids unnecessary medicalization, and takes into account women's roles as caregivers and their patterns and preferences in obtaining health care (see, for example, Ballem & Women's Health Planning Project Steering Committee, 2000; Cory, 2007; Greaves, Poole, & Cormier, 2002).

Culturally Safe

Around the world, health promotion interventions must grapple with recognition of the influences of colonization and migration on women's identities and health as critically important. Health promoters need to be aware of their own cultural identity and socio-historical location in relation to service recipients, as well as of their attitudes and ways of conceptualizing health, wellness, and parenting. Respect for women's cultural location and taking onto account their values and preferences in any health promotion encounter is important, as is accommodation of a woman's interest in culturally based healing (see, for example, Aboriginal Nurses Association of Canada, Canadian Association of Schools of Nursing, & Canadian Nurses Association, 2009; Ball, 2008; Hanson, 2009).

Trauma-Informed

Experiences of gender-based violence and trauma are fundamentally linked to women's physical and mental health problems. In many settings, experiences of current partner violence and symptoms of past trauma are often overlooked, and interactions with service providers themselves can be re-traumatizing. Importantly, trauma-informed systems and services do not depend on disclosures of trauma but rather take into account the influence of trauma and violence on health; understand trauma-related symptoms as attempts to cope; and integrate this knowledge into all aspects of service delivery, policy, and service organization (see, for example, Harris & Fallot, 2001; Poole & Greaves, 2012; Varcoe, 2008).

Harm Reduction–Oriented

Harm-reducing initiatives are pragmatic; help with immediate goals; provide a variety of options and supports for improving health; and focus not only on attainment of narrow goals related to change in a specific health behaviour (such as abstinence from tobacco use), but rather on facilitating change in the full range of influences and harms associated with that health behaviour (see, for example, Mehrabadi et al., 2008; Poole, Urquhart, & Talbot, 2010; Shannon et al., 2008).

Strengths-Based

A strengths-based approach is health-focused, not deficit-oriented. It involves a fundamental shift in the conceptualization of health promotion as it explicitly recognizes the positive efforts and factors in women's lives that can be built upon to further improve health. It extends the focus of health promotion to include secondary prevention and harm reduction, and actively considers what is working well for girls and women and what resources can be supported, enhanced, or made available to them. It transforms stereotypes of women as weak, sick, and fragile to those of women who can grow and thrive and recognize their own strengths (see, for example, Gottlieb, 2013; Norman, 2000; Watkins, 2002).

Revisiting the Continuum

Several chapters in this book make reference to the idea of the continuum of potential actions on gender and health depicted in Figure 1.2 (page 22). This illustration shows an array of approaches along a continuum, from gender inequity to gender equity, identifying approaches ranging from those that are gender-unequal to gender-blind to gender-sensitive to gender-specific to gender-transformative. To understand this continuum and its implications for health promotion research, policy, and practice, it helps to review the features of each approach. Though not universally agreed upon, we find the following definitions usefully articulated and illustrated in WHO (2010).

Gender-Unequal

Gender-unequal initiatives perpetuate gender inequalities by reinforcing unbalanced gender norms, roles, and relations. Typically, one sex will be privileged over another and this leads to that sex enjoying more rights, privileges, opportunities, and resources than the other, whether it be information, services, or opportunities for decision making. For example, a program might be available only to people who are able to pay a fee; given that women generally have fewer economic resources, they might not be able to access the program as easily as men.

Gender-Blind

Gender-blind programs ignore gender norms, roles, and relations and may therefore reinforce gender-based discrimination, biases, and stereotypes. The most common argument for gender-blind initiatives is that they are "fair" because they treat everyone the same, but by ignoring structured barriers faced by some program participants, the program may contribute to inequities. Technologies may also be gender-blind. For example, a report on gender inequities in science and technologies documented how car seat belts are not routinely tested using models that simulate adult women, particularly pregnant women. As a result, women, who are smaller on average than men, have been described as "out-of-position" drivers because they sit closer to the steering wheel than men do (see Schiebinger, 2011, p. 6).

Gender-Sensitive

Gender-sensitive programs acknowledge and consider gender norms, roles, and inequalities but do not necessarily include action to address them. For example, a program to reduce maternal–child transmission of HIV would likely acknowledge that women may not have the status, rights, nor decision-making authority to practise safer sex, insist upon the use of condoms, or adopt safer child-feeding strategies, though they would be encouraged to do so nonetheless (World Health Organization, 2009).

Gender-Specific

Gender-specific programs acknowledge that gender norms, roles, and relations exist and have an impact on access to or control over resources. This may mean targeting a program specifically at women or men, and accommodating gender norms but not working to address or change them. Programs that provide child-minding and offer women-only spaces can be gender-specific but not necessarily gender-transformative because they do not challenge why women are responsible for children when they need their own health care or why mixed spaces are unsafe or deemed unsuitable for women. While obviously an important approach, gender-specific programs do not necessarily address the root causes of gender imbalances in power, resources, or opportunities.

Gender-Transformative

Gender transformation is a relative concept that seeks to shift gender roles and relations closer to gender equity in a given context. Gender-transformative approaches actively strive to examine, question, and change rigid gender structures and imbalance of power as a means of reaching health and gender equity objectives (Rottach et al., 2009). Since gender equity is likely never fully attained, gender transformation is an ongoing process. What is transformative in one context, however, may not be transformative in another. Gender transformation involves identifying the ways that gender discrimination, inequality, or oppression operate in a particular situation and taking feasible steps toward improving these conditions, even if the result would still be considered regressive by the standards of another situation (Rottach et al., 2009). Gender transformation is therefore possible in every context, from the most repressive to the most progressive.

Illustrating the Continuum: Heart Health Promotion Campaigns for Women
As described in greater detail in Chapter 7, cardiovascular disease has long been considered a men's health problem, and awareness programs, research, and clinical innovations historically focused largely on men. But in recent years, governments and heart health advocacy organizations have begun to generate media campaigns to raise the awareness of women about their risks for heart disease. At the Australian Women's Health Conference in Sydney in May 2013, we showed three videos that are available online and argued that they represent examples of three major approaches to health promotion and gender commonly seen. The first video depicted death by heart disease as a stalker of women with the tag line, "Death Loves the Ladies." This campaign generated some controversy and critique, particularly among bloggers (for example, Hodge, 2011). By exploiting women's fears of rape and sexual violence, this film was quite literally horrifying—it used fear-mongering, gendered imagery, and associations to generate the message that women should be afraid of heart disease.

In contrast, a second video plays on different gendered stereotypes. Using well-known television and film stars, the video depicts morning preparations in a het-ero-normative, First World household. While the mother attempts to get her family ready for school and work, she displays the symptoms of a heart attack but does not recognize them and tries to carry on with making lunches, feeding her children, and getting everyone out the door. As she starts to show evidence of shortness of breath, sweating, and pain, her young son shows her a list of symptoms of a heart attack on a cell phone and convinces her to call emergency services. In describing her experience, she refers to it as "just a little heart attack" and, learning that an ambulance could be there in about three minutes, she surveys the disorder of her household and asks if they could delay their arrival a bit, presumably to allow her time to clean up. In contrast to the previous video, which plays on women's fear, this video plays on different gender norms, including depicting the woman as ignorant of the symptoms of heart disease, worried about the appearance of her home rather than her health, and continuing to fulfill her responsibilities as a mother despite feeling ill, among other things. Perhaps because it accommodates gender norms and stereotypes and featured well-known actors, this film has generated less controversy than the first.

The third video involves a montage of images of diverse women in a multiplicity of settings. The voice-over describes the multiple meanings of heart for women, including its significance as an expression of emotional bonds and connection, and explicitly talks about women's risks for heart disease as arising from sex and gender differences. The video celebrates women's diversity, resilience, activity, and connectedness as resources for improving women's heart health. In these ways, this piece goes some way toward transforming both heart health education itself and also how women and girls see themselves, the possibilities for their lives, and the value of their health. We suggest that this example of heart health promotion has some of the ingredients of gender-transformative health promotion.

Conclusion

Various international declarations and agreements call for gender equality and its integration or mainstreaming within the health field, including the Beijing Declaration and accompanying Platform for Action from the 1995 Fourth World Conference on Women. However, to date, health promotion policies and practices have not sufficiently ensured that all peoples—both women and men—can have equal opportunities to achieve health (Epp, 1986). In addressing women's health issues, health promotion has typically lacked attention to components needed to tackle inequities produced by gendered structures and norms.

In 2007, the report of the Women and Gender Equity Knowledge Network (Sen & Östlin, 2007), established to contribute to the WHO Commission on Social Determinants of Health, argued that gender inequality is among the most influential of the social determinants of health and that "because of the numbers of people involved and the magnitude of the problems, taking action to improve gender equity in health and to address women's rights to health is one of the most direct and potent ways to reduce health inequities and ensure effective use of health resources" (p. 1). Health promotion that does not take account of the social and environmental issues that affect health—such as income disparities, lack of power in household decision making, or gendered social roles—and that continues to locate responsibility for health within the individual will not be able to adequately address the key pressures on health in general and on women's health in particular. Indeed, Östlin, Eckermann, Mishra, Nkewane, and Wallstam (2006) assert that even though knowledge about the impact of gender on health inequities is increasing, this knowledge has not been translated into effective programs and policies: "The lack of translation of knowledge about gender inequities in health promotion interventions leads to misallocated resources and weakened potential for success" (p. 26).

A gender-transformative approach will have to redress the tendency in health promotion to focus on women largely in their reproductive and caregiving roles and instead embrace a comprehensive view of women's health that recognizes how women's lives and experiences affect their health. With respect to interventions, we will need to more consistently question universalistic, one-size-fits-all approaches, and devise, tailor, and implement approaches that take gender, other determinants of health, and their interactions into account. A gender-transformative approach to health promotion will also pay close attention to the tone and nature of messaging that is used to engage and inform women. Instead of messages deliberately or inadvertently playing to women's fears, sexualizing women, or treating women as a homogeneous group, gender-transformative health promotion helps put power—as knowledge, as choice, and as opportunity—into women's hands.

NOTE

1   This chapter represents the work of many individuals. First, we want to acknowledge the other members of the PhiWomen research team who participated in countless discussions related to this framework over the years and who pushed us to articulate our vision as clearly as possible: Jan Christilaw, Karin Humphries, Beth Jackson, Pamela Ponic, and Lynne Young. We also want to thank the members of our project Advisory Group, who brought critical wisdom from practice to our table: Paola Ardiles, Petra Begnell, Rose Durey, Joan Geber, Irving Rootman, and Elizabeth Whynot. Over the years, a number of staff and students supported this work and contributed their own vision and insights, including Sirad Deria, Karen Gelb, Natalie Hemsing, Phoebe Long, and Brenda Kent. Lauren Bialystok and Pam Ponic also both worked with us at various points, contributing to theoretical papers. Sue Mills served as the New Investigator on the team and was an important contributor to early discussions of the framework.

   We are indebted to the individuals who served as key informants, completed the online survey, and participated in our virtual focus groups—your input confirmed we were on the right track. Finally, we wish to thank our partners and colleagues—past and present—at Women's Health Victoria, in Melbourne, Australia, who have been an inspiration to us over the years and who helped bring an international perspective to our consultation on the framework.

REFERENCES

Aboriginal Nurses Association of Canada, Canadian Association of Schools of Nursing, & Canadian Nurses Association. (2009). *Cultural competence and cultural safety in nursing education: A framework for First Nations, Inuit, and Métis nursing.* Ottawa: Aboriginal Nurses Association of Canada.

Ball, J. (2008). *Cultural safety in practice with children, families, and communities.* Retrieved from www.ecdip.org/culturalsafety/

Ballem, P., & Women's Health Planning Project Steering Committee. (2000, January). *Women's Health Planning Project final report.* Vancouver: Vancouver/Richmond Health Board.

Barker, F., Hulme, P., & Iversen, M. (Eds.). (1994). *Colonial discourse, postcolonial theory.* Manchester: Manchester University Press.

Bazeley, P. (2007). *Qualitative data analysis with NVivo.* London: Sage Publications.

Benoit, C., & Shumka, L. (2009). *Gendering the health determinants framework: Why girls and women's health matters.* Vancouver: Women's Health Research Network.

Browne, A., Varcoe, C., Wong, S., Smye, V., Lavoie, J., Littlejohn, D., & … Lennox, S. (2012). Closing the health equity gap: Evidence-based strategies for primary health care organizations. *International Journal for Equity in Health, 11*(59), 1–15. doi:10.1186/1475-9276-11-59

Cohen, M. (1998). Towards a framework for women's health. *Patient Education & Counselling, 33*(3), 187–196.

Collins, P. H. (1989). The social construction of black feminist thought. *Signs: Journal of Women in Culture and Society, 14*(4): 745–773.

Commission on Social Determinants of Health. (2008). *Closing the gap in a generation: Health equity through action on the social determinants of health.* Final Report of the Commission on Social Determinants of Health. Geneva: World Health Organization.

Cory, J. (2007). *Women-centred care: A curriculum for health providers.* Vancouver: Vancouver Coastal Health Authority, BC Women's Hospital and Health Care.

Crenshaw, K. (1989). Demarginalizing the intersection of race and sex: A black feminist critique of antidiscrimination doctrine, feminist theory, and antiracist politics. *University of Chicago Legal Forum,* 139–167.

Daykin, N., & Naidoo, J. (1995). Feminist critiques of health promotion. In R. Bunton, S. Nettleton, & R. Burrows (Eds.), *The sociology of health promotion: Critical analyses of consumption, lifestyle, and risk* (pp. 59–69). London: Routledge.

Doyal, L. (1995). *What makes women sick? Gender and the political economy of health.* Basingstoke & London: Macmillan.

Epp, J. (1986). *Achieving health for all: A framework for health promotion.* Ottawa: Health and Welfare Canada.

Gaventa, Y. (1980). *Power and powerlessness: Quiescence and rebellion in an Appalachian valley.* Urbana: University of Illinois Press.

Gelb, K., Pederson, A., & Greaves, L. (2012). How have health promotion frameworks considered gender? *Health Promotion International, 27*(4), 445–452. doi:10.1093/heapro/dar08

Gottlieb, L. N. (Ed.). (2013). *Strengths-based nursing care: Health and healing for person and family.* New York: Springer.

Greaves, L. (2004). *Women-centred health research: A strategy for BC Women's.* Vancouver: BC Women's Hospital and Health Centre.

Greaves, L., & Ballem, P. (2001). *Fusion: A model for integrated health research.* Vancouver: British Columbia Centre of Excellence for Women's Health. Retrieved from www.bccewh.bc.ca/publications-resources/documents/fusionreport.pdf

Greaves, L., Poole, N., & Cormier, R. (2002). *Fetal alcohol syndrome and women's health: Setting a women-centred research agenda.* Vancouver: British Columbia Centre of Excellence for Women's Health.

Gupta, G. R. (2000). *Gender, sexuality, and HIV/AIDS: The what, the why, and the how.* Plenary address at the 13th International AIDS Conference, Durban, South Africa. Retrieved from www.un.org/womenwatch/daw/csw/hivaids/Gupta.htm

Gupta, G. R., & Weiss, E. (1993). *Women and AIDS: Developing a new health strategy.* Washington, DC: International Center for Research on Women.

Hankivsky, O., Reid, C., Cormier, R. A., Varcoe, C., Clark, N., Benoit, C., & Brotman, S. (2010). Exploring the promises of intersectionality for advancing women's health research. *International Journal for Equity in Health, 9*(5), 5–20.

Hanson, G. (2009). A relational approach to cultural competence. In G. G. Valaskakis, M. Dion Stout, & E. Guimond (Eds.), *Restoring the balance: First Nations women, community, and culture.* Winnipeg: University of Manitoba Press.

Harris, M., & Fallot, R. D. (2001). *Using trauma theory to design service systems.* San Francisco: Jossey Bass.

Hodge, J. (2011, July 8). Do edgy Heart and Stroke Foundation ads go too far? Retrieved from www.huffingtonpost.ca/jarrah-hodge/heart-and-stroke-foundation-ads_b_1093016.html

Johnson, J., Greaves, L., & Repta, R. (2007). *Better science with sex and gender: A primer for health research.* Vancouver: Women's Health Research Network.

Keleher, H. (2004). Why build a health promotion evidence base about gender? *Health Promotion International, 19*(3), 277–279.

Kelly, L. (2008). Women's health in Canada: Critical perspectives on theory and practice. *Affilia: Journal of Women & Social Work, 23*(4), 408–409.

Kirby, S. L., Greaves, L., & Reid, C. (2006). *Experience research social change: Methods beyond the mainstream* (2nd ed.). Peterborough, ON: Broadview Press.

Kitzinger, J. (1994). The methodology of focus groups: The importance of interaction between research participants. *Sociology of Health & Illness, 16*(1), 103–121.

Krieger, N. (2003). Genders, sexes, and health: What are the connections—and why does it matter? *International Journal of Epidemiology, 32,* 652–657.

Lewin, K. (1951). *Field theory in social science: Selected theoretical papers.* New York: Harper & Row.

Marmot, M. (2007). Achieving health equity: From root causes to fair outcomes. *The Lancet, 370*(9593), 1153–1163.

McCall, L. (2005). The complexity of intersectionality. *Signs: Journal of Women in Culture and Society, 3*(3), 1771–1800.

Mehrabadi, A., Craib, K. J. P., Patterson, K., Adam, W., Moniruzzaman, A., Ward-Burkitt, B., … Spittal, P. M. (2008). The Cedar Project: A comparison of HIV-related vulnerabilities amongst young Aboriginal women surviving drug use and sex work in two Canadian cities. *International Journal of Drug Policy, 19*(2), 159–168.

Miles, A. (Ed.). (2013). *Women in a globalizing world: Transforming equality, development, diversity, and peace.* Toronto: Inanna Press.

Moya, P. M. L. (2002). *Learning from experience: Minority identities, multicultural studies.* Berkeley: University of California Press.

Norman, E. (2000). Introduction: The strengths perspective and resiliency enhancement—a natural partnership. In E. Norman (Ed.), *Resiliency enhancement: Putting the strengths perspective into social work practice* (pp. 1–18). New York: Columbia University Press.

Östlin, P., Eckermann, E., Mishra, U., Nkowane, M., & Wallstam, E. (2006). Gender and health promotion: A multisectoral policy approach. *Health Promotion International, 21*(1), 25–35.

Pederson, A., Haworth-Brockman, M., Clow, B., Isfeld, H., & Liwander, A. (2013). *Rethinking women and healthy living in Canada.* Vancouver: British Columbia Centre of Excellence for Women's Health.

Petersen, A., & Lupton, D. (1996). *The new public health: Health and self in the age of risk.* London: Allen & Unwin, Sydney & Sage.

Ponic, P., & Frisby, W. (2010). Unpacking assumptions about "inclusion" in community-based health promotion: Perspectives of women living in poverty. *Qualitative Health Research, 20*(11), 1519–1531.

Poole, N. (2008). How can consciousness raising principles inform modern knowledge translation practices in women's health? *Canadian Journal of Nursing Research, 40*(2), 77–93.

Poole, N., & Greaves, L. (Eds.). (2012). *Becoming trauma informed.* Toronto: Centre for Addiction and Mental Health.

Poole, N., Urquhart, C., & Talbot, C. (2010). Women-centred harm reduction. *Gendering the National Framework Series: Vol. 4.* Vancouver: British Columbia Centre of Excellence for Women's Health.

Raphael, D. (Ed.). (2004). *Social determinants of health: Canadian perspectives.* Toronto: Canadian Scholars' Press Inc.

Reid, C., Tom, A., & Frisby, W. (2006). Finding the "action" in feminist participatory action research. *Action Research, 4*(3), 315–332.

Reid, C., Pederson, A., & Dupéré, S. (2007). Addressing diversity in health promotion: Implications of women's health and intersectional theory. In M. O'Neill, A. Pederson, S. Dupéré, & I. Rootman (Eds.), *Health promotion in Canada: Critical perspectives* (2nd ed., pp. 75–89). Toronto: Canadian Scholars' Press Inc.

Reid, C., Pederson, A., & Dupéré, S. (2012). Addressing diversity and inequities in health promotion: The implications of intersectional theory. In I. Rootman, S. Dupéré, A. Pederson, & M. O'Neill (Eds.), *Health promotion in Canada: Critical perspectives on practice* (3rd ed., pp. 54–66). Toronto: Canadian Scholars' Press Inc.

Ridgeway, C. L. (2009). Framed before we know it: How gender shapes social relations. *Gender & Society, 23*(2), 145–160.

Risman, B. J. (2004). Gender as a social structure: Theory wrestling with activism. *Gender & Society, 18*(4), 429–450.

Robert Wood Johnson Foundation. (2010). *A new way to talk about the social determinants of health.* New York: Robert Wood Johnson Foundation. Retrieved from www.rwjf.org/content/dam/farm/reports/reports/2010/rwjf63023

Rootman, I., Dupéré, S., Pederson, A., & O'Neill, M. (Eds.). (2012). *Health promotion in Canada: Critical perspectives on practice* (3rd ed.). Toronto: Canadian Scholars' Press Inc.

Rottach, E., Schuler, R., & Hardee, K. (2009). *Gender perspectives improve reproductive health outcomes.* Washington, DC: PRB for the IGWG and USAIDS.

Rycroft-Malone, J., Seers, K., Titchen, A., Harvey, G., Kitson, A. L., & McCormack, B. (2004). What counts as evidence in evidence-based practice? *Journal of Advanced Nursing, 47*(1), 81–90.

Sadan, E. (1997). *Empowerment and community planning: Theory and practice of people-focused social solutions.* Tel Aviv: Hakibbutz Hameuchad Publishers.

Saunders, P. (1990). *Social class and stratification.* London: Routledge.

Schiebinger, L. (2011). *Progressing toward gender-responsive science and technology.* Paper presented at the Interactive Expert Panel on Key Policy Initiatives and Capacity-Building on Gender Mainstreaming: Focus on Science and Technology. United Nations Commission on the Status of Women, 55th Session, February 22–March 4. Retrieved from www.un.org/womenwatch/daw/csw/csw55/panels/Panel1-Schiebinger-Londa.pdf

Sen, G., & Östlin, P. (2007). *Unequal, unfair, ineffective, and inefficient. Gender inequity in health: Why it exists and how we can change it.* Final report to the WHO Commission on Social Determinants of Health, Women and Gender Equity Knowledge Network. Geneva: World Health Organization.

Sen, G., & Östlin, P. (2010). Gender as a social determinant of health: Evidence, policies, and innovations. In G. Sen & P. Östlin (Eds.), *Gender equity in health: The shifting frontiers of evidence and action* (pp. 1–46). New York & London: Routledge.

Shannon, K., Kerr, T., Allinott, S., Chettiar, J., Shoveller, J., & Tyndall, M. (2008). Social and structural violence and policing in mitigating HIV risk of drug-using women in survival sex work. *Social Science and Medicine, 66*(4), 911–921. doi:10.1016/j.drugpo.2007.11.024

Tolman, C. W., Cherry, F., van Hezewijk, R., & Lubke, I. (Eds.). (1996). Problems of theoretical psychology—ISTP 1995. Captus University Publications. Retrieved from www.captus.com/information/catalogue/book.asp?Book+Number=174

Varcoe, C. (2008). Inequality, violence, and women's health. In B. S. Bolaria & H. D. Dickinson (Eds.), *Health, illness, and health care in Canada* (4th ed., pp. 259–282). Toronto: Nelson.

Watkins, M. L. (2002). Listening to girls: A study in resilience. In R. R. Greene (Ed.), *Resiliency: An integrated approach to practice, policy, and research* (pp. 115–131). Washington, DC: NASW Press.

World Health Organization. (1986). *Ottawa Charter for health promotion.* Retrieved from www.who.int/hpr/NPH/docs/ottawa_charter_hp.pdf

World Health Organization. (2009). *Integrating gender into HIV/AIDS programmes in the health sector: Tool to improve responsiveness to women's needs.* Geneva: Author.

World Health Organization. (2010). *Gender, women, and primary health care renewal: A discussion paper.* Geneva: Author.

World Health Organization. (2011). Evidence for gender responsive actions to prevent and manage overweight and obesity. Young people's health as a whole-of-society response. Copenhagen: WHO Regional Office for Europe. Retrieved from www.euro.who.int/en/health-topics/health-determinants/gender/publications/2012/young-peoples-health-as-a-whole-of-society-response-series/evidence-for-gender-responsive-actions-to-prevent-and-manage-overweight-and-obesity

2

Power and Empowerment in Health Promotion for Women

Pamela Ponic, Lorraine Greaves, Ann Pederson, and Lynne Young

Health promotion operates across multiple domains. Broadly speaking, it includes high-level frameworks, such as the Ottawa Charter, that define key principles and areas of action; local, regional, and state-wide polices that direct action; on-the-ground programs and projects in a variety of substantive areas, including physical activity, substance use, housing, and chronic-disease management; and professional practices by health professionals such as physicians and nurses. As a field of practice, policy, and research, health promotion is dedicated to "enabling people to increase control over, and to improve, their health" (World Health Organization, 1986, p. 1). "Increasing control" is explicitly linked to the notion of power, such that individuals and social groups have the agency and resources necessary to shape the social, political, and economic conditions for health as well as manage their personal health practices. Given women's overall relative lack of power compared to men in patriarchal societies, the notion of power is critically important to a new, gender-transformative approach to health promotion.

While the concept of power is embedded in some frameworks and policies, it is not always clearly articulated. Rather, the primary response in health promotion are attempts to facilitate the empowerment of marginalized social groups, including women, through on-the-ground programs and projects (Boutilier, Cleverly, & Labonte, 2000; Champeau & Shaw, 2002; Gutierrez & Lewis, 2005; Wallerstein, 1992; Wong, Zimmerman, & Parker, 2010). Using a variety of community-engagement, consciousness-raising, and educational strategies, such empowerment approaches typically aim to improve marginalized groups' ability to influence factors that determine their health, including health promotion programming and their own health behaviours. For example, Frisby, Reid, and Ponic (2007) described how a community-engagement approach to recreation provision fostered a collaborative process through which a diverse group of women living in poverty designed and implemented their own programming. They chose the recreation activities they felt would benefit them, organized activities with the support of paid service providers, and participated in them—all as a means to promote their health. While such empowerment approaches have been shown to be beneficial for participants during the length of time-limited projects, questions remain about their ability to fundamentally improve health over the long term unless the structural conditions (e.g., poverty, housing, systemic violence) that foster women's disempowerment are addressed (Frohlich, Ross, & Richmond, 2006; Kar, Pascual, & Chickering, 1999; Ponic, 2007; Reid, Pederson, & Dupéré, 2007). These questions point to the need to consider more deeply how power implicates the relationships between individual and social determinants of health, particularly for women.

Laverack (2004) suggests that health promoters typically have only a superficial understanding of power and how it implicates health and health promotion processes. That health promoters tend to under-conceptualize power is particularly problematic for women's health. Feminist thinkers in health promotion have long noted that women tend to be assigned responsibility for individual, family, and community health promotion without the power to enable it, as gendered and related systems of power limit women's ability to create changes in health behaviours and in the broader structural factors that determine health (Daykin & Naidoo, 1995; Doyal, 2000; Östlin, Eckermann, Mishra, Nkowane, & Wallstam, 2007). This dilemma creates an oppressive situation for women and exploits their gender-defined roles. Linking women's health to issues of power requires a broad and contextualized understanding of women's health:

> Women's health involves their emotional, social and physical well-being and is determined by the social, political and economic context of their lives, as well as by biology. This broad definition of women's health recognizes the validity of women's life experiences and women's own beliefs about and experiences of health. Every woman should be provided with the opportunity to achieve, sustain and maintain health, as defined by the woman herself, to her full potential. (Phillips, 1995, pp. 507–508)

This definition highlights multiple dimensions of women's health and the contexts within which it is situated, as well as the importance of a woman's control or power over defining her own health. Throughout this chapter we highlight gendered power relations and their role in shaping women's health and illness. This focus does not imply that all women experience gender in the same way, as we recognize that gender is but one axis of power that interacts with many others, in particular, race, class, and sexual orientation (Hankivsky et al., 2010). Rather than neglecting or diminishing variations among women, we mean to highlight that gendered power relations play a critical role in all women's social and health outcomes, albeit in different ways.

Explicit definitions and theories of power and empowerment are under-articulated in health promotion literature and practice generally, and, given the prevalence of uneven gendered power relations, in women's health promotion more specifically. There is minimal exploration of the interplay between power, women's health, and health promotion strategies. Reid et al. (2007) state that "we must have a theory of power if we are to understand health inequities and redress them" (p. 84). Critical theorizing of power is also necessary to avoid developing health promotion interventions and practices that continue to exploit and maintain traditional gender relations by making women responsible for health promotion without the power to enact it (Bottorff et al., 2010; Daykin & Naidoo, 1995; Interagency Gender Working Group, 2004). Failure to consider gendered power relations will perpetuate and exacerbate, rather than remediate, women's poor health and health inequities (Benoit & Shumka, 2009; Reid, Pederson, & Dupéré, 2012).

Our objectives in this chapter are to illustrate the potential of critically informed health promotion by outlining a theoretical perspective that helps to illuminate gendered power relations, explore how this perspective can inform empowerment strategies in health promotion, and discuss implications for the development of creating effective health promotion for women. Recognizing that the concept of power is complex, as is the task of promoting women's health and reducing gendered health inequities, we renew calls for the integration of critical theoretical perspectives in health promotion practice, research, and policy-making (Carroll, 2012; Labonte, Polanyi, Muhajarine, McIntosh, & Williams, 2005; Poland, 1998; Potvin, Gendron, Bilodeau, & Chabot, 2005). Power has been conceptualized in a number of disciplines and examined through a variety of lenses, such as modernist, critical feminist, post-colonial, and post-structuralist (Allen, 2008; Foucault, 1977; Gandhi, 1998; Giddens, 1984; Lukes, 2005). While there is no commonly agreed-upon definition or theory of power, there seems to be an explicit understanding in critical social thinking that power implicates all social structures, relationships, and individual actions. Critical theoretical perspectives are fundamentally concerned with uncovering socially constructed assumptions, practices, and institutionalized structures that create systems of power, privilege, and oppression, including racism, patriarchy, hetero-normativity, and the global political economy (Kincheloe & McLaren, 2000; Morrow & Browne, 1994). Critical feminist perspectives further focus on how such systems of power affect women's lives across their diverse social locations (Cancian, 1991; Collins, 2000; Fonow & Cook, 2005; Frisby, Maguire, & Reid, 2009). While we are not suggesting that a unified view of power for health promotion be articulated, we do suggest that given its centrality as part of socially constructed relations, health promoters need to critically engage with ideas and concepts of power.

Theoretical Perspectives on Power

Power is in large part a function of the relationship between structure and agency, which are central concepts in critical theories and have particular importance to health promotion because they inform ongoing debates in the field about where to locate responsibility for health—at broader social levels (i.e., structure) or individual, behavioural levels (i.e., agency) (Frohlich & Potvin, 2010; Godin, 2007; Minkler, 1999). Anthony Giddens, a contemporary British sociologist, articulated a seminal perspective on structure and agency (Giddens, 1984). In Giddens's duality of structure theory, he does not give primacy to either structure or agency as the central feature influencing social life and health. Rather, his main premise is that structure and agency are in constant interaction with each other and mutually reinforcing; structures shape possibilities for agency, and agency in turn creates and recreates structures (Giddens, 1984). Giddens defines structures as social procedures—assumptions, discourses, and ideologies—and institutionalized resources—material, regulatory, and interpersonal—while agency is the capacity for action (Cohen, 1989).

Power determines the structure-agency duality; it influences the degree to which structures enable or inhibit agency for individuals and social groups, as well as the possibilities for individuals and social groups to influence the creation and recreation of structures (Ponic, 2000). Giddens (1984) defines power as the ability to act to achieve desired ends or to make a difference. Power is something that individuals enact rather than have, albeit to different degrees, based on the ways in which structures enable or hinder a person's ability to act toward desired ends. Structures are not power per se; rather, they are "power tools" that enhance or limit agency and therefore facilitate or limit a person's power (Ponic, 2000).

Power is also relational: the degree to which a person is able to achieve desired ends is determined in relation to others' abilities to do so. Based on interpretations of Foucault's body of work, post-structuralist feminists envision power as a relational force rather than a fixed entity (Kesby, 2005; Ristock & Pennell, 1996).

Foucault (1977) has best articulated a ... perspective on power as productive and relational. Rather than repressive power being monolithic or a resource to be possessed, he conceptualizes power as built into a web of discourses and practices found in institutions, communities, and families that is exercised through actions in a multiplicity of relationships. These power relationships are inherently unstable and therefore open to challenge. (Wallerstein & Duran, 2003, p. 38)

Like Giddens, post-structuralists explicitly link power with action. Power is exercised in and through social relations and is a persistent feature of society whether or not we are conscious of it (Dominelli, 2005; Weedon, 1999). Power relations connect individuals and groups as active agents who experience and exercise it (English, 2006). Foucault (1982) further suggests that systemic power relations, such as patriarchal relations, are a product of "actions upon actions" over time that manifest between social groups and create and recreate systems of privilege, oppression, and domination (Young, 1990). As noted above, power relations are not set in stone as agents have the capacity to create and resist change, albeit to different degrees based on structural conditions (Giddens, 1984; Laverack & Labonte, 2008). As such, power is situational, in that our capacity for power is relative to the capacity of those with whom we are relating in a particular circumstance as shaped by social locations.

Power is fundamentally a productive force. A dominant conception of power in Western societies is predicated on the notion of power-over, such that to meet one's ends a person needs to dominate or have control over others. This perspective is based in patriarchal, colonialist, and other hierarchical understandings of how individuals relate to one another. According to Kesby (2005), such enactments of power emanate "from the top-down and from the centre outward" (p. 2040), using productive force to maintain relations of control and domination. Power is thus understood to be a capacity that you either have or don't have and "thinking is dichotomous—you win or you lose" (Teske, 2000, p. 108). In this model, the power of those who occupy privileged social locations is maintained through material, authoritative, and ideological structures (Giddens, 1984; McCall, 2005). Mohanty (2004) suggests that "the major problem with such a definition of power is that it locks all revolutionary struggles into binary structures—possessing power versus being powerless" (p. 39).

In contrast, feminist activists and thinkers have articulated positive and creative perspectives on power that are action-oriented and expansive through the concepts of power-to, power-with, and power-for. These perspectives are built on the assumption that although power is not equally facilitated by dominant structures, all people have the capacity for power in enabling rather than dominating manners (hooks, 2000; Ristock & Pennell, 1996). By working in collective and mutually supportive partnerships, power can be created with one another, a process that can aid "power-to" take action and initiate change (Teske, 2000; Tett, 2005). Such critical feminist perspectives illustrate how relational aspects of power can support alternative or more egalitarian relationships and resist practices of oppression and domination (Collins, 2000; hooks, 2000).

Gender is a central axis around which power operates. Gender refers to a system of social practices that prescribe femaleness and maleness in society (Johnson, Greaves, & Repta, 2007). Broom (2008) suggests that

> embodied individuals are shaped by gendered institutions and social practices, and at the same time, they question, revise, and resist those forces. *Gender entails both structure and agency.* It manifests at all levels of analysis, from the individual to the global. (italics added; p. 4)

Gender is a manifestation of power based on the degree to which gendered structures differently and inequitably facilitate the agency of males in relation to the agency of females—individually or as social groups—to reach productive ends. Importantly, gendered power relations are in constant interaction with race, class, hetero-normativity, and other systems of power that shape how different women experience gendered power. In the context of women's health and health promotion, social determinants of health such as income, education, age, or housing, along with the policies and practices through which they are provided, structure women's agency and health behaviours. In health promotion terms, the theoretical concepts of power and agency most often manifest through efforts toward empowerment.

A Critical Look at Empowerment

Empowerment is central to health promotion. While there is no agreed-upon or consistently used definition of empowerment (Kabeer, 1999), the core concept underlying it is "enhanced control over life circumstances" (Ehrhardt, Sawires, McGovern, Peacock, & Weston, 2009; Kar et al., 1999). This is directly in line with the Ottawa Charter definition of health promotion and is linked to Giddens's definition of power as the ability to achieve desired ends. Given its centrality, it is important to bring a critical lens to how empowerment is understood and employed in health promotion so as not to exacerbate the very power relations that empowerment strategies seek to address, particularly when working with members of marginalized social groups (Ponic, 2007; Potvin et al., 2005; Zimmerman, 1995). Many health promotion interventions are built on the assumption that it is the responsibility of professionals to "empower" their clients, as if power is something that can be bestowed, given, or transferred (Rappaport, 1987, 1995). However, as power is not "a thing" but is the capacity for action, the attempt to "empower" someone is an example of power-over that reinforces rather than mitigates dominant power relations and is based on the assumption that those living on the margins are "powerless" and in need of help from those with power to intervene (Buchanan, 2006; Cornish & Ghosh, 2007).

In comparison, when we begin with an understanding of power as relational, empowerment is understood as embedded in systems of relative privilege and oppression (Allen, 2008; Kabeer, 1999). Aboriginal organizer Lily Walker succinctly summarizes this important point by saying "If you are here to help me, then you are wasting my time. But if you come because your liberation is bound up in mine, then let us begin" (Laverack, 2004, p. 138). This perspective invokes the notions of power-with and power-to as acts that emerge through relationship and collective learning. VanderPlaat (1999) outlines such a notion of relational empowerment:

> In a relational approach to empowerment, everyone involved, regardless of position of power and privilege, recognizes that he or she is both an agent and a subject in the empowerment process. The ability to be empowering or to support someone else's capacity to be empowering grows out of the mutual recognition that all of us can contribute to the construction of knowledge and social change but that, in that process, all of us have a lot to learn. In a truly empowering process, everyone changes. Empowerment is always mutual. (p. 778)

In this light, empowerment is more of a collective than an individual process. It seeks to remedy broader power relations rather than focus on change in select individuals. In fact, Allen (2008) suggests that collective empowerment is a necessary condition for the possibility for individual empowerment.

Yet it is important to remember that empowerment concepts—be they relational, collective, or individual—are not solely dependent upon action. The capacity to act or make a difference is always shaped by structural conditions that differentially privilege the power of some over others, particularly across gender and other oppressive systems (Bunjun et al., 2006; Giddens, 1984; Young, 1990). In her reading and critique of Iris Marion Young's work on power and social justice, Allen (2008) suggests that "empowerment must be understood in terms of social, cultural, economic, and political relations that foster and promote ... self-determination and self-development" (pp. 165–166). In this light, the most important strategies to foster empowerment for improved health may be in addressing the broader structural conditions that shape possibilities for individual and community change and control. Ehrhardt et al. (2009) suggest that the aim of health promotion and health equity interventions should be economic, educational, social, and political empowerment.

This approach to empowerment is not focused on attempting to change individual health behaviours; rather, it attends to broader social determinants of health and the root causes of health inequities (Raphael, 2006). Lack of attention to broader social conditions and the social determinants of health can generate "empowerment" strategies that download responsibility for health promotion to those with the least power to realize it, a tension that reflects the long-standing feminist critique of how traditional approaches to health promotion exploit women's gender roles and exacerbate women's oppression (Daykin & Naidoo, 1995; Östlin et al., 2007; Reid et al., 2007).

Implications for Gender-Transformative Health Promotion for Women

This chapter has described a critical theoretical perspective on power as the ability to take action toward desired ends, differentially facilitated by structural conditions embedded in social relationships—and thus enacted through relational practices—and a productive force. Together, these ideas have a number of implications for the creation of gender-transformative health promotion for women.

Health promotion initiatives and practice must be informed by the concept that gendered power is a central feature of all social structures and relationships, and centrally influence women's health. Therefore, empowerment must be re-emphasized as the key underlying principle of all health promotion domains rather than a specific strategy unto itself in targeted community-development projects. To promote women's health, this means understanding and addressing the ways in which systems of power intersect across axes of gender, race, class, sexual orientation, physical ability, and age (among others) to differentially shape women's health and social locations (Hankivsky et al., 2010; Reid et al., 2012). Doing so requires attention to the gendered nature of the social determinants of health such as income, education, and housing, and questioning the appropriateness of targeting women as vectors of change in family and community health promotion interventions or assigning women responsibilities for health promotion that increase inequities (Pederson & Donner, 2007).

Given an understanding of the dual relationship between structure and agency, health promotion interventions should aim to create and transform structures—at social, organizational, community, and interpersonal levels—that facilitate women's agency (Frohlich & Potvin, 2010; Ponic & Frisby, 2010). While enabling positive health behaviours is certainly important, a critical perspective on power would further suggest that efforts be made to facilitate women's ability to influence the creation and transformation of the broader structures that determine their health.

This means enabling women's capacity for economic control, political advocacy, and public participation, and destabilizing gendered structures and systems.

Relational perspectives on power point to the need to actively reflect upon and negotiate the diverse and fluid relationships of privilege and oppression in all health promotion settings. Feminist researchers promote the use of reflexivity as a tool to systematically reflect upon our own power and social location, and how it implicates relationships and processes of working across difference (Shope, 2006; Williams & Lykes, 2003). In a health promotion context, reflexivity means explicitly naming, confronting, and navigating the power relations among multiple stakeholders and collaborators, including intersectoral partners, health professionals and patients, and participants working together in group or community settings (Boutilier & Mason, 2007). It also means taking the context within which health promotion operates into account at all times, including the social location of all involved and how it manifests in given situations (Poland, Krupa, & McCall, 2009; Varcoe, Hankivsky, & Morrow, 2007). As it relates to women's health, this means understanding how gender, race, class, education, age, and other systems of privilege and oppression impact women's involvement in health promotion. For women who are marginalized by race and class, this may mean attending to such day-to-day issues as child care, transportation, stigma, and discrimination when creating on-the-ground programs to support them. For women working within a health institution, it means recognizing how gendered bureaucracies may silence their voices in policy-making processes.

Finally, the perspectives on power we describe point to the need for collaborative approaches to health promotion practice, policy-making, and research that harness women's individual and collective power in a positive manner. Combining the strengths and resources that individuals, families, community members, health care professionals, social service providers, government policy-makers, and researchers bring to health promotion domains at all levels is a first step in building individual and collective capacity to facilitate change in the structures that shape health and possibilities for health promotion (Labonte, 2005). Building such partnerships can be challenging when working across differences and power imbalances, but doing so also creates the potential for mutual learning, growth, and the collective action necessary to make a difference in women's health and social inequities (Ponic, Reid, & Frisby, 2010).

Conclusion

> Power cannot be avoided … it must be worked with.
>
> —M. Kesby, "Retheorizing Empowerment-Through-Participation as a Performance in Space: Beyond Tyranny"

BOX 2.1: **TRAUMA-INFORMED PRACTICE IN PHYSICAL ACTIVITY**

Trauma-informed practice (TIP) in physical activity exemplifies how issues of gendered power and empowerment can be accounted for in health promotion. TIP is an innovative health care and health promotion strategy that takes understandings of trauma and violence into account in all phases of program design and delivery (Poole & Greaves, 2012). It recognizes, for example, that women who have experienced violence and trauma often feel unsafe and disempowered in their bodies and that dominant approaches to physical activity provision can actually mirror systems of violence and may thus be potentially re-traumatizing (Weissbecker & Clark, 2007). Finding appropriate and effective ways for women who have experienced violence and trauma to be physically active is important not only to ensure that all women can reap the health-promoting benefits of physical activity, but also because research shows that safe embodied experiences are effective in healing from trauma (Spinazzola, Rhodes, Emerson, Earle, & Monroe, 2011).

TIP in physical activity addresses an explicit problem related to gendered power—violence against women—which is a serious worldwide issue (World Health Organization, 2005). Trauma is both the experience of and response to violence and can result in a range of symptoms that compromise women's ability to be physically active, including avoidance of stimuli associated with the traumatic event(s), estrangement, hyper-vigilance, and an exaggerated startle response (Covington, 2008). Many women become disempowered as a result of the power-over domination they experienced when abused. TIP in physical activity takes these experiences into account by creating safe environments (i.e., structures) where women can experience control (e.g., agency) in their bodies.

Relational empowerment is an integral part of TIP in physical activity in that providers recognize their relationship to participants is crucial in creating safe environments. Trauma-sensitive yoga is a prime example (Emerson, Sharma, Chaudhry, & Turner, 2009). ["Trauma-sensitive" is one among varying types and applications of TIP in physical activity (Ponic, Pederson, & Ng, in review).] In trauma-sensitive yoga classes, yoga teachers avoid power-over language and actions in recognition that they could recreate traumatizing experiences. For example, every instruction given by a teacher is framed in the form of an invitation rather than a directive to avoid replicating domineering language: "I invite you to put your hand on your hip if that feels good for you" versus "Put your hand on your hip." Trauma-sensitive yoga teachers do not touch participants to assist with poses nor do they walk around class standing over participants on mats. These changes may seem subtle but are profound for traumatized individuals, because the choice of how to move their bodies is their own and teachers are teaching in a power-with and power-to manner.

> Other empowering aspects of TIP in physical activity can include no requirements to disclose or discuss experiences of violence and adaptations in the rules and/or purposes of the activity to accommodate the needs of traumatized participants. Again, each of these shifts is aimed at creating safe environments where women can regain a sense of control over their bodies and lives in the context of violence and trauma. Taking power explicitly into account in these ways can transform gendered power relations and health promotion for women.

Working from clearly articulated definitions and theories of power is central to creating effective health promotion for women. Based on the critical perspectives outlined here, working effectively with power means maintaining the principle of empowerment in all health promotion domains; focusing on the creation and transformation of structures and elements that enable women's ability to control their own health and the social conditions that shape it; actively and reflexively negotiating relationships of power, privilege, and oppression in all health promotion activities; and working collaboratively across sectors, disciplines, and social locations to mobilize our collective power toward improved health and social justice. Taking power into account in a serious and meaningful way means asking ourselves if health promotion practices and interventions exploit, accommodate, or transform power relations (Interagency Gender Working Group, 2004) and taking action to transform gendered power relations in an explicit manner. Moving in these directions is imperative so that health promotion processes avoid recreating and exacerbating gendered health and social inequities, and strive to improve health for women.

REFERENCES

Allen, A. (2008). Power and the politics of difference: Oppression, empowerment, and transnational justice. *Hypatia, 23*(3), 156–172.

Benoit, C., & Shumka, L. (2009). *Gendering the health determinants framework: Why girls' and women's health matters.* Vancouver: Women's Health Research Network.

Bottorff, J. L., Oliffe, J. L., Kelly, M. T., Greaves, L., Johnson, J. L., Ponic, P., & Chan, A. (2010). Men's business, women's work: Gender influences and fathers' smoking. *Sociology of Health & Illness, 32*(4), 583–596.

Boutilier, M., Cleverly, S., & Labonte, R. (2000). Community as a setting for health promotion. In B. D. Poland, L. W. Green, & I. Rootman (Eds.), *Settings for health promotion: Linking theory and practice* (pp. 250–287). Thousand Oaks, CA: Sage Publications.

Boutilier, M., & Mason, R. (2007). The reflexive practitioner in health promotion: From reflection to reflexivity. In M. O'Neill, A. Pederson, S. Dupéré, & I. Rootman (Eds.),

Health promotion in Canada: Critical perspectives (2nd ed., pp. 301–316). Toronto: Canadian Scholars' Press Inc.

Broom, D. (2008). Gender in/and/of health inequalities. *Australian Journal of Social Issues, 43*(1), 11–28.

Buchanan, D. R. (2006). A new ethic for health promotion: Reflections on a philosophy for health education in the 21st century. *Health Education & Behaviour, 33*(3), 290–304.

Bunjun, B., Lee, J., Lenon, S., Martin, L., Torres, S., & Waller, M. K. (2006). *Intersectional feminist frameworks: An emerging vision.* Ottawa: Canadian Research Institute for the Advancement of Women.

Cancian, F. (1991). Feminist science: Methodologies that challenge inequality. *Gender & Society, 6*(4), 623–642.

Carroll, S. (2012). Social theory and health promotion. In I. Rootman, S. Dupéré, A. Pederson, and M. O'Neill (Eds.), *Health promotion in Canada: Critical perspectives on practice* (3rd ed., pp. 33–53). Toronto: Canadian Scholars' Press Inc.

Champeau, D. A., & Shaw, S. A. (2002). Power, empowerment, and critical consciousness in community collaboration: Lessons from an advisory panel for an HIV awareness media campaign for women. *Women & Health, 36*(3), 31–50.

Cohen, I. (1989). *Structuration theory: Anthony Giddens and the constitution of social life.* New York: St. Martin's Press.

Cohen, M. (1998). Towards a framework for women's health. *Patient Education and Counseling, 33*(3), 187–196.

Collins, P. H. (2000). *Black feminist thought: Knowledge, consciousness, and the politics of empowerment* (2nd ed.). New York: Routledge.

Cornish, F., & Ghosh, R. (2007). The necessary contradictions of "community-led" health promotion: A case study of HIV prevention in an Indian red light district. *Social Science & Medicine, 64*(2), 496–507.

Covington, S. S. (2008). Women and addiction: A trauma-informed approach. *Journal of Psychoactive Drugs, 40*(Supp. 5), 377–385.

Daykin, N., & Naidoo, J. (1995). Feminist critiques of health promotion. In R. Bunton, S. Nettleton, & R. Burrows (Eds.), *The sociology of health promotion: Critical analyses of consumption, lifestyle, and risk* (pp. 59–69). London: Routledge.

Dominelli, L. (2005). Social inclusion in research: Reflecting on a research project involving young mothers in care. *International Journal of Social Welfare, 14*(1), 13–22.

Doyal, L. (2000). Gender equity in health: Debates and dilemmas. *Social Science and Medicine, 51*(6), 931–939.

Ehrhardt, A. A., Sawires, S., McGovern, T., Peacock, D., & Weston, M. (2009). Gender, empowerment, and health: What is it? How does it work? *Journal of Acquired Immune Deficiency Syndrome, 51*(3), 96–105.

Emerson, D., Sharma, R., Chaudhry, S., & Turner, J. (2009). Trauma-sensitive yoga: Principles, practice, and research. *International Journal of Yoga Therapy, 19*, 123–128.

English, L. M. (2006). A Foucauldian reading of learning in feminist, nonprofit organizations. *Adult Education Quarterly, 56*(2), 85–101.

Fonow, M. M., & Cook, J. A. (2005). Feminist methodology: New applications in the academy and public policy. *Signs: Journal of Women in Culture and Society, 30*(4), 2211–2236.

Foucault, M. (1977). *Power/knowledge: Selected interviews & other writings 1972–1977.* New
York: Pantheon Books.

Foucault, M. (1982). The subject and power. In H. Dreyfus & P. Rabinow (Eds.), *Michel
Foucault: Beyond structuralism and hermeneutics* (pp. 208–226). Chicago: University of
Chicago Press.

Frisby, W., Maguire, P., & Reid, C. (2009). The "f" word has everything to do with it:
How feminist theories inform action research. *Action Research, 7*(1), 13–29.

Frisby, W., Reid, C., & Ponic, P. (2007). Leveling the playing field: Promoting the health
of poor women through a community development approach to recreation. In P. White
& K. Young (Eds.), *Sport and gender in Canada* (2nd ed., pp. 120–136). Don Mills, ON:
Oxford University Press.

Frohlich, K. L., & Potvin, L. (2010). Structure or agency? The importance of both for
addressing social inequalities in health. *International Journal of Epidemiology, 39*(2), 378–379.

Frohlich, K. L., Ross, N., & Richmond, C. (2006). Health disparities in Canada today: Some
evidence and a theoretical framework. *Health Policy, 79*(2–3), 132–143. doi:10.1016/j.
healthpol.2005.12.010

Gandhi, L. (1998). *Postcolonial theory: A critical introduction.* New York: Columbia University
Press.

Giddens, A. (1984). *Constitution of society: Outline of the theory of structuration.* Berkeley:
University of California Press.

Godin, G. (2007). Has the individual vanished from Canadian health promotion? In M.
O'Neil, A. Pederson, S. Dupéré, & I. Rootman (Eds.), *Health promotion in Canada: Critical
perspectives* (2nd ed., pp. 367–370). Toronto: Canadian Scholars' Press Inc.

Gutierrez, L., & Lewis, E. (2005). Education, participation, and capacity building in community organizing and women of colour. In M. Minkler (Ed.), *Community organizing
& community building for health* (2nd ed., pp. 216–229). New Brunswick, NJ: Rutgers
University Press.

Hankivsky, O., Reid, C., Cormier, R., Varcoe, C., Clark, N., Benoit, C., & Brotman,
S. (2010). Exploring the promises of intersectionality for advancing women's health
research. *International Journal for Equity in Health, 9*(5), 5–20.

hooks, b. (2000). *Feminist theory: From margin to center* (2nd ed.). Cambridge, MA: South
End Press.

Interagency Gender Working Group. (2004). *The "So what?" report. A look at whether integrating a gender focus into programs makes a difference in outcomes.* Washington, DC: Population
Reference Bureau.

Johnson, J., Greaves, L., & Repta, R. (2007). *Better science with sex and gender: A primer for
health research.* Vancouver: BC Women's Health Research Network.

Kabeer, N. (1999). Resources, agency, achievements: Reflections on the measurement of women's empowerment. *Development and Change, 30,* 435–464.

Kar, S. B, Pascual, C. A., & Chickering, K. L. (1999). Empowerment of women for health promotion: A meta analysis. *Social Science and Medicine, 49*(11), 1431–1460.

Kesby, M. (2005). Retheorizing empowerment-through-participation as a performance in space: Beyond tyranny. *Signs: Journal of Women in Culture & Society, 30*(4), 2037–2065.

Kincheloe, J. L., & McLaren, P. (2000). Rethinking critical theory and qualitative research. In N. K. Denzin & Y. S. Lincoln (Eds.), *Handbook of qualitative research* (pp. 279–313). Thousand Oaks, CA: Sage Publications.

Labonte, R. (2005). Community, community development, and the forming of authentic partnerships: Some critical reflections. In M. Minkler (Ed.), *Community organizing & community building for health* (2nd ed., pp. 82–96). New Brunswick, NJ: Rutgers University Press.

Labonte, R., Polanyi, M., Muhajarine, N., McIntosh, T., & Williams, A. (2005). Beyond the divides: Towards critical population health research. *Critical Public Health, 15*(1), 5–17.

Laverack, G. (2004). *Health promotion practice: Power & empowerment.* Thousand Oaks, CA: Sage Publications.

Laverack, G., & Labonte, R. (2008). *Health promotion in action: From local to global empowerment.* New York: Palgrave Macmillan.

Lukes, S. (2005). *Power: A radical view* (2nd ed.). New York: Palgrave Macmillan.

McCall, L. (2005). The complexity of intersectionality. *Signs: Journal of Women in Culture and Society, 30*(3), 1771–1880.

Minkler, M. (1999). Personal responsibility for health? A review of the arguments and the evidence at century's end. *Health Education & Behaviour, 26*(1), 121–140.

Mohanty, C. T. (2004). Feminism without borders: Decolonizing theory, practicing solidarity. Durham, NC: Duke University Press.

Morrow, R. A., & Browne, D. D. (1994). *Critical theory and methodology.* Thousand Oaks, CA: Sage Publications.

Östlin, P., Eckermann, E., Mishra, U. S., Nkowane, M., & Wallstam, E. (2007). Gender and health promotion: A multisectoral policy approach. *Health Promotion International, 2*(S1), 25–35.

Pederson, A., & Donner, L. (2007). Beyond vessels and vectors: Reflections on women and primary health care reform in Canada. *Pan American Journal of Public Health, 21*(2/3): 145–154.

Phillips, S. (1995). The social context of women's health: Goals and objectives for medical education. *Canadian Medical Association Journal, 152*(4), 507–511.

Poland, B. (1998, November 5–6). *Social inequalities, social exclusion, and health: A critical social science perspective on health promotion theory, research, and practice.* Paper presented at the Health Promotion Research: Status and Progress Symposium, Bergen, Norway.

Poland, B., Krupa, G., & McCall, D. (2009). Setting for health promotion: An analytic framework to guide intervention design and implementation. *Health Promotion Practice, 10*(4), 505–516.

Ponic, P. (2000). A herstory, a legacy: The Canadian Fitness and Amateur Sport Branch's Women's Program. *Avante, 6*(1), 48–61.

Ponic, P. (2007). Embracing complexity in community-based health promotion: Inclusion, power, and women's health (Doctoral dissertation). University of British Columbia, Vancouver, BC.

Ponic, P., & Frisby, W. (2010). Unpacking assumptions about "inclusion" in community-based health promotion: Perspectives of women living in poverty. *Qualitative Health Research, 20*(11), 1519–1531.

Ponic, P., Pederson, A., & Ng, C. (in review). Bringing trauma-informed practice to physical activity for marginalized women: Implications for health promotion. *Health Promotion International.*

Ponic, P., Reid, C., & Frisby, W. (2010). Cultivating the power of partnerships in feminist participatory action research in women's health. *Nursing Inquiry, 17*(4), 324–335.

Poole, N., & Greaves, L. (2012). *Becoming trauma informed.* Toronto: Centre for Addiction and Mental Health.

Potvin, L., Gendron, S., Bilodeau, A., & Chabot, P. (2005). Integrating social theory into public health practice. *American Journal of Public Health, 95*(4), 591–595.

Raphael, D. (2006). Social determinants of health: Present status, unanswered questions, and future directions. *International Journal of Health Services, 36*(4), 651–677.

Rappaport, J. (1987). Terms of empowerment/exemplars of prevention: Toward a theory of community psychology. *American Journal of Community Psychology, 15*(2), 121–147.

Rappaport, J. (1995). Empowerment meets narrative: Listening to stories and creating settings. *American Journal of Community Psychology, 23*(5), 795–807.

Reid, C., Pederson, A., & Dupéré, S. (2007). Addressing diversity in health promotion: Implications of women's health and intersectionality theory. In M. O'Neill, A. Pederson, S. Dupéré, & I. Rootman (Eds.), *Health promotion in Canada: Critical perspectives* (2nd ed., pp. 75–89). Toronto: Canadian Scholars' Press Inc.

Reid, C., Pederson, A., & Dupéré, S. (2012). Addressing diversity and inequities in health promotion: The implications of intersectionality theory. In I. Rootman, S. Dupéré, A. Pederson, and M. O'Neill (Eds.), *Health promotion in Canada: Critical perspectives on practice* (3rd ed., pp. 54–66). Toronto: Canadian Scholars' Press Inc.

Ristock, J., & Pennell, J. (1996). *Community research as empowerment: Feminist links, postmodern interruptions.* Toronto: Oxford University Press.

Shope, J. H. (2006). "You can't cross a river without getting wet": A feminist standpoint on the dilemmas of cross-cultural research. *Qualitative Inquiry, 12*(1), 163–184.

Spinazzola, J., Rhodes, A. M., Emerson, D., Earle, E., & Monroe, K. (2011). Application of yoga in residential treatment of traumatized youth. *Journal of the American Psychiatric Nurses Association, 17*(6), 431–444.

Teske, R. L. (2000). The butterfly effect. In R. L. Teske & M. A. Tetreault (Eds.), *Conscious acts and the politics of social change: Feminist approaches to social movements, community, and power* (Vol. 1, pp. 107–123). Columbia: University of South Carolina Press.

Tett, L. (2005). Partnerships, community groups, and social inclusion. *Studies in Continuing Education, 27*(1), 1–15.

VanderPlaat, M. (1999). Locating the feminist scholar: Relational empowerment and social activism. *Qualitative Health Research, 9*(6), 773–785.

Varcoe, C., Hankivsky, O., & Morrow, M. (2007). Introduction: Beyond gender matters. In M. Morrow, O. Hankivsky, & C. Varcoe (Eds.), *Women's health in Canada: Critical perspectives on theory and policy* (pp. 3–30). Toronto: University of Toronto Press.

Wallerstein, N. (1992). Powerlessness, empowerment, and health. Implications for health promotion programs. *American Journal of Health Promotion, 6*(3), 197–205.

Wallerstein, N., & Duran, B. (2003). The conceptual, historical, and practice roots of community based participatory research and related participatory traditions. In M. Minkler & N. Wallerstein (Eds.), *Community-based participatory research for health* (pp. 27–52). San Francisco: Jossey-Bass.

Weedon, C. (1999). *Feminist practice and poststructuralist theory* (2nd ed.). Oxford: Blackwell Publishers.

Weissbecker, I., & Clark, C. (2007).The impact of violence and abuse: Can trauma-informed treatment make a difference? *Journal of Community Psychology, 35*(7), 909–923.

Williams, J., & Lykes, M. B. (2003). Bridging theory and practice: Using reflexive cycles in feminist participatory action research. *Feminism & Psychology, 13*(3), 287–294.

Wong, N., Zimmerman, M., & Parker, E. (2010). A typology of youth participation and empowerment for child and adolescent health promotion. *American Journal of Community Psychology, 46*(1/2), 100–114.

World Health Organization. (1986). *Ottawa Charter for health promotion*. Ottawa: Author.

World Health Organization. (2005). WHO multi-country study on women's health and domestic violence against women: Summary report of initial results on prevalence, health outcomes, and women's responses. Geneva: Author.

Young, I. M. (1990). *Justice and the politics of difference*. Princeton, NJ: Princeton University Press.

Zimmerman, M. (1995). Psychological empowerment: Issues and illustrations. *American Journal of Community Psychology, 23*(5), 581–599.

3 Diversifying Health Promotion

Colleen Reid, Ann Pederson, and Sophie Dupéré

Theory is a tool to think with.

—Dorothy Smith[1]

Introduction

Many have argued that health promotion's theoretical base is still largely dominated by biomedical, psychological, and behavioural models, and call for the development of more social theories (Potvin, Gendron, Bilodeau, & Chabot, 2005) and expanded academic alliances to enrich its theoretical base (Ziglio, Hagard, & Griffiths, 2000). Vigilance is required, however, to ensure that the exchange of concepts and theories between disciplines is done rigorously. While interdisciplinary exchanges can be potentially enriching, such "transfers" from one field to another frequently occur without an in-depth understanding of their theoretical and epistemological basis, as has been the case with the introduction of the concept of social capital into public health (Forbes & Wainwright, 2001; see Moore, Haines, Hawe, & Shiell, 2006 for a full discussion of the theoretical and policy implications of mistranslating the concept "social capital"). Of any concept or theory, it should be asked: Whose is it? How is it constructed and reconstructed? Whose interests does it serve? (Noffke, 1998). As humans we always operate from a theoretical position, whether implicit or explicit. What is fundamentally important is that we continue to ask and answer these questions while becoming increasingly explicit about naming our theoretical positions and, in turn, how concepts become operationalized in our research, practice, and policy.

In this chapter we argue that health promotion could learn from more dialogue and exchange with feminist scholarship by presenting intersectionality as an important theoretical contribution from women's studies and other fields (McCall,

2005; Weber & Parra-Medina, 2003) that could help health promotion grapple with diversity and the persistence of health inequities. Through drawing mainly on developments in the field of women's health over the past 40 years, we propose intersectionality as a contemporary approach that could increase the theoretical rigour and enhance health promotion practice and policy both within and beyond women's health. We caution, however, against a superficial adoption of intersectional theory into health promotion research and practice, arguing instead that health promotion advocates should adopt a critical stance toward the contributions that intersectional theory offers to the field, and deliberately seek opportunities to test and refine the theory from the perspective of health promotion research, practice, and policy.

Limitations of Current Approaches to Health Promotion in Addressing Persistent Health Inequities: The Case of Gender

A number of important concerns persist in Canadian society about the effects of gender (Canadian Feminist Alliance for International Action, 2003). Examples include: the high percentage of Canadian women who live in poverty and report poor health status; the persistence of violence against Canadian women; the diminished status of immigrant and refugee women; the vulnerability of Aboriginal women who are the "poorest of the poor"; or the educational underachievement of boys, to name a few. With its continual focus on lifestyle change—despite rhetoric addressing the elements of the Ottawa Charter—health promotion may have contributed to the persistence of health inequities by perpetuating the advantages that certain groups in Canadian society have in accessing information, organizing themselves for change, and creating the conditions to support healthier living.

Twenty years ago, British sociologists Daykin and Naidoo (1995) suggested that health promotion rested on and perpetuated certain aspects of gender inequities (Pederson et al., 2010). In particular, they argued that health promotion held women responsible for their own health and the health of others, and employed the techniques of health education and social marketing to encourage women to adopt healthy lifestyles without regard for the individual and structural constraints of power, income, race, and education—among others—that limited women's ability to take action on health issues. Since then, scholars have recognized that health promotion has contributed to gender inequities in other ways. These include perpetuating a confusion regarding the differences between sex and gender (see Box 3.1) and the tendency to see both as dichotomies (Clow, Pederson, Haworth-Brockman, & Bernier, 2009); failing to recognize gender as a social determinant of health (Benoit et al., 2009); homogenizing and isolating social categories such as gender, class, and ethnicity rather than focusing on power relations and associated values such as social justice (Reid, Ponic, Hara, Kaweesi, & Ledrew, 2011); and contributing to an overall ambiguity regarding theoretical approaches and underpinnings with respect to health inequities (Hankivsky et al., 2010).

Recently, the World Health Organization (WHO) has taken a step toward addressing health inequities. The final report of the Commission on Social Determinants of Health, *Closing the Gap in a Generation: Health Equity Through Action on the Social Determinants of Health* (CSDH, 2008), argues that many persistent and avoidable health inequities remain between and within countries. The report outlines a global agenda for health equity with three overarching recommendations, none of which refers to increasing individual health-promoting behaviours. Instead, the report recommends: (1) improving daily living conditions; (2) tackling the inequitable distribution of power, money, and resources; and (3) measuring and understanding the problem and assessing the impact of action. Within these recommendations, an essential action highlighted by the report pertains to addressing gender inequities that are seen as unfair, ineffective, and inefficient. "By supporting gender equity, governments, donors, international organizations and civil society can improve the lives of millions of girls and women and their families" (CSDH, 2008, p. 16).

However, the WHO Commission's report is generally thin on specific recommendations for addressing inequities related to gender and offers only a partial view of the contribution of gender to health. The WHO report offers a framework that identifies gender as an intermediate factor shaped by other more fundamental ones such as socio-economic status and policy as well as cultural and societal norms and values. Other scholars have argued, however, that gender must be understood as a fundamental determinant of health that structures access to key resources. Benoit and Shumka (2009) are proponents of such a view and suggest that sex and gender shape access to education, employment, child care, safe neighbourhoods, and health services—themselves determinants of health. Importantly, Benoit and Shumka's framework identifies other key aspects of social location such as social class, race, ethnicity, age, immigrant status, and geographic location as fundamental determinants of health as well. Together these determinants shape access to resources and ultimately health behaviours and morbidity and mortality. Understanding the relationships among the determinants of health is important for action to reduce health inequities arising from gender. It is critical that action be taken to tackle gender-related inequities and their consequences both directly and indirectly to reduce the resulting health inequities. That is, action should be taken to reduce gender-related inequities themselves, rather than simply expecting action on other factors to trickle down to improve gender-related inequities. Health promotion research and practice in Canada therefore needs to take bold action (Raphael, 2008).

Theoretical innovations to improve knowledge and praxis, such as the uptake of recommendations arising from Benoit and Shumka (2009), are needed to enable us to embrace the complex interplay of health determinants and to understand how they intersect and mutually reinforce each other.

Lessons from the Women's Health Movement

The women's health movement and health promotion share important core values, priorities, and approaches to practice. Those in the women's health field have long embraced a positive conceptualization of health (Thurston & O'Connor, 1996) and perceived health as a continuum that extends throughout the life cycle and that is critically and intimately related to the conditions under which women live. Moreover, women's health activists and scholars have long recognized the link between the social location of a person or a group and their health, and advocated for both individual and community empowerment to improve health (see, for example, Morrow, Hankivsky, & Varcoe, 2007; Armstrong & Deadman, 2009).[2]

Questions asked early in the women's health movement that continue to inform women's health research and gender and health research can be instructive for health promotion theory and praxis. For over four decades this broad field has grappled with substantive challenges, including: raising consciousness around "the personal is political"; drawing attention to the increasing medicalization of women's health and loss of control over health decision making: debating the distinct influences and interactions between biology and social structure; examining the uniqueness of women's issues versus the many diversities and differences among women; and understanding the relevance of gender to men's experiences while expanding analytic categories to understand diverse men's and women's experiences.

 BOX 3.1: DISTINGUISHING SEX AND GENDER

Sex is "a multidimensional biological construct that encompasses anatomy, physiology, genes, and hormones that together create a human 'package' that affects how we are labelled" (Johnson, Greaves, & Repta, 2007, pp. 4–5). *Gender* is "a social construct that is culturally based and historically specific [and] refers to the socially prescribed and experienced dimensions of 'femaleness' or 'maleness' in a society, and is manifested at many levels" (ibid., p. 5).

Disentangling sex and gender, describing the interactions of sex and gender and their effects, and situating this analysis in the context of other oppressions have become increasingly important to understanding women's health (Greaves, 2009). Johnson, Greaves, and Repta (2007) argue that including the concepts of sex and gender in research leads to a variety of benefits, such as the increased rigour and validity of research, cost savings, greater social justice, and the potential to save lives. It makes important political statements as well. For example, the arguments embedded in a sex- and gender-based analysis reflect the values of inclusiveness and equity, and are based on historical claims for redress for women (Greaves, 2009).

Indeed, while we posit that advances in the field of women's health can be instructive to health promotion and critique health promotion's slow uptake of theories and concepts, the field of gender and women's health has been marred by some limitations. While theoretical advances are sophisticated and complex, there remains a tendency to essentialize the category of "woman," to see gender as primarily affecting women, and to ignore or pay scant attention to men and masculinities. As well, there are those who would argue that some women's health advocates give too much primacy to gender over other key social determinants of health (Hankivsky et al., 2010), or fail to recognize and acknowledge this as a limitation in their work.[3]

The Potential Contributions of Intersectional Theory: Expanding Understandings and Approaches

Many argue that gender is distinct from but interactive with other social features like social class or race/ethnicity. All these social factors combine to determine power relations in society that lead not only to inequities between women and men, but also to inequities among different groups of women and different groups of men (Östlin, George, & Sen, 2003).

Intersectional theory is based on the idea that "different dimensions of social life cannot be separated into discrete or pure strands" (Brah & Phoenix, 2004, p. 76). When attempting to understand social inequities, an intersectional analysis focuses on social relationships of power instead of focusing on access to resources. An intersectional analysis examines social experiences and how they intersect at multiple forms of oppression, and what happens at these intersections (McCall, 2005).

Intersectional theory was developed most prominently by black feminist social scientists emphasizing the simultaneous production of race, class, and gender inequity, such that in any given situation, the unique contribution of one factor might be difficult to measure (Collins, 1989; Fonow & Cook, 1991). This approach—an alternative to earlier models that assumed that advantage and disadvantage simply accumulate to produce "double jeopardy"—suggests that the content and implications of gender and race as socially constructed categories vary as a function of each other (Mullings & Schulz, 2006). For example, whiteness and blackness are

BOX 3.2: **INTERSECTIONALITY**

Intersectionality is a new paradigm that brings to the forefront the complexity of social locations and experiences for understanding differences in health needs and outcomes. It refers to "the interaction between gender, race and other categories of difference in individual lives, social practices, institutional arrangements, and cultural ideologies and the outcomes of these interactions in terms of power" (Davis, 2008, p. 68). The following are key assumptions of intersectionality:

1. The pursuit of social justice is the main objective.
2. The conceptualization of identity that resists essentializing one group or assuming shared similar perspectives.
3. The recognition that social categories of difference, such as gender, race, age, and so on, are complex, fluid, and flexible.
4. Power and a consideration of systems of domination are central to the analysis.

Source: Hankivsky & Cormier (2009).

gendered, and masculinity and femininity are "raced" within particular cultural contexts. Hence it is often difficult to pinpoint how the interaction, articulation, and simultaneity of race, class, and gender affect women and men in their daily lives, and the ways in which these forms of inequity interact in specific situations to condition health (Mullings & Schulz, 2006).

Intersectional theory suggests that we need to move beyond seeing ourselves and others as single points in some specified set of dichotomies: male or female, white or black, straight or gay, scholar or activist, powerful or powerless. Rather, "we need to imagine ourselves as existing at the intersection of multiple identities, all of which influence one another and together shape our continually changing experience and interactions" (Brydon-Miller, 2004, p. 9). Intersectional scholarship arose primarily to better understand and address the multiple dimensions of social inequity, including class, race/ethnicity, gender, sexual orientation, age, and disability. Intersectionality is an analytical tool and framework that can be used both at micro and macro levels. At a micro level, it aims to understand the effects of structural inequities on individual lives by focusing on the interplay between social categories and multiple sources of power and privilege. At a macro level, it seeks to understand how multiple power systems (i.e., institutions) are implicated in the production, organization, and sustainability of inequities. It provides a social structural analysis of inequity (Bilge, 2009).

What distinguishes intersectionality from a social-determinants-of-health approach is that an intersectional analysis does not seek to simply add categories to one another (e.g., gender, race, class, sexuality) but instead strives to understand what is created and experienced at the intersection of two or more categories (Hankivsky et al., 2010). In so doing, it recognizes the multi-dimensional and relational nature of social locations and places lived experiences, social forces, and overlapping systems of discrimination and subordination at the centre of analysis (Hannan, 2001). In this way an intersectionality analysis captures several levels of difference (Hankivsky et al., 2010).

While the flexibility of intersectionality may be beneficial in some respects, its elasticity may lend itself to the theory's superficial appropriation. Some argue that it has been used in a reductionist and simplistic way. For example, it has not always been accompanied by an analysis that is actually intersectional (Knapp, 2005). There has also been a tendency to use intersectionality in "micro-level" analyses that focus on the narration of social identities to the exclusion of macro socio-structural analyses of inequities (Collins, 2009, cited by Bilge, 2009). Other authors raise cautions about its use and have highlighted potential limits to its ability to explain power (see Bilge, 2009). Indeed, intersectional theory is still in its early stages of development and further theoretical and methodological development is needed. Nevertheless, we feel that greater consideration of the theory of intersectionality could enhance the ability of health promotion to recognize and address diversity in research, policy, and practice.

Intersectionality:
A Theory to Guide Health Promotion Research and Practice

Intersectional frameworks have much to offer health promotion research and practice. For example, intersectionality can help us see through and beyond defined population groups, targeted settings, and specific health issues. It can move us beyond taken-for-granted assumptions and expectations that have characterized much of health promotion to date. For instance, Matsuda (1991) writes of "asking the other question": "When I see something that looks racist, I ask 'Where is the patriarchy in this?' When I see something that looks sexist, I ask, 'Where is the heterosexism in this?'" (p. 1189). In a recent study conducted by Reid et al. (2011) that involved South Asian and Aboriginal women, they "asked the other question" and adopted research strategies and an analytic sharpness to prevent them from seeing these women's experiences as the product of their gender or ethnicity alone. Indeed, "if we fail to ask the other question, what assumptions are being made, and what is lost?" (Reid et al., 2011, p. 104).

A few authors (Cole, 2008; Hankivsky & Cormier, 2009; Hankivsky et al., 2010; Weber, 2007) provide some useful questions for conducting an intersectional analysis that can deepen the typical questions asked of health promotion practice and research:

- Who is the target population for the study or intervention? Why was this group chosen, and how do they identify themselves? Who is being compared to whom? Why?
- What issues are of central importance to the researchers, practitioners, and people themselves? How were they identified? Are issues of domination and exploitation being examined? How will the issue of power be at the centre of all analyses?
- How will human commonalities and differences be recognized without resorting to broad generalizations, stereotypical categories, or obliviousness to historical and contemporary patterns of inequity?
- How do researchers and practitioners ensure that they are not seeing what they want to see?
- Are the perspectives of all key stakeholder groups such as policy-makers, grassroots activists, and community groups, including multiply oppressed communities, represented?
- Is the research or intervention framed within the current cultural, societal, and/or situational context?

Posing these questions in health promotion research and practice will improve the work conducted: the range of the issues raised will be broader and dealt with in more depth, the nature of the work conducted will expand, and new and previously unexamined dimensions of both will shift the kinds of issues raised in the work as well as change the nature of health promotion itself.

While posing these questions is an important step forward for health promotion research and practice, we must be mindful that by virtue of intersectionality's complexity, it is a challenging framework to work with: there is no "one-size-fits-all" approach (for specific examples, see Hankivsky et al., 2010).

Implications for Health Promotion Practice

Even as intersectionality continues to advance as a theory and methodology, we want to consider the challenge of "operationalizing" an intersectional analysis to further and enhance the practice of health promotion. In order to consider this challenge, we asked ourselves, "What would interventions look like, or how would they be different, if we applied an intersectional analysis? What might this mean for health promotion practice?" We developed the following insights and invite health promotion researchers and practitioners to join this conversation:

- *Change outlook on individual characteristics:* An intersectional analysis would shift our focus from "immutable" individual characteristics (e.g., sex, ethnicity) to "mutable social realities" (e.g., those that can be targeted by intervention). Gender and race are not simply biological categories but also social ones (Krieger, 2003). Rather than adopting rigid categories of "populations," we would focus on the interplay between and among social categories.
- *Reframe the concept of health:* An expanded conception of health would include refocusing on a broad framework of social relations and would locate health in families and communities and not only in individual bodies. This is consistent with contemporary reflections on the health promotion field (see Chapter 2) as well as intersectional analyses.
- *Shift the focus of intervention:* An intersectional analysis invites us to target not only the individual but also to take into consideration and even address explicitly social structures, social processes, and the underlying relationships of power. This will involve developing more upstream interventions and policies (i.e., taking action on the "causes of the causes"—the macro determinants of health such as poverty) (see Chapter 7) and adopting ecological (see Chapter 5) and multi-sectoral approaches. Additionally, an intersectional analysis would deepen understandings of health by adopting a framework of power and oppression and conceptualizing alternative health interventions.
- *Recognize multiple and diverse perspectives through holistic and community-based approaches:* A holistic perspective invites us to examine social experiences, how they intersect at multiple strands of oppression, and what happens at these intersections (McCall, 2005). It encourages us to bring together multiple and diverse stakeholders and to view research and practice as mutual and reciprocal. Holistic and community-based approaches foster the broad-based participation of stakeholders, inter-sectoral practice, the creation of coalitions and strategic alliances, and increased forms of activism. Additionally, such approaches will help operationalize intersectionality in terms of unpacking the "nuts and bolts" of running an initiative or research project.
- *Encourage reflexive practice:* Intersectional theory invites us to pay attention to social processes, social dynamics, and the role of power in producing and sustaining social inequities. It also encourages the researcher-practitioner to connect her or his personal and political identities, and to become

aware of her or his own power and privilege. Adopting a reflexive practice (see Chapter 11) can help prevent health researchers and practitioners from unknowingly perpetuating, sustaining, and reinforcing harmful stereotypes (Reid & Herbert, 2005).

These recommendations are consistent, we believe, with most of the advice given elsewhere in this book about how to strengthen the foundations of health promotion to enhance its effectiveness.

Conclusion

To address the mounting critiques of the atheoretical nature of health promotion research and practices, as well as calls for health promotion, public health, and health science researchers to increase the theoretical rigour of their work to better inform and direct practice and policy, we advocate intersectional theory because it challenges us to think about conceptualizations of the content, context, and boundaries of social groups (Mullings & Schulz, 2006). Yet we see two important challenges—to push health promotion researchers, practitioners, educators, and advocates to understand the complexity and diversity of health through an intersectional analysis, and to develop strategies for moving a more theoretically informed health promotion into the mainstream. There is an opportunity and appetite for health promotion to pay attention to the more nuanced and complex understandings of health inequities, and of women's and men's health, that have been recently advanced by many feminist and intersectional scholars. Intersectional analysis reminds health promotion researchers, theoreticians, and practitioners that we must have a theory of power if we are to understand health inequities and redress them. The field of health promotion in turn reminds intersectional scholars that ongoing attention is needed to adapting intersectional frameworks for policy development and day-to-day practice. Health promotion's tradition of action and engagement can be useful to those who may get caught up in critique and theorizing at the expense of practice. By learning from each other, the fields of health promotion and intersectionality can both contribute to reducing health disparities and improving health.

NOTES

1 Dorothy E. Smith is professor of sociology and the author of *The Everyday World as Problematic: A Feminist Sociology* and *The Conceptual Practices of Power*. She has written about prevailing discourses of sociology, political economy, philosophy, popular culture, and feminist theory and practice. She is reputed to have made this point in her presentations.

2   Recently feminist and intersectionality scholars have acknowledged the importance of understanding gender—the experience of being feminine or masculine—for both women and men. However, the women's health movement arose from examinations of women's experiences of health and health care. Some examples used in this chapter come from the women's health movement and therefore focus only on women's health.

3   To essentialize is to apply a homogenizing view of a fixed category that specifies the "essential" properties or characteristics of all women (Ristock & Pennell, 1996).

REFERENCES

Armstrong, P., & Deadman, J. (Eds.). (2009). *Women's health: Intersections of policy, research, and practice*. Toronto: Women's Press.

Benoit, C., & Shumka, L. (2009). *Gendering the health determinants framework: Why girls' and women's health matters*. Vancouver: Women's Health Research Network.

Benoit, C., Shumka, L., Phillips, R., Hallgrímsdóttir, H., Kobayashi, K., Hankivsky, O., ... & Brief, E. (2009). Explaining the health gap between girls and women in Canada. *Sociological Research Online, 14*(5). Retrieved from www.socresonline.org.uk/14/5/9.html

Bilge, S. (2009). Théorisations feminists de l'intersectionnalité. *Diogène, 1*(225), 70–88.

Brah, A., & Phoenix, A. (2004). Ain't I a woman? Revisiting intersectionality. *Journal of International Women's Studies, 5*(3), 75–86.

Brydon-Miller, M. (2004). The terrifying truth: Interrogating systems of power and privilege and choosing to act. In M. Brydon-Miller, P. Maguire, & A. McIntyre (Eds.), *Traveling companions: Feminism, teaching, and action research* (pp. 3–19). Westport: Praeger.

Canadian Feminist Alliance for International Action. (2003). *Canada's failure to act: Women's inequality deepens*. Ottawa: Canadian Feminist Alliance for International Action. Retrieved from www.fafia-afai.org/en/node/164

Clow, B., Pederson, A., Haworth-Brockman, M., & Bernier, J. (2009). *Rising to the challenge: Sex- and gender-based analysis for health planning, policy, and research in Canada*. Halifax: Atlantic Centre of Excellence for Women's Health.

Cole, E. (2008). Coalitions as a model for intersectionality: From practice to theory. *Sex Roles, 59*(5–6), 443–453.

Collins, P. H. (1989). The social construction of black feminist thought. *Signs: Journal of Women in Culture and Society, 14*(4), 745–773.

CSDH. (2008). *Closing the gap in a generation: Health equity through action on the social determinants of health*. Geneva: World Health Organization. Retrieved from http://whqlibdoc.who.int/hq/2008/WHO_IER_CSDH_08.1_eng.pdf

Davis, K. (2008). Intersectionality as buzzword: A sociology of science perspective on what makes a feminist theory successful. *Feminist Theory, 9*(1), 67–85.

Daykin, N., & Naidoo, J. (1995). Feminist critiques of health promotion. In R. Bunton, S. Nettleton, & R. Burrows (Eds.), *The sociology of health promotion: Critical analyses of consumption, lifestyle, and risk* (pp. 59–69). London & New York: Routledge.

Fonow, M. M., & Cook, J. A. (1991). Back to the future: A look at the second wave of feminist epistemology and methodology. In M. M. Fonow & J. A. Cook (Eds.), *Beyond methodology: Feminist scholarship as lived research* (pp. 1–15). Bloomington: Indiana University Press.

Forbes, A., & Wainwright, S. P. (2001). On the methodological, theoretical, and philosophical context of health inequalities research: A critique. *Social Science and Medicine, 53*(6), 801–816.

Greaves, L. (2009). Women, gender, and health research. In P. Armstrong & J. Deadman (Eds.), *Women's health: Intersections of policy, research, and practice* (pp. 3–20). Toronto: Women's Press.

Hankivsky, O., & Cormier, R. (with De Merich, D.) (2009). *Intersectionality: Moving women's health research and policy forward.* Vancouver: Women's Health Research Network. doi:10.1186/1475-9276-9-5

Hankivsky, O., Reid, C., Varcoe, C., Clark, N., Benoit, C., & Brotman, S. (2010). Exploring the promises of intersectionality for advancing women's health research. *International Journal for Equity in Health, 9*(5). Retrieved from www.equityhealthj.com/content/9/1/5

Hannan, C. (2001). Gender mainstreaming—a strategy for promoting gender equality: With particular focus on HIV/AIDS and racism. Paper presented at the NGO Consultation in preparation for the 45th Session of the Commission on the Status of Women. NYU Medical Centre, New York.

Johnson, J., Greaves, L., & Repta, R. (2007). *Better science with sex and gender: A primer for health research.* Vancouver: Women's Health Research Network.

Knapp, G. (2005). Race, class, gender: Reclaiming baggage in fast travelling theories. *European Journal of Women's Studies, 12*(3), 249–265.

Krieger, N. (2003). Genders, sexes, and health: What are the connections—and why does it matter? *International Journal of Epidemiology, 32*(4), 652–657.

Matsuda, M. J. (1991). Beside my sister, facing the enemy: Legal theory out of coalition. *Stanford Law Review, 43*(6), 1183–1192.

McCall, L. (2005). The complexity of intersectionality. *Signs: Journal of Women in Culture and Society, 30*(3), 1771–1800.

Moore, S., Haines, V., Hawe, P., & Shiell, A. (2006). Lost in translation: A genealogy of the "social capital" concept in public health. *Journal of Epidemiology and Community Health, 60*(8), 729–734.

Morrow, M., Hankivsky, O., & Varcoe, C. (Eds.). (2007). *Women's health in Canada: Critical perspectives on theory and policy.* Toronto: University of Toronto Press.

Mullings, L., & Schulz, A. J. (2006). Intersectionality and health: An introduction. In A. J. Schulz & L. Mullings (Eds.), *Gender, race, class, and health: Intersectional approaches* (pp. 3–17). San Francisco: Jossey-Bass.

Noffke, S. (1998). *What's a nice theory like yours doing in a practice like this? And other impertinent questions about practitioner research.* Keynote address presented at the 2nd International Practitioner Research Conference, Sydney, Australia.

Östlin, P., George, A., & Sen, G. (2003). Gender, health, and equity: The intersections. In R. Hofrichter (Ed.), *Health and social justice: Politics, ideology, and inequity in the distribution of disease* (pp. 132–156). San Francisco: Jossey-Bass.

Pederson, A., Ponic, P., Greaves, L., Mills, S., Christilaw, J., Frisby, W., ... & Young, L. (2010). Igniting an agenda for health promotion for women: Critical perspectives, evidence-based practice, and innovative knowledge translation. *Canadian Journal of Public Health, 101*(3), 259 –261.

Potvin, L., Gendron, S., Bilodeau, A., & Chabot, P. (2005). Integrating social theory into public health practice. *American Journal of Public Health, 95*(4), 591–595.

Raphael, D. (2008). Grasping at straws: A recent history of health promotion in Canada. *Critical Public Health, 18*(4), 483–495.

Reid, C., & Herbert, C. (2005). "Welfare moms and welfare bums": Revisiting poverty as a social determinant of health. *Health Sociology Review, 14*(2), 161–173.

Reid, C., Ponic, P., Hara, L., Kaweesi, C., & Ledrew, R. (2011). Performing intersectionality: The mutuality of intersectional analysis and feminist participatory action research. In O. Hankivsky (Ed.), *Health inequities in Canada: Intersectional frameworks and practices* (pp. 92–111). Vancouver: UBC Press.

Ristock, J. L., & Pennell, J. (1996). *Community research as empowerment: Feminist links, postmodern interruptions.* Toronto: Oxford University Press.

Thurston, W. E., & O'Connor, M. (1996, August 9–11). *Health promotion for women: A Canadian perspective.* Paper prepared for the Canada–USA Women's Health Forum, Ottawa.

Weber, L. (2007). *Through a fly's eyes: Addressing diversity in our creative, research, and scholarly endeavours.* Paper presented at the inaugural celebration of GREAT Day (Geneseo Recognizing Excellence, Achievement, and Talent), State University of New York at Geneseo, Geneseo, NY.

Weber, L., & Parra-Medina, D. (2003). Intersectionality and women's health: Charting a path to eliminating health disparities. In M. T. Segal & V. Demos (Eds.), *Gender perspectives on health and medicine: Key themes* (pp. 181–230). London: Elsevier.

Ziglio, E., Hagard, S., & Griffiths, J. (2000). Health promotion development in Europe: Achievements and challenges. *Health Promotion International, 15*(2), 143–154.

PART 2

4 Igniting Global Tobacco Control

Natalie Hemsing and Lorraine Greaves

Introduction

The use of tobacco is a leading cause of death globally, and given its addictive qualities, it is particularly difficult to stop once started. Both tobacco use and the promotion of tobacco products have long been gendered. In addition, recent evidence suggests that women are more biologically susceptible to health damage from smoking than men, whether for cancers, heart disease, or chronic illnesses (Huxley & Woodward, 2011; Parajuli et al., 2013). Indeed, all of the patterns of uptake, consumption levels, and products used have typically been different for women and men, with women generally taking up tobacco later than men in any given population. In part, this is because over the latter half of the twentieth century the tobacco industry mounted gender-specific marketing, advertising, and product development initiatives in developed countries to appeal to girls and women and, most importantly, to shift gendered social norms to create a female market and increase the number of women who smoke.

In this century, the focus of tobacco marketing, and consequently tobacco control, has been on women in low- and middle-income countries, where women's rates of smoking are still low and far lower than those of men, but where their rates of exposure to tobacco smoke are high. However, rates of women's tobacco use are rising, and could form an explosive public health issue for women this century in a range of countries around the world. Not surprisingly, this trend has been preceded by the tobacco industry's shift of attention from the high-income countries to the low- and middle-income countries in cultivation, manufacturing, promotion, and advertising.

What has been the health promotion response to both incipient female smoking and well-established trends and patterns? And how do these efforts fit into the wider project of tobacco control? This chapter investigates these questions with a view to developing gender-transformative tobacco control. We argue that, unlike the tobacco industry, tobacco control efforts have been fundamentally gender-blind. With increasing evidence of high smoking prevalence among socially disadvantaged groups of women, and increasing tobacco use and production in low- and middle-income countries, this approach needs to change.

The global prevalence of smoking among men has peaked and is slowly declining, yet tobacco use among women is on the rise (Mackay, Eriksen, & Shafey, 2006). Smoking rates among women and men are similar in high-income countries, including Canada, the United States, Australia, and those of Wsestern Europe, while in low- and middle-income countries, smoking rates among women are much lower than among men (Hitchman & Fong, 2011; Mackay & Amos, 2003). Tobacco-control policies aimed at prevention, protection, de-normalization, and cessation—the pillars of tobacco control—have decreased overall smoking prevalence within high-income countries, yet these reductions have not been evenly experienced (Graham, Inskip, Francis, & Harman, 2006). In high-income countries, where women have a longer history of tobacco use, disadvantaged groups of women (with lower education, income, etc.) are more likely to smoke (Amos, Greaves, Nichter, & Bloch, 2011; Berridge & Loughlin, 2005). For example, at 18 percent, the overall prevalence of smoking is relatively low in Canada when compared to other countries, yet tobacco use remains high among specific subgroups of the population, including young women and men (CTUMS, 2010), Aboriginal peoples (Health Canada, 2007), and particularly Aboriginal teenage girls (Assembly of First Nations RHS National Team, 2007). Similarly, while smoking rates have decreased among higher socio-economic groups in England since the 1960s, inequalities in tobacco use are evident, with tobacco use now much greater among those with lower income and education or those in manual unskilled employment (Giskes et al., 2007). Disadvantaged groups of women may be both more vulnerable to tobacco use and encounter greater challenges in reducing or quitting smoking, as well as reducing their exposure to second-hand smoke (Greaves & Jategaonkar, 2006). Low-income women may, for example, have greater exposure to second-hand smoke and less power to manage their exposure to second-hand smoke both at work and at home (Greaves & Hemsing, 2009).

In the majority of low- and middle-income countries, smoking rates for women are below 5 percent (Amos et al., 2011). In countries where smoking rates among men are high, women face considerable health risk due to exposure to second-hand smoke from their partners (Greaves, Jategaonkar, & Sanchez, 2006). But the gap in smoking rates between women and men in low- and middle-income countries is shrinking, and it is anticipated that this trend will continue (Hitchman & Fong, 2011). Recent data from youth in 151 countries reveal that 7 percent of adolescent girls and 12 percent of adolescent boys smoke, and in some countries the smoking rates are comparable (World Health Organization, 2010), making tobacco use among girls, boys, and young men and women a key global health promotion issue.

Rising smoking rates among women have been linked to: changes in social norms regarding women's smoking; the tobacco industry's advertising targeting women, which typically frames smoking as a sign of empowerment; upward shifts in women's socio-economic status; and the relative lack of women-specific cessation programs and health education programs, particularly for women in developing countries (Amos et al., 2011; Hitchman & Fong, 2011; Mackay & Amos, 2003). With the growing population in low- and middle-income countries, even if the increase in smoking among women can be halted, there will be an increase in the absolute number of women smokers (Mackay & Amos, 2003). In addition to the growing concerns of tobacco use and smoke exposure for women in low-income countries is the issue of tobacco cultivation, which is increasingly being relocated to these countries, where women and children suffer serious health and economic consequences (Greaves et al., 2006).

These trends are critically important as they indicate the gender and equity considerations that affect both past and future trends in women's tobacco use, and pertain to both the emergence of smoking among women and girls in low- and middle-income countries as well as the shift in smoking to disadvantaged groups of women in high-income countries. Tobacco strategies and responses that are not tailored to these specific contexts may be less likely to result in either further reductions in tobacco use or short-circuiting the epidemic in low- and middle-income countries. Given these evolving trends of use, exposure, growing, and marketing of tobacco, both gender and equity need to be integrated into tobacco policy and program and research initiatives. In particular, they need to be integrated into health promotion activities and to reflect the multi-faceted effects of tobacco, not only on health, but also on women's social and economic status. As such, comprehensive approaches that also seek to improve women's equality are imperative, so the need for gender-transformative health promotion initiatives in tobacco control is critical.

History of Tobacco Control

Early evidence emerged in the 1950s and 1960s regarding the association of smoking with cancer and cardiovascular diseases, lung cancer, and total death rates (Hammond & Horn, 1958; Jacobson, Wasserman, & Anderson, 1997; Warner & Mendez, 2010). However, this evidence came from research conducted with male participants and findings were targeted toward men. The first U.S. Surgeon General's report on smoking and health in 1964 provided evidence on the deleterious effects of tobacco and in particular linked smoking with lung cancer, chronic bronchitis, and coronary disease, and increased death rates from chronic bronchitis and emphysema (Jacobson et al., 1997), but it too focused primarily on men's health. For example, the report states that "cigarette smoking is causally related to lung cancer in men … the data for women, though less extensive, point in the same direction" (United States Surgeon General's Advisory Committee on Smoking and Health, 1964, p. 37). Since men initiated smoking before women, they were also first to experience the health effects, so studies did not explore gender differences (Greaves, 2007a). As noted by Bobbie Jacobson, in the 1960s and 1970s, issues related to women's smoking were neither seen nor heard (Jacobson, 1992). The focus of tobacco control on males and male bodies affected programming, research, and treatment of tobacco-related diseases, leading to gender-blind tobacco control where sex-specific and gender-related factors were ignored and unaccounted for.

The tobacco industry had no such reluctance about addressing gender, and has had a long history of using a gender-sensitive and gender-specific approach to tobacco marketing. Gender-based stereotyping and imagery have long been used to portray masculine ideals of strength and independence, while marketing for women has typically focused on glamour, sexuality, and liberation (Greaves, 2007b). The links between freedom, empowerment, equality, and tobacco were forged beginning in the 1920s, when efforts were made to develop the women's market for tobacco by encouraging tobacco use among women in developed countries. In particular, Edward Bernays, nephew of Sigmund Freud, who is often referred to as the "father of public relations," was hired by the American Tobacco Company to help expand the female market by normalizing women smoking in public (ibid.). Bernays hired debutantes to smoke in public at the 1929 Easter Sunday Parade in New York to protest for women's equality while smoking their "torches of freedom," garnering massive national publicity and debate (ibid., 1996). The tobacco industry has continued to target women since then by using feminist images and slogans in brand promotion (Ernster, Kaufman, Nichter, & Yoon, 2000; Greaves, 1996; Toll & Ling, 2005), developing light and low-smoke products to appeal to women's health concerns (Carpenter, Wayne, & Connolly, 2005; Ernster et al., 2000), and developing brand imagery to match female smoking trends, such as uptake by young working-class women (Simpson, 2007; Barbeau, Leavy-Sperounis, & Balbach, 2004). More recently, in low- and middle-income countries, the tobacco industry has also connected women's smoking with liberation (Amos & Haglund, 2000), glamour, independence, and sexuality (Ernster et al., 2000).

Belatedly, tobacco control responders awakened to the gendered nature of tobacco use, trends, cessation patterns, and marketing. In developed countries, the focus began to shift from completely male-centred tobacco control to the inclusion of women in about 1970. However, the earliest tobacco control initiatives for women focused entirely on the time of pregnancy (Greaves, 1996; Greaves & Barr, 2000; Jacobson, 1986), marking the tobacco control response to women's smoking until the 1980s. Beginning in the 1980s, health promotion and tobacco control efforts were critiqued by women writers and doctors for their gender-blind and/or gender-exploitive tobacco control response, highlighting the stark contrast between the tobacco industry's long history of women-specific marketing and the almost completely non-gendered tobacco control efforts (Graham, 1993; Greaves, 1996; Jacobson, 1981, 1986). In the 1980s, passive smoking was also increasingly identified as a health issue for women (Hirayama, 2000). Smoking also began to be connected to women's social status and relative social disadvantage, led largely by the work of Graham, who demonstrated that tobacco use among lone mothers was a means of coping with disadvantage (Graham, 1993).

Meetings and conferences addressing women and smoking were first held in the early 1980s, and calls were made to improve tobacco control policies and initiatives for women (Jacobson, 1992). In 1990, the International Network of Women Against Tobacco (INWAT) was launched at the Perth World Conference on Tobacco and Health. INWAT is aimed at reducing tobacco use among women and girls and continues to provide a key hub for communications, advocacy, and the dissemination of information related to women and tobacco (see www.inwat.org). In 1999, the international conference on Tobacco and Health in Kobe, Japan, focused on women and youth, resulting in the development of the Kobe Declaration, which identified the need to halt the tobacco epidemic among women and youth (Ernster et al., 2000). In 2002, the Framework Convention on Tobacco Control (WHO–FCTC), the first international public health treaty, was finalized; it contains a strong statement regarding the inclusion of gender in its preamble, along with arguing for sensitivity to indigenous populations (World Health Organization, 2003).

Tobacco control is now regarded as a key model of comprehensive policy because it encompasses a host of different measures, including prevention, cessation, regulation, taxation, trade and agricultural policy, advertising bans, and location restrictions, among other policies. In 2008, the World Health Organization defined six key elements of a comprehensive tobacco control strategy to support the guidelines of the FCTC. These are captured by the mnemonic "MPOWER" and include: "Monitor tobacco use and prevention policies; Protect people from tobacco smoke; Offer help to quit tobacco use; Warn about the dangers of tobacco; Enforce bans on tobacco advertising, promotion and sponsorship; and Raise taxes on tobacco"

(Samet & Yoon, 2010). This comprehensive approach to tobacco control is promising in its capacity to target global tobacco production, distribution, consumption, and exposure. While it is possible to integrate a gender equality lens within each of these tobacco control measures (ibid.), this has yet to be fully articulated.

Gender-Exploitative and Gender-Accommodating Tobacco Control Approaches

While there is potential to apply a gender lens at each level of tobacco control policy, tobacco control initiatives that lack this perspective also hold the potential to further marginalize women by exploiting or accommodating gender and power differences. Prior to discussing some of the key gender and equity concerns within tobacco control and opportunities for addressing these issues with gender-transformative initiatives, we will provide examples of gender-exploiting and gender-accommodating approaches to tobacco control and the potential harms associated with each.

Gender-Exploitative

While the tobacco industry has clearly exploited gender relations to market cigarettes to women, there are also examples from within tobacco control of the exploitation of gender relations. In particular, fetus-centric approaches to smoking during pregnancy have been exploitative by marginalizing or ignoring women's health. An early example comes from the Health Education Council (HEC) in England in 1973, which worked with advertising agency Saatchi and Saatchi to target smoking among mothers. One of the advertisements from this campaign featured a naked and pregnant woman smoking with the caption: "Is it fair to force your baby to smoke cigarettes?" (Berridge & Loughlin, 2005). The gendered nature of this advertisement went even further. As noted by Berridge and Loughlin, the

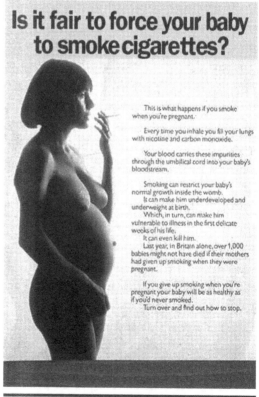

FIGURE 4.1: Poster from the 1973–1974 Health Education Council Campaign

Source: Health Education Council, England

at-risk fetus was clearly male; the HEC press release noted that "Mums-to-be will be told that smoking can restrict the baby's growth, make him underdeveloped and underweight at birth and even kill him" (Berridge & Loughlin, 2005, p. 335).

This campaign heightened women's inequality by both sexualizing and objectifying them and minimizing the importance of women's health while highlighting their smoking behaviour and its effect on the fetus/baby. Almost 20 years later, a recent anti-smoking advertisement from the Regional Cancer Centre in India used a picture of a woman's naked breast with a cigarette butt in place of her nipple, with the caption "Women who smoke feed more than just milk to their children" (Regional Cancer Centre, 2008).

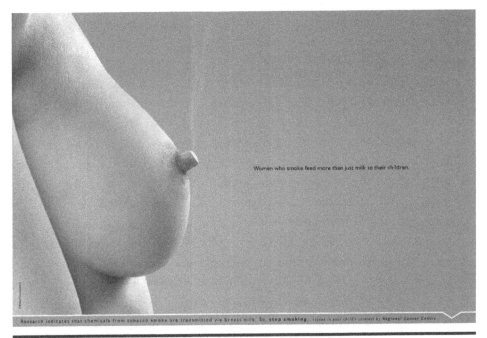

Women who smoke feed more than just milk to their children.

Research indicates that chemicals from tobacco smoke are transmitted via breast milk. So, stop smoking. Issued in your child's interest by Regional Cancer Centre.

FIGURE 4.2: Regional Cancer Centre of India Anti-smoking Campaign
Source: Bhadra Communications

But perhaps the most striking gender-exploitative health promotion campaign was a 1972 American Cancer Society (ACS) advertisement featuring an "unattractive" older woman smoking, with the caption "Smoking is very glamorous." This ad, using a realistic black-and-white photo, clearly exploits an objectifying beauty norm in getting the tobacco control message across to women (Viralworthy, 2010). This theme has been particularly persistent: when in a welcome move World No Tobacco Day in 2012 focused on women, its tag line was "Smoking is ugly," a full 40 years after the ACS poster first appeared.

Gender-Accommodating

Women's gendered roles may also be accommodated by tobacco control efforts that focus on women in the traditional roles of nurturer, caregiver, or reproducer. Oaks describes how anti-smoking campaigns aimed at pregnant women have often used "dominant, traditional (white, middle-class) ideas about motherhood" and women's purported maternal nature along with fetal images to encourage women to "protect their babies-to-be" (Oaks, 2000, p. 74). For example, the slogan of the American Lung Association from 1983–88 was "Because You Love Your Baby ... There's Never Been a Better Time to Quit," which equated smoking with a lack of caring, while quitting smoking was associated with maternal caring (Oaks, 2000). These early initiatives accommodate the reproductive roles of women. The harmful effects of smoking on the fetus/baby or child are emphasized, while concern for women smokers is centred on them only as "vessels" or "vectors" and not on their own health (Greaves & Poole, 2005).

There are also multiple examples of messages that employ notions of motherhood and maternal care to urge mothers not to smoke around their children. One example is an anti-smoking advertisement from the South Dakota Department of Health, which portrays a mother buckling her children in the back seat of the car, and then climbing into the driver's seat and lighting up a cigarette, accompanied by the message "You have the choice to smoke, your children don't" (South Dakota Department of Health, 2009). More shocking is an anti-smoking advertisement from Australia, which depicts a mother serving her children tar and chemicals for dinner while a male narrator announces the effects of second-hand smoke on children (Quit Harming Others, 2008). Both of these campaigns are based upon stereotypical ideas of maternal responsibility, locating women solely within the domestic sphere as the guardians of their children's health. Researchers have heavily critiqued approaches that marginalize women's health and focus on women's responsibility as caretakers for delegitimizing women's health in and of itself; for increasing stigma, shame, and guilt among pregnant smokers; and for lacking effectiveness (with most women relapsing in the postpartum period) (Greaves & Barr, 2000; Greaves & Poole, 2005; Jacobson, 1986).

In addition to mass media campaigns aimed at prevention, cessation, and protection from second-hand smoke, the focus in tobacco control on the health of the fetus or child is reflected in the majority of interventions available for pregnant women who smoke. For example, comprehensive reviews of interventions for pregnant smokers astonishingly revealed that measures of women's health were missing from these interventions, indicative of the relative undervaluing of women's health when compared to the potential impact on fetal or children's health (Greaves et al., 2003; Greaves et al., 2011).

Gender and Equity Issues in Tobacco Control

Issues of equity and gender have become critically important in program and policy responses to women and tobacco. While women's health, socio-economic status, and political empowerment have long been entangled in tobacco use, advertising, marketing, exposure, and production, these factors are now blatant and foremost in measuring and responding to the impact of tobacco on women in the current century. In the long term, the health consequences of tobacco use result in women's diminished economic status and potential gender equity (Greaves et al., 2006). It has been observed that the narrowing of socio-economic gaps between women and men typically corresponds with a narrowing of gender differences in women's smoking rates (Hitchman & Fong, 2011). However, smoking continues to be associated with poverty, with poorer and more socially disadvantaged subgroups in both developed and developing countries typically exhibiting the highest smoking rates (Greaves, 2007b). Women continue to occupy a lower social and economic status relative to men in both developed and developing countries, and experience greater discrimination in employment, less representation in decision-making in both public and private, and are at a much greater risk of gender-based violence (Greaves, 2007b).

Women's health and status are affected by tobacco use indirectly as well. Since men take up smoking first and there are higher rates of male smokers in most countries, tobacco use exacerbates poverty by reducing family income due to spending on tobacco products, reducing the health and economic potential of men who smoke and exposing women and children to second-hand smoke (Greaves et al., 2006). Women's health and economic status are further challenged by the specific and, in some instances, greater health consequences that women experience from smoking and smoke exposure. For example, emerging evidence suggests there are differences between women and men in the stage, type, and severity of lung diseases, although further sex- and gender-based research is required to examine these differences (ibid.). In developing countries, where women already face high levels of disease, food insecurity, and malnutrition, tobacco use by women or men intensifies both health and economic inequalities.

Women's status is also affected by their involvement in tobacco production and processing. As global production has shifted from the Americas to Asia and Africa, gendered and negative health and economic consequences have emerged that negatively affect women, regardless of their smoking status. The use of land for tobacco limits available space for food production and contributes to environmental degradation, and tobacco workers are often exposed to harmful chemicals (particularly in poor countries with fewer environmental regulations) and exploitive labour practices (Greaves et al., 2006). Women and children in particular are often the source of cheap or unpaid labour and, due to unequal power relations in the household, are less likely to benefit from any profits earned (ibid.). Children may also lose the opportunity for education due to their involvement in tobacco farming or production, particularly girls, who are less likely to receive education in developing countries (ibid.). In addition, through their involvement in tobacco harvesting and farming, women are at greater risk for illness, cancers, birth defects, and liver disease (Greaves, 2007b). While the tobacco industry typically frames tobacco production as a source of economic viability, in essence tobacco farming leads to greater health and economic inequalities, with the profits going to multinational tobacco corporations rather than small farmers. A gender- and equity-oriented approach to tobacco control policies, research, and programming is critical to respond to the social, economic, and health consequences of tobacco use, exposure, and production, especially for women.

What Can Be Done to Improve Health Promotion and Tobacco Control?

The WHO's Framework Convention on Tobacco Control (FCTC) identifies tobacco control among women and girls and the inclusion of gender sensitivity as key issues, making this treaty a key support in exploring how to improve the response of tobacco control for women (Greaves, 2007b). Indeed, there are many opportunities for integrating gender into the policies and actions emerging from the FCTC (ibid.). These range from understanding gendered responses to policies and programs in health education, to gendering cessation and prevention initiatives. The challenge, however, is to rise above the easy exploitation of gender-related factors, such as assumptions about body image or independence, to linking health promotion and tobacco control to more gender-transformative and affirming principles and goals. Tobacco control initiatives are particularly hampered in this regard by the agenda that has been consistently and repeatedly set over many decades by the tobacco industry in its blatant linkage of "liberation" and "freedom" to tobacco use among women. This linkage, perhaps most famously epitomized by Philip Morris's tag line "You've come a long way, baby," has proven to be an insidious and persistent myth that has permeated assumptions held by health providers, political leaders, and epidemiologists. This has been a dangerous linkage, leading to the identification of "protective factors" against uptake of tobacco, such as religiosity and low income (Bradby & Williams, 2006; Islam & Johnson, 2003).

In order to develop more advanced, progressive, gender-transformative tobacco control that values improving women's and girls' status as much as reducing and preventing tobacco use, more evidence, imagination, and creativity among health promoters are required. On the evidence side, ongoing and consistent gender analyses of the differential effects of tobacco policies for diverse groups of women and men are required (Greaves, 2007b). For example, evidence on the specific gendered responses to policies such as sales restrictions (WHO-FCTC Article 16), taxation (WHO-FCTC Article 6), and smoking location restrictions (WHO-FCTC Article 8) is needed on which to base gendered responses that respect and advance women's status, income levels, and labour force participation. On the intervention side, similar gender- and diversity-sensitive prevention and cessation approaches are also required to respond to sex-based differences in tobacco use and gender- and diversity-based influences on behaviours, attitudes, and practices associated with tobacco use to develop appropriate tailored responses.

The extension of tobacco cultivation and production to low- and middle-income countries requires ensuring that girls and women have economic security and educational and employment alternatives to tobacco production (Greaves, 2007b). Public education and information campaigns require parallel women's education programs to address their greater rates of illiteracy (Greaves & Tungohan, 2007). Implementing advertising bans and enhancing media literacy among girls and women to reduce the impact of tobacco advertising is required, particularly in developing countries where there are fewer regulations on advertising, sponsorship, and promotions, and women are increasingly being targeted by tobacco advertising (Greaves, 2007b; Greaves & Tungohan, 2007). Specifically, campaigns that expose the tobacco industry's exploitation of women can underpin transformative health promotion programs, including empowerment and skills training in both developing and developed countries to enable girls and women to more powerfully and effectively manage tobacco use and exposure (ibid.). Underlying all of this is the dire need to generate a different kind of evidence by increasing research among high-risk groups; improving research capacity in developing countries; fostering multidisciplinary and participatory research; addressing the research bias toward men; and increasing the examination of sex and gender influences and differences in the use, effects, and control of tobacco (Greaves, 2007b).

What would these improvements lead to? The focus in tobacco control has typically been on changing the behaviour of smokers, "unlinked to social settings, structures, lived experience or health equity concerns" (Greaves, 2007b, p. 122). But this has been a very limited approach in tobacco control and indeed in health promotion more generally. Gender, socio-economic status, race/ethnicity, and location, as well as experiences such as trauma/violence and mental health issues, all contribute to tobacco use and quitting rates, and influence the impact of overarching policies and specific program interventions. A much more holistic approach to health is required that aims to reduce women's vulnerability to tobacco use by addressing social, housing, and economic inequalities via policy reforms and providing empowering and transformative tailored responses.

For example, prevention and reduction/cessation strategies are required that more adequately respond to the complex reasons for women's smoking or challenges in quitting smoking. Gender-sensitive smoking prevention may include empowerment groups for girls to encourage positive self-image without tobacco use (Amos et al., 2011). Research among Aboriginal adolescent girls reveals the need for prevention programs that include the wider community and cessation programs that are trauma-sensitive (de Finney et al., 2013). Across the world, empowerment and skill-building programs are required to enable women to manage their exposure to second-hand smoke (Amos et al., 2011). These initiatives will need to address women's lack of power in households as compared to men's, as well as placing responsibility for maintaining healthy, tobacco-free homes on mostly male smokers.

Perhaps most critical to generating gender-transformative health promotion on tobacco is the need to directly challenge the connotation of tobacco use in girls and women with progress and freedom. Significant global counter-advertising is needed that integrates messages of "freedom," "liberation," and "control" to override the long-time and highly exploitative association of tobacco use with women's liberation (Greaves et al., 2006). Linked to this is specific intervention in tobacco-producing countries, where there is a dire need for culturally sensitive information and education campaigns for women that address exploitative working practices and health consequences, labour regulations, and healthier, economically viable alternatives to tobacco production.

None of these shifts in approach will be accomplished quickly or easily, but all are sorely needed to address the convergence of gender and equity concerns in tobacco use, exposure, and production. The large and emergent group of female smokers in low- and middle-income countries demands this approach. Current evidence indicates that varied subpopulations of women respond differently to price and taxation, sales restrictions, and location restrictions (Greaves & Jategaonkar, 2006). However, tobacco control policies have largely lacked integration of gendered roles, social context, unequal power relations affecting women in relationships and workplaces, and differences in access to resources and social support (ibid.). Indeed, smoking location restrictions have been critiqued for their potential stigmatization of socially disadvantaged groups, including women and men who are poor, or who have mental health or substance use issues (Bell, Salmon, Bowers, Bell, & McCullough, 2010; Greaves & Hemsing, 2009; Hemsing, Greaves, Poole, & Bottorff, 2012). A shift from the individual level to broader social structural issues affecting tobacco use is required. For example, Graham argues that social disadvantage, in particular what she terms "biographies of disadvantage," must be addressed to adequately address tobacco use (Graham et al., 2006). Tobacco control policies need to be extended to include economic and social policies that shape tobacco use and cessation. In short, an equity-oriented policy approach is required to decrease smoking in women who are vulnerable to smoking that would include tailored policies and programs that reflect social justice principles, assist in eroding social-structural inequalities of health, and more tightly link tobacco policy to a human rights and women's rights agenda.

There have been some important equity initiatives within tobacco control research, particularly work conducted by the Tobacco Research Network on Disparities (TReND) in the United States, a multidisciplinary team of researchers dedicated to examining and eliminating health disparities related to tobacco (see www. tobaccodisparities.org). However, equity initiatives tend to focus on socio-economic status rather than gender; further research and tobacco control initiatives that combine equity and gender to address the emerging markets and global trends are required. This form of approach would integrate principles of improving women's status with improving tobacco control, taking care to transform women's status and gender relations along with reducing tobacco use, and explicitly not exploiting unequal gender relations in order to achieve tobacco control goals (Greaves, 2007b, 2014; Greaves & Tungohan, 2007). A number of additional women's empowerment indicators may be important to draw on and apply to tobacco control, such as levels of domestic and decision-making power and the quality of household and couple dynamics. There is also an ongoing need to fully integrate sex, gender, and diversity-based analysis in developing the evidence base for tailoring tobacco control. Further research is required to explore the intersection of gender with other factors, including race/ethnicity, class, and education and how these shape tobacco use (Greaves, 2007a).

Participatory and collaborative approaches that prioritize equitable involvement of research participants are also required to examine smoking and vulnerability more adequately (Amos et al., 2011). In developing countries, further gender- and diversity-sensitive research is required to examine the social context of women's tobacco use and exposure (Greaves et al., 2006).

Gender-Transformative Tobacco Control

Gender-transformative tobacco control has the dual goal of improving women's health and socio-economic status while the same time as reducing tobacco use or exposure. Blending these two goals will clearly advance women's health as well as circumstances by focusing not only on changes to smoking behaviour but also on changes to structures that encourage or contribute to tobacco use or exposure. For example, tobacco control may be most effective if linked with improving social determinants of health, such as access to housing or child care, or engaging women in planning interventions, addressing stigmatization, or improving media literacy among girls.

Transforming gender relations through tobacco control requires a more comprehensive approach to tobacco control that integrates social justice issues and includes examination of the gendered consequences of policies (Greaves, 2014; Greaves & Tungohan, 2007). While gender-transformative approaches to tobacco control are relatively few and concentrated largely in developed countries, there are several that seek to both reduce women's smoking while improving women's equality. Start Thinking About Reducing Secondhand Smoke (STARSS), developed by Action on Women's Addictions-Research and Education (AWARE), a health promotion group in Canada, is one example (AWARE, n.d.). This approach provides tips and worksheets to support mothers in managing their tobacco use. It is not focused on cessation, but rather on supporting women to take small steps toward managing second-hand smoke in the home. The approach supports women in identifying both the positive and negative roles that tobacco plays in their lives, and uses a non-judgmental harm reduction approach to engage and empower women.

The research conducted and materials developed by Families Eliminating and Controlling Tobacco (FACET) provide another example of a gender-transformative approach to tobacco control. The "Couples and Smoking: What You Need to Know When You Are Pregnant" booklet provides information to support women and their partners to reduce or quit smoking, but focuses on the dynamics between partners that influences smoking and cessation, highlighting and identifying some of the negative dynamics that can affect pregnant women, and offering tips on reducing their impact. It also

The Guide to STARSS Strategies

Start Thinking About Reducing Secondhand Smoke

A harm reduction support strategy for low-income moms who smoke

FIGURE 4.3: Start Thinking about Reducing Second-Hand Smoke

Source: Action on Women's Addictions-Research and Education (AWARE)

aims to reduce stigma and shame associated with smoking during pregnancy, and offers harm reduction strategies for women who are unable to quit (Bottorff, Carey, Poole, Greaves, & Urquhart, 2008). In contrast to fetus-centric approaches discussed previously, this multi-faceted approach to smoking during pregnancy recognizes the realistic aspects of couple dynamics and the positive and negative roles of both partners in reduction/cessation, and overall, it values women's health. This resource takes aim at gender relations, with a view to not only exposing their links to tobacco cessation during pregnancy and after birth, but to empowering women in particular to address them in a transformative, change-oriented, and empowering manner.

Finally, *Liberation! Helping Women Quit Smoking: A Brief Tobacco-Intervention Guide*, developed by the British Columbia Centre of Excellence for Women's Health (BCCEWH), provides guidelines for engaging in a conversation with women about tobacco use and reduction or cessation (Urquhart, Jasiura, Poole, Nathoo, & Greaves, 2012). These guidelines focus on providing reduction or cessation support that is individualized or tailored, women-centred, and holistic, and that integrates social justice issues. This guide emphasizes the connection between smoking and other forms of disadvantage, including mental health issues, violence and trauma, low socio-economic status, and other addictions. Tips are offered for service providers to engage in a conversation about smoking with women that is trauma-sensitive, empowering, reduces stigma, and is tailored to women's needs and experiences.

Couples and Smoking

What You Need to Know When You are Pregnant

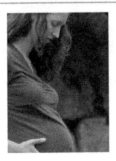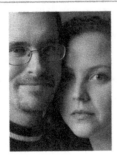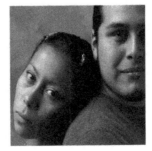

FIGURE 4.4: Couples and Smoking Guide

Source: Families Eliminating and Controlling Tobacco (FACET), http://www.facet.ubc.ca

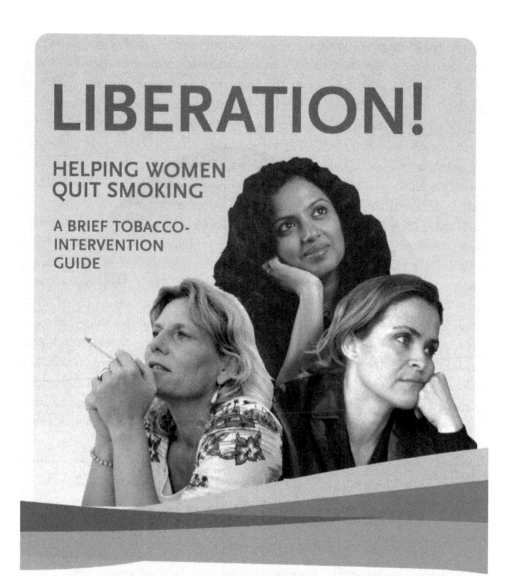

LIBERATION!

HELPING WOMEN QUIT SMOKING

A BRIEF TOBACCO-INTERVENTION GUIDE

Prepared by Cristine Urquhart, Frances Jasiura, Nancy Poole, Tasnim Nathoo and Lorraine Greaves

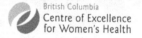

British Columbia
Centre of Excellence
for Women's Health

FIGURE 4.5: *Liberation!* Guide

Source: British Columbia Centre of Excellence for Women's Health (BCCEWH)

Again, the goal of this guide is to empower women and providers in understanding the complexities of tobacco use and the difficulty in quitting, and to offer respectful and realistic advice for intervening in positive ways.

While these approaches are promising, many more gender-transforma-tive policy, program, and research approaches are required to address tobacco prevention, reduction/cessation, and protection. This is particularly true in some low- and middle-income countries where tobacco use is just taking hold among women, but exposure to tobacco use is high and there is often no gender-sensitive tobacco control. In these settings, establishing approaches that are gender-trans-formative—as opposed to gender-exploitative or accommodating—could enhance the impact of tobacco control and potentially short-circuit the trajectory of the tobacco epidemic among girls and women, saving countless lives and resources over the next century.

Conclusions

While the tobacco industry has a long history of integrating gender into tobacco marketing, tobacco control has been largely gender-blind. There has been a histor-ical bias in tobacco control toward men, and when issues related to women's tobacco use surfaced, these were largely related to pregnancy and the effects of smoking on a fetus. But the shift in tobacco use in high-income countries to disadvantaged groups of girls and women, and a simultaneous increase in tobacco use and production among girls and women in developing countries, necessitates a more nuanced and thoughtful approach to tobacco control. This requires a shift from an individual-level focus of tobacco control to a more comprehensive examination of the social, eco-nomic, and political contexts of smoking, smoke exposure, and tobacco cultivation. Essential to improving women's health status are gender-transformative approaches that simultaneously improve women's status while addressing tobacco-related issues such as tobacco cessation. While a few promising approaches have been developed in high-income countries, the *Liberation!* guide in particular has been focus-tested internationally and has the potential to ignite a more global gender-transformative approach to tobacco control. Generating more tobacco control initiatives within health promotion that explicitly question, challenge, and transform gendered social norms along with reducing or preventing the use of tobacco is a key challenge for the twenty-first century (Greaves, 2014).

REFERENCES

Amos, A., Greaves, L., Nichter, M., & Bloch, M. (2011). Women and tobacco: A call for including gender in tobacco control research, policy, and practice. *Tobacco Control, 21*(2), 236–243.

Amos, A., & Haglund, M. (2000). From social taboo to "torch of freedom": The marketing of cigarettes to women. *Tobacco Control, 9*(1), 3–8.

Assembly of First Nations RHS National Team. (2007). *RHS Our Voice, Our Survey, Our Reality: Selected Results from RHS Phase 1.* Ottawa: Assembly of First Nations.

AWARE. STARSS [Start Thinking About Reducing Secondhand Smoke]. n.d. Retrieved from www.aware.on.ca/starss

Barbeau, E. M., Leavy-Sperounis, A., & Balbach, E. D. (2004). Smoking, social class, and gender: What can public health learn from the tobacco industry about disparities in smoking? *Tobacco Control, 13*(2), 115–120.

Bell, K., Salmon, A., Bowers, M., Bell, J., & McCullough, L. (2010). Smoking, stigma, and tobacco "denormalization": Further reflections on the use of stigma as a public health tool. A commentary on *Social Science & Medicine's* Stigma, Prejudice, Discrimination, and Health Special Issue, *67*(3). *Social Science & Medicine, 70*(6), 795–799.

Berridge, V., & Loughlin, K. (2005). Smoking and the new health education in Britain. *American Journal of Public Health, 95*(6), 956–964.

Bottorff, J. L., Carey, J., Poole, N., Greaves, L., & Urquhart, C. (2008). *Couples and smoking: What you need to know when you are pregnant.* Vancouver: British Columbia Centre of Excellence for Women's Health, Institute for Healthy Living and Chronic Disease Prevention, NEXUS.

Bradby, H., & Williams, R. (2006). Is religion or culture the key feature in changes in substance use after leaving school? Young Punjabis and a comparison group in Glasgow. *Ethnicity & Health, 11*(3), 307–324.

Brandt, A. M. (1996). Recruiting women smokers: The engineering of consent. *Journal of the American Medical Women's Association, 51*(1–2), 63–66.

Carpenter, C. M., Wayne, G. F., & Connolly, G. N. (2005). Designing cigarettes for women: New findings from the tobacco industry documents. *Addiction, 100*(6), 837–851.

CTUMS. (2010). *Canadian Tobacco Use Monitoring Survey (CTUMS) 2010.* Ottawa: Author.

de Finney, S., Greaves, L., Janyst, P., Hemsing, N., Jategaonkar, N., Browne, A. ... Poole, N. (2013). "I had to grow up pretty quickly": Cultural and gender contexts of Aboriginal girls' smoking. *Pimatisiwin, 11*(2), 151–170.

Ernster, V., Kaufman, N., Nichter, M. J. S., & Yoon, S. (2000). Women and tobacco: Moving from policy to action. *Bulletin of the World Health Organization, 78*(7), 89–101.

Giskes, K., Kunst, A. E., Ariza, C., Benach, J., Borrell, C., Helmert, U. ... Mackenbach, J. P. (2007). Applying an equity lens to tobacco-control policies and their uptake in six Western-European countries. *Journal of Public Health Policy, 28*(2), 261–280.

Graham, H. (1993). *When life's a drag: Women, smoking, and disadvantage.* University of Warwick: Great Britain Department of Health.

Graham, H., Inskip, H. M., Francis, B., & Harman, J. (2006). Pathways of disadvantage and smoking careers: Evidence and policy implications. *Journal of Epidemiology and Community Health, 60*(Supp. 2), ii7–ii12.

Greaves, L. (1996). *Smoke screen: Women's smoking and social control.* Halifax: Fernwood Publishing.

Greaves, L. (2007a). Gender, equity, and tobacco control. *Health Sociology Review, 16*(2), 115–129.

Greaves, L. (2007b). *Sifting the evidence: Gender and tobacco control.* Geneva: World Health Organization.

Greaves, L. (2014). Can tobacco control be transformative? Reducing gender inequity and tobacco use among vulnerable populations. *International Journal of Environmental Research and Public Health, 11*(1), 792–803.

Greaves, L., & Barr, V. (2000). *Filtered policy: Women and tobacco in Canada.* Vancouver: Women's Health Bureau, Health Canada.

Greaves, L., Cormier, R., Devries, K., Bottorff, J., Johnson, J., Kirkland, S., & Aboussafy, D. (2003). *A best practices review of smoking cessation interventions for pregnant and postpartum girls and women.* Vancouver: British Columbia Centre of Excellence for Women's Health.

Greaves, L., & Hemsing, N. (2009). Sex, gender, diversity, and second-hand smoke policies: Implications for disadvantaged women. *American Journal of Preventive Medicine, 37*(Supp. 2), S131–137.

Greaves, L., & Jategaonkar, N. (2006). Tobacco policies and vulnerable girls and women: Toward a framework for gender sensitive policy development. *Journal of Epidemiology and Community Health, 60*(Supp. 2), ii57–ii65.

Greaves, L., Jategaonkar, N., & Sanchez, S. (2006). Turning a new leaf: Women, tobacco, and the future. Vancouver: British Columbia Centre of Excellence for Women's Health (BCCEWH) and International Network of Women Against Tobacco (INWAT).

Greaves L., & Poole, N. (2005). Victimized or validated? Responses to substance-using pregnant women. *Canadian Woman Studies Journal, 24*(1), 87–95.

Greaves, L., Poole, N., Okoli, C. T. C., Hemsing, N., Qu, A., Bialystok, L., & O'Leary, R. (2011). *Expecting to quit: A best practices review of smoking cessation interventions for pregnant and post-partum women* (2nd ed.). Vancouver: British Columbia Centre of Excellence for Women's Health.

Greaves, L., & Tungohan, E. (2007). Engendering tobacco control: Using an international public health treaty to reduce smoking and empower women. *Tobacco Control, 16*(3), 148–150.

Hammond, C., & Horn, D. (1958, March 15). Smoking and death rates: Report on forty-four months of follow up of 187,783 men. *Journal of the American Medical Association, 166*(11), 1294–1308.

Health Canada. (2007). *First Nations, Inuit, and Aboriginal health: Tobacco.* Retrieved from www.hc-sc.gc.ca/fniah-spnia/substan/tobac-taba/index-eng.php

Hemsing, N., Greaves, L., Poole, N., & Bottorff, J. L. (2012). Reshuffling and relocating: The gendered and income-related differential effects of restricting smoking locations. [Article ID 907832]. *Journal of Environmental and Public Health.* doi:10.1155/2012/907832

Hirayama, T. (2000). Non-smoking wives of heavy smokers have a higher risk of lung cancer: A study from Japan. *Bulletin of the World Health Organization, 78*(7), 940–942.

Hitchman, S. C., & Fong, G. T. (2011). Gender empowerment and female-to-male smoking prevalence ratios. *Bulletin of the World Health Organization, 89*(3), 195–202.

Huxley, R. R., & Woodward, M. (2011). Cigarette smoking as a risk factor for coronary heart disease in women compared with men: A systematic review and meta-analysis of prospective cohort studies. *The Lancet, 378*(9799), 1297–1305.

Islam, S. M. S., & Johnson, C. A. (2003). Correlates of smoking behavior among Muslim Arab-American adolescents. *Ethnicity & Health, 8*(4), 319–337.

Jacobson, B. (1981). *The ladykillers: Why smoking is a feminist issue.* London: Pluto Press.

Jacobson, B. (1986). *Beating the ladykillers: Women and smoking.* London: Pluto Press.

Jacobson, B. (1992). Putting women in the picture. *Tobacco Control, 1*(2), 123–125.

Jacobson, P., Wasserman, J., & Anderson, J. (1997). Historical overview of tobacco legislation and regulation. *Journal of Social Issues, 53*(1), 75–95.

Mackay, J., & Amos, A. (2003). Women and tobacco. *Respirology, 8*(2), 123–130.

Mackay, J., Eriksen, M., & Shafey, O. (2006). *The tobacco atlas.* Geneva: World Health Organization.

Oaks, L. (2000). Smoke-filled wombs and fragile fetuses: The social politics of fetal representation. *Signs, 26*(1), 63–108.

Parajuli, R., Bjerkaas, E., Tverdal, A., Selmer, R., Le Marchand, L., Weiderpass, E., & Gram, I. T. (2013). The increased risk of colon cancer due to cigarette smoking may be greater in women than men. *Cancer Epidemiology Biomarkers & Prevention, 22*(5), 862–871.

Quit Harming Others. (2008). *Smoking harms children.* Retrieved from www.youtube.com/watch?v=nXN3eWg0pi8

Regional Cancer Centre. (2008). *Women who smoke feed more than just milk to their children ad.* Retrieved from http://adsoftheworld.com/media/print/regional_cancer_centre_breast?size=original

Samet, J. M., & Yoon, S.-Y. E. (2010). *Gender, women, and the tobacco epidemic.* Geneva: World Health Organization.

Simpson, D. (2007). USA: Camel for women. *Tobacco Control, 16*(3), 167–168.

South Dakota Department of Health. (2009). *Smoking mom.* Retrieved from www.youtube.com/watch?v=dbkZoaGJUNk&list=PLF2472A2F283EC9E1&index=12

Toll, B. A., & Ling, P. M. (2005). The Virginia Slims identity crisis: An inside look at tobacco industry marketing to women. *Tobacco Control, 14*(3), 172–180.

United States Surgeon General's Advisory Committee on Smoking and Health. (1964). *Smoking and health: Report of the Advisory Committee to the Surgeon General of the Public Health Service.* Washington, DC: U.S. Department of Health, Education and Welfare.

Urquhart, C., Jasiura, F., Poole, N., Nathoo, T., & Greaves, L. (2012). *Liberation! Helping women quit smoking: A brief tobacco-intervention guide.* Vancouver: British Columbia Centre of Excellence for Women's Health.

Viralworthy. (2010, February 18). *Smoking is very glamorous.* Retrieved from http://viralworthy.com/post/396739823/smoking-is-very-glamorous

Warner, K. E., & Mendez, D. (2010). Tobacco control policy in developed countries: Yesterday, today, and tomorrow. *Nicotine and Tobacco Research, 12*(9), 876–887.

World Health Organization. (2003). *WHO Framework Convention on Tobacco Control.* Geneva: World Health Organization.

World Health Organization. (2010). *World No Tobacco Day 2010.* Retrieved from www.who.int/tobacco/wntd/2010/announcement/en

5 Recalculating Risk: An Opportunity for Gender-Transformative Alcohol Education for Girls and Women

Lauren Bialystok, Nancy Poole, Lorraine Greaves, and Gerald Thomas

Introduction

Alcohol consumption has been a key target of health promotion efforts, and for good reason. Drinking in excess of low-risk guidelines has high social costs, yet alcohol use in Canada is not a rare phenomenon but a nearly universal one, and at-risk or binge drinking is common. But both the measurement of and the response to at-risk drinking have been gender-blind. Over the years, estimates of at-risk drinking from some high-profile national surveys have been made without taking sex and gender into account, resulting in serious underestimation of at-risk drinking levels among girls and women in Canada, and the proliferation of gender-blind alcohol education and health promotion. In this chapter we recalculate the data, integrating both sex and gender into an assessment of alcohol consumption, which radically reframes the scope of the problem of at-risk drinking by girls and women. This recalculation substantially changes the scale of this public health problem and sets the stage for a new approach to alcohol-related health promotion for women. We then review social influences on girls' and women's drinking and the interplay between gendered alcohol advertising and the health promotion responses it provokes. Finally, we conclude by pointing toward promising practices for reducing at-risk drinking among girls and women using principles of gender-transformative health promotion.

Historically, health promotion efforts have paid little attention to the intersection of gender and other determinants of alcohol use. Instead, concern about fetal alcohol spectrum disorder (FASD) has prompted an inordinate focus on the drinking habits of pregnant women and, more generally, women of child-bearing age. The approach has been to warn all pregnant women of the dangers of alcohol consumption and to castigate those who do not avoid it altogether. The assumption is that, regardless of one's previous drinking habits and personal pressures, one can and ought to stop drinking completely for the duration of pregnancy. Alcohol use during pregnancy, however, is strongly linked to patterns of drinking across the lifespan, which are in turn affected by a host of social determinants, personal circumstances, and genetic influences. Hence, addressing at-risk drinking when developing effective health promotion requires more attention to the range of factors affecting girls' and women's use of alcohol prior to and during their child-bearing years. In particular, this challenge requires a commitment to women's health before, during, and after pregnancy as key to efforts to protect fetal health.

In order to make recommendations for gender-transformative alcohol-related health promotion, we analyzed data about Canadian women's drinking patterns during their child-bearing years (15–44). Taking sex and gender into consideration when examining these data results in significantly higher estimates of the prevalence of risky drinking and supports calls for a new approach to alcohol messaging. Considering sex-related factors is critical because, drink for drink, alcohol is riskier for women than it is for men. Gender-related factors help to explain why women drink and what kinds of information and support they need to drink in less risky ways. Finally, considerations of emergent trends and patterns among different groups of women more finely focus the need for gender-sensitive and, ultimately, gender-transformative health promotion to reduce at-risk drinking among girls and women.

Sex, Gender, and Alcohol: Recalculating the Risks, Harms, and Costs

The evidence used to measure alcohol consumption and develop policy and programmatic responses has not always factored in the role of sex as a physiological determinant of alcohol-related risk. This is a significant oversight. The negative health impacts of alcohol on women's bodies are more severe than those on men's and include certain sex-specific consequences. For example, drinking among women and girls has been connected to breast cancer (Chen et al., 2011; Li et al., 2010), obesity and depression (Farhat, Iannotti, & Simons-Morton, 2010; McCarty et al., 2009), and reproductive health problems (Nolen-Hoeksema, 2004). Even when controlling for blood alcohol content, studies have found that women experience greater cognitive and motor impairment from drinking than men (ibid.). Over the long term, women who drink alcohol are at greater risk of liver damage, heart problems, and brain damage than men who consume the same amounts of alcohol. Further, women transition from regular use to alcohol abuse more quickly than their male counterparts (National Institute on Alcohol Abuse and Alcoholism, 2004).

The interaction between alcohol and physiology suggests that women are predisposed to greater alcohol-related harms than men, assuming equal consumption. Historically, women's consumption has been lower than men's, and efforts to curb risky drinking at a population level have not attended to sex differences, or have simply assumed that any additional risks that women faced would be balanced by their lower consumption levels (Greaves & Poole, 2008). However, the historical gender difference between rates of past-year drinking for men and women is shrinking. As Figure 5.1 shows, the gap in prevalence of past-year alcohol use between men and women has decreased from 12 percent in 1989 to less than 8 percent in 2009–2010. In addition, heavy drinking (defined by Statistics Canada, in a non-sex-specific way, as five or more drinks per occasion) is slowly increasing among women while it is more stable for men (Figure 5.2), and rates of risky drinking are highest for women in their peak fertility years (Figure 5.3).

These trends are alarming and require a fresh approach to health promotion regarding alcohol use among women and girls. All these data corroborate the claim that efforts to reduce risky drinking should pay attention to gendered trends in alcohol consumption. Even so, these figures are based on a definition of "risky drinking"

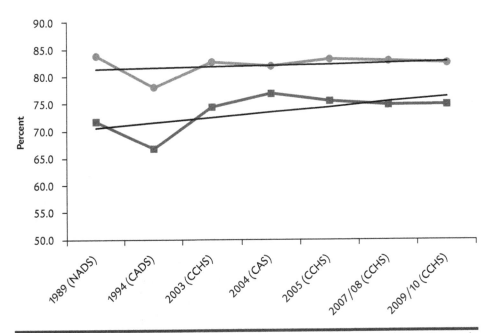

FIGURE 5.1: Long-Term Trends in Prevalence of Past-Year Alcohol Use, General Household Population Age 15+, Canada

Source: Adlaf, Begin, & Sawka (2005); Eliany, Giesbrecht, & Nelson (1990); Health Canada (1995); Statistics Canada (2011).

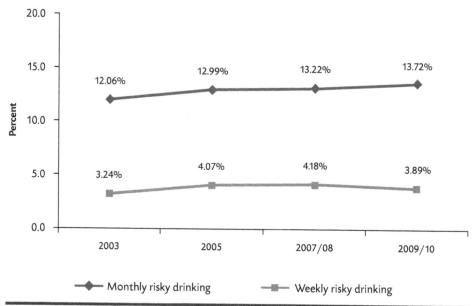

FIGURE 5.2: Trends in Percentage of Female Current (Past-Year) Drinkers Reporting Risky Drinking (5+ Drinks/Occasion) Monthly or More Often, General Household Population Age 15+, Canada*

*Between 2001 and 2005, the CCHS collected data biannually from a sample of approximately 130,000 Canadians. Since 2007, however, data have been collected annually from approximately 65,000 respondents with results from two years (e.g., 2009/10) pooled to improve statistical power when findings are reported.

Source: Statistics Canada (2011).

that is undifferentiated by sex. Although four or more drinks in one sitting is the sex-specific criterion recommended in Canada's Low-Risk Drinking Guidelines to describe high-risk drinking for women, the Canadian Community Health Survey (CCHS) uses five or more drinks for both men and women. But this difference of one drink per sitting makes a crucial difference to women's health. Preliminary analysis comparing the proportion of current (past-year) drinking women who report four or more drinks per occasion once a month or more in the past year, and women who report five or more drinks per occasion once a month or more in the past year from four national surveys (Adlaf, Begin, & Sawks, 2005; Health Canada, n.d. a, n.d. b, n.d. c) suggests that lowering the threshold by one drink per occasion increases the estimated prevalence of risky drinking by almost 50 percent for women of child-bearing age (see Appendix 5A on page 107 for details). This difference is astounding and highlights the danger of not paying sufficient attention to sex-related differences in the calculation of the scope of women's risky drinking. Further, this gross underestimation of women's alcohol-related risk has potentially

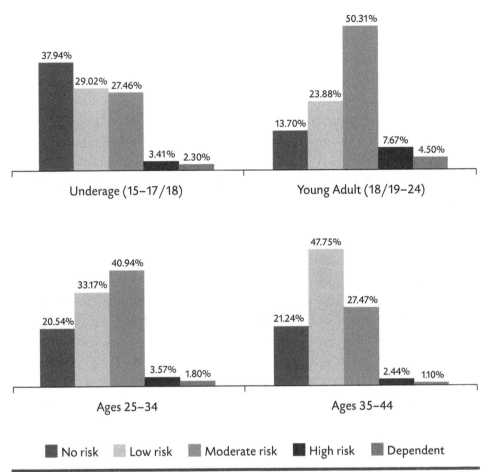

FIGURE 5.3: Distribution of Alcohol-Related Risk, Females Age 15–44, Canada, 2009 and 2010 (Pooled Data for the CCHS Component)

Note: No risk = No alcohol use in past year; Low risk = No 5+ days in past year; Moderate risk = 5+ drinks three times or less a month in past year; High risk = 5+ drinks weekly or more often in past year; Dependent = Endorsing three or more of seven symptoms associated with alcohol dependence. The seven symptoms assessed were: (1) drunk or hungover at work, school, or while caring for children; (2) alcohol taken in larger amounts or over longer periods than intended; (3) in a situation while drunk/hungover that increased chance of injury; (4) increased tolerance; (5) a month or more when a great deal of time was spent getting drunk; (6) emotional/psychological problems because of alcohol use; (7) strong desire or urge to drink could not be resisted.

Source: Statistics Canada (n.d., 2011); Tjepkema (2004).

justified inadequate and gender-blind health promotion practices.

There may also be insufficient attention paid to women who are at moderate risk of alcohol-related harms because of the phenomenon known as the prevention paradox. This is the paradox wherein a large number of people exposed to a small risk can account for more harms on a population level than a small number exposed to a high risk (Rose, Khaw, & Marmot, 2008). Research from Canada suggests that the comparatively large number of people who occasionally drink to excess account for at least half of the harms and costs associated with drinking (Rehm et al., 2006). In Figure 5.3, even if a large number of women move to the "high-risk" category with the adjustment of the per-sitting consumption guidelines from five or more to four or more, there is still a large group of women who are at moderate risk and who may be overlooked by typical targeted campaigns to reduce alcohol risks. Principles of gender-transformative health promotion practice—such as being strengths-based, equity-oriented, and harm reduction–oriented—are very relevant to reaching women at all levels of risk and recognizing their agency regarding drinking and other health-related decisions.

Once the data are analyzed with recognition of sex- and gender-related factors, it is clear that at-risk drinking by women of child-bearing age is a large and growing concern in Canada. Over the long term, the rate of growth of alcohol use by women is higher than that for men, so the gap in consumption between the genders is narrowing over time (Figure 5.1). In addition, both occasional and regular at-risk drinking is increasing for women of child-bearing age across Canada, and the distribution of alcohol-related risk in women ages 18/19–44 clearly embodies the prevention paradox (i.e., a large number of women exposed to moderate alcohol-related risk). This means that efforts to reduce alcohol-related risk must necessarily include both policy interventions to lower consumption across the population and programmatic interventions to address the needs of the relatively smaller number of women who drink in high-risk patterns. To date, with few exceptions, health promotion and prevention efforts related to alcohol have not met that challenge (Poole, Urquhart, & Gonneau, 2010).

Gendered Influences on Women's Drinking and Gendered Responses

Combining an awareness of sex (the physiological effects of alcohol on women) with attention to the trend of rising consumption among women of child-bearing age crystallizes the importance of alcohol-related health promotion designed specifically for women. But in order to create such health promotion, it is imperative to understand the gendered influences that account for women's drinking patterns and the pressures they encounter when trying to reduce their consumption.

Women drink less than men on the whole, but this simple comparison masks powerful gendered influences that contribute to women's alcohol use. There are important risk factors and influences on drinking among women that have not been appropriately incorporated into health promotion efforts. For example, risky drinking and drinking during pregnancy are significantly more common among young women (Walker, Al-Sahab, Islam, & Tamim, 2011), women who smoke or use drugs (Gladstone, Levy, Nulman, & Koren, 1997; Walker et al., 2011), and women who have experienced violence (Logan, Walker, Cole, & Leukefeld, 2002; Martin, Beaumont, & Kupper, 2003). Higher socio-economic status and educational attainment predict more frequent drinking, but lower socio-economic status and educational attainment predict heavier drinking (Ahmad, Flight, Singh, Poole, & Dell, 2008). Drinking is correlated to psychological issues, but not necessarily the same ones in women as in men: whereas men are more likely to use alcohol for sensation-seeking or escapism (Nolen-Hoeksema, 2004), women are more likely to use it to cope with depression or low self-esteem (Amaro, Blake, Schwartz, & Flinchbaugh, 2001; CASA, 2003; Fillmore et al., 1997). Drinking among girls and women is also associated with disordered eating (McCreary Centre Society, 2010; Stewart & Brown, 2007).

Across all these populations, notions of femininity interact with personal circumstances to inform how much women drink, what they drink, and when. The relationship between gender roles and drinking behaviours is complex. On the one hand, "it is often argued that the main reason women do not drink more than men is that the social sanctions against drinking are greater for women than for men" (Nolen-Hoeksema, 2004, p. 987). However, there is also evidence that women's reasons for choosing to drink are informed by notions of femininity. For example, young women in particular may associate drinking with sexual attractiveness or availability, and therefore drink to convey messages to potential romantic partners.

Experiences of violence and trauma are important predictors of alcohol use, risky drinking, and dependency among women and girls, and as such trauma-informed health promotion responses need pioneering. Girls who have experienced abuse at any point in their lives tend to use alcohol and other substances earlier, more often, and at more dangerous levels than other girls (CASA, 2003). Intimate partner violence is also a strong predictor of women's drinking during pregnancy, and indeed often emerges for the first time during pregnancy (Amaro, Fried, Cabral, & Zuckerman, 1990). These correlations reflect the pressures on women that can make it harder to respond to health advice or health promotion messaging. Indeed, across all ethnic, socio-economic, and age groups, intimate partner violence (IPV) is a strong risk factor for heavy drinking, and a condition that is usually immune to quick behaviour modification. Consuming alcohol may perform an adaptive function in the lives of women experiencing violence, despite its detrimental health effects. It may help dull the pain of abuse, or provide reliability and comfort, or dim the memories of abusive experiences. It makes sense that some women are not necessarily capable of or interested in reducing or eliminating alcohol without sensitive, non-judgmental guidance, a harm reduction and women-centred approach, and the provision of guidance toward adopting alternate coping mechanisms. These approaches need to be incorporated into alcohol health promotion responses.

These gendered associations with drinking are exacerbated by the most pervasive influence on drinking of all: alcohol advertising. Both women and men—but particularly younger women and men—are affected by ubiquitous advertising for alcohol and media messages about the social statuses afforded by different types of drinking. Jean Kilbourne (1999) argues that "alcohol advertising is really our main form of alcohol education" (Devereaux, 2003, p. 18). Over a decade ago, the alcohol industry already spent $3 billion a year on advertising, much of it directed at youth; college students spend more money on alcohol than on books (Kilbourne, 1999). Alcohol-related health promotion is perpetually playing catch-up to an industry that is vastly better funded and more culturally savvy.

Alcohol marketing is one of the most conspicuously gendered and sexually suggestive cultural phenomena today. Most alcohol advertisements or representations of drinking (e.g., on television, in film, etc.) associate drinking with men's sexual potency or attractiveness or, more recently, with women's sexual enjoyment or "liberation." In advertisements geared at men, alcohol is sometimes presented as a replacement for sex itself.[1] Even alcohol advertisements that are putatively targeted at women make use of women's sexuality as a marketing strategy, reinforcing the suspicion that almost everything is geared toward the supposed appetites of heterosexual men.[2]

With such gender-exploitative images serving as the benchmark in alcohol messaging, there is an urgent need for gender-transformative health promotion directed at women and men, yet some alcohol companies are pre-empting this type of women-centred health promotion by exploiting gender in their advertising in order to stimulate greater alcohol consumption by women. Alcohol products are now linked with weight loss, sexiness, popularity, and other "feminine" goals (CASA, 2003; Media Smarts, n.d.). Specific brands of alcohol try to appeal to girls' tastes by masking the alcohol content with sugary mixers; this makes drinking more palatable, which can result in faster inebriation (CASA, 2003), and may promote earlier uptake of drinking (ibid.). In a series for the *Toronto Star*, a leading newspaper in Canada, journalist Ann Dowsett Johnston described how the alcohol industry is marketing directly to women with drinks such as Girls' Night Out, MommyJuice wines, Mike's Pink Hard Lemonade, and coolers in flavours that are considered more "feminine" such as kiwi mango (Johnston, 2011). "Low-calorie" drinks such as Skinnygirl wine have been created and marketed specifically to women who are presumed to be concerned with caloric intake (Crosariol, 2013). Such influences are at least partially responsible for recent increases in alcohol consumption by women.

Advertisements for alcohol products targeted at women are at times just as gender-exploitative as the conventional women-as-sex-object images, but more surreptitious because they masquerade as empowering. An example is MommyJuice (http://mommyjuicewines.com), which is significantly cheaper than most brands of wine. It is intended to appeal to the "supermom" who seamlessly juggles everyone else's needs and therefore "deserves" a glass of wine at the end of a hectic day.

Other brands appear to subvert the androcentric orientation of most alcohol advertising by pitching their product as a tonic for women's physical discomfort ("PMS isn't anything a good vodka cocktail and a cupcake can't cure" [Van Gogh Blue Vodka]) or even as the women's equivalent of sexual satisfaction in a bottle ("What's Your O-Face" [Three-O Vodka]). All of this "alcohol education" is intended to recruit and earn the allegiance of women consumers, with little regard for the health consequences of drinking, much less those consequences that are more severe among women.

Many health promotion efforts have, unfortunately, taken their lead from these types of messages, encouraging women to reduce risky drinking by underlining the negative aesthetic effects of consumption. For example, a "drinking mirror" phone application encourages women to "drop a glass size" by foregoing the extra calories contained in their alcoholic beverages. It allows the mobile phone user to take a photo of herself and then adjust the "mirror" according to how many drinks she consumes in order to see the premature aging and decrease in beauty that these drinks will supposedly cost her. Similarly, the UK Drinkaware health promotion campaign messaging highlights the amount of calories in alcoholic drinks, with handy facts such as "a glass of wine has similar calories to a slice of cake" and "the average wine drinker consumes 2,000 extra calories each month [or] 184 bags of crisps a year." The American Medical Association, in turn, provides information about the health impacts of alcohol use by young women while using a sexualized image similar to those used in alcohol industry advertising (see Figure 5.4).

These messages simultaneously provide relevant health information and exploit gendered pressure for beauty and thinness, aware that it is likely the motivation for beauty and thinness that will capture the public's attention.

While there is an important health imperative to consume nutritious foods and beverages, the prescription to not "drink yourself fat,"[3] whether applied to sugary sodas or vodka cocktails, reinforces gendered anxieties in a bid to change individual behaviour without regard for the unhealthy cultural and systemic structures that sustain it. Even women who take the fat fear-mongering seriously may not curb their drinking, but in fact adopt even riskier behaviours in response. For example, the use of weight concern to educate about the health impacts of alcohol use can lead to the "drunkorexia"

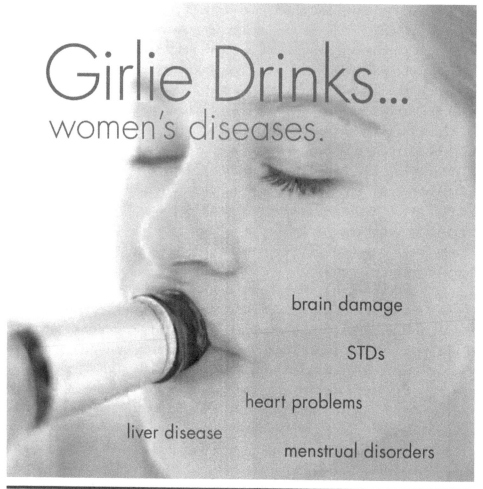

FIGURE 5.4: American Medical Association Poster: Girlie Drinks, Women's Diseases

Source: www.AlcoholPolicyMD.com.

phenomenon, whereby (largely) college-age women have reported starving themselves during the day and/or over-exercising so they could drink at night, thus netting the same number of daily calories and also getting drunk faster (Beller, 2013).

Health promotion campaigns directed to pregnant women are often particularly blind to influences on women's drinking, and instead emphasize women's individual responsibility (see Figure 5.5) and their drinking in pregnancy with a lack of love for their children. In addition, it is common for fetal alcohol spectrum disorder (FASD) prevention campaigns to use photos depicting naked pregnant women and emphasizing the womb, thus increasing the focus on fetal health without addressing women's health needs (see Figure 5.5).

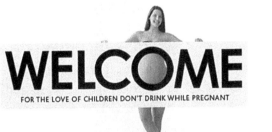

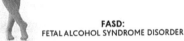

FIGURE 5.5: Poster about FASD Prevention

Source: FASworld Toronto.

Given that not only alcohol advertising but also health campaigns may inadvertently or consciously exploit damaging gender stereotypes, all sides of the issue, both causes and responses, need to be assessed using the framework in order to create transformative responses.

Conclusion: Gender-Transformative Alcohol Education and Health Promotion

Recalculations of at-risk drinking among women and heightened awareness of the factors affecting women's alcohol use underscore the urgency of creating more inspired and gender-sensitive health promotion. Health promoters have done an inadequate job thus far of identifying which women are drinking at risky levels and why. Considering this evidence and applying best practices from other areas of health care and health promotion could help reach women in a meaningful and supportive way, rather than blanketing all women with stern messages about individual responsibility and the threat alcohol poses to their waistlines. While there have been some encouraging programs that promote girls' empowerment (Girls Action Foundation, 2010; Hossfeld, 2008; LeCroy, 2008), address under-age drinking (CCSA, 2012; Stigler, Neusel, & Perry, 2012), and explore factors influencing risky drinking among college students (LaBrie, Thompson, Huchting, Lac, & Buckley, 2007), there has been a troubling dearth of alcohol education and health promotion that consciously empowers girls and women to make choices out of concern for their health and comprehensive well-being.

One example of a promising alcohol education campaign directed at young women is the Queensland, Australia, short commercial (available on YouTube) called "Becky's not drinking tonight." It depicts a young woman casually announcing her intention to not drink and then satirizes the imagined fallout: sports stadiums full of strangers gasping in disbelief, the United Nations issuing a statement, and so on. It ends with the young woman saying, "They'll get over it" and the tagline, "Make up your own mind about drinking." This type of health promotion is encouraging because it taps into some of the pressures, real or imagined, affecting young women who are in the highest-risk age group for binge drinking, and shows that a young woman can be empowered to challenge social conventions. However, it also shows the young woman who chooses not to drink as necessarily staying home alone.

Gender-transformative health promotion approaches would ensure that health messages are based on evidence showing the influences of sex and gender on alcohol-related harms and offer messages tailored to high-risk groups of women in a supportive, woman-centred way. Education and empowerment need to occur on a number of fronts simultaneously. There is a need to draw women's attention to the exploitative messages about thinness in alcohol advertising rather than simply countering them with similar techniques. The health risks of excessive drinking need to be communicated without reframing them as failures of femininity. As well, the health risks of drinking during pregnancy need to be communicated in ways that do not focus exclusively on individual responsibility and that shame women who have difficulty stopping or curtailing their substance use. Approaches that enhance social support among women, such as in the health promotion poster in Figure 5.6, are promising. Third, approaches that address the adaptive function of drinking for women in vulnerable circumstances would be a basis for sympathetic and empowering health promotion that takes into account real life issues that make risky drinking more likely, such as violence, poverty, racism, and depression. Finally, programs that emphasize the power of girls and women to make health-promoting decisions and to be critical consumers of both alcohol advertising and alcohol-related health promotion

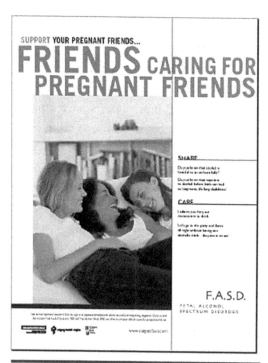

FIGURE 5.6: Friends Caring for Pregnant Friends Poster

Source: Calgary Fetal Alcohol Network (http://calgary-fasd.com/cfan-initiatives/circle-of-friends).

could have potentially longer-lasting effects than any individual instance of alcohol education. Young women, for instance, could be empowered to question the assumed equation between drinking and popularity to counteract the relentless external messages put out by alcohol industry.

As well as the recalculation of girls' and women's risk, research is needed to further enhance understanding of the range of the intersecting factors that affect their drinking patterns. This analysis would assess the impact of these factors on drinking throughout the life course of women in their child-bearing years and inform the development of policies and programs to reduce alcohol-related risk across the population.

Alcohol has been correctly identified as a prime target for health promotion efforts, but its history of sex- and gender-blindness means that this area of health promotion has missed numerous opportunities to be more effective and positive for women. This has been exacerbated by non-sex-specific calculations of at-risk drinking that have underpinned gender-blind health promotion. Gender-transformative health promotion would not only empower women to change drinking behaviours and empower themselves through critique of alcohol marketing, but it would, more radically, inspire and direct more structural changes to reduce the negative influences and factors affecting women's alcohol use.

Appendix 5A

Comparison of Four or More and Five or More Drinks Per Occasion as a Measure of Risky Drinking for Women of Child-bearing Age

Data from four national surveys were used to compare the percentage of current (past-year) drinking women who said they drank four or more drinks per occasion once a month or more often in the past year and those who said they drank five or more drinks per occasion once a month or more in the past year to assess the potential effect on estimates of prevalence of risky drinking of women in their child-bearing years. Results are depicted in Table 5.1.

Method

Sample: Women who drank at least once in the past year. Data elements used: (1) Women who reported four or more drinks per occasion monthly or more often in the past year based on the question: How often in the past 12 months have you had four or more drinks on one occasion (alc5f or AHEAVYMN in CADUMS and alc5a or AHEAVYMN in 2004 CAS)? (2) Women who reported five or more drinks per occasion monthly or more often in the past year based on the question: How often in the past 12 months have you had five or more drinks on one occasion

TABLE 5.1: Comparison of Percentage of Current (Past-Year) Drinking Women in the Household Population Reporting 4+ Drinks Per Occasion and Those Reporting 5+ Drinks Per Occasion Once a Month or More, Canada, 2004, 2008, 2009, 2010

Age	CADUMS 2010			CADUMS 2009			CADUMS 2008			CAS 2004			Average % Difference
	4+	5+	% Difference †	4+	5+	% Difference †	4+	5+	% Difference †	4+	5+	% Difference †	
Underage	29.3 (±7.2)	17.3 (±6.3)	69.36	24.0 (±12.3)	12.5 (±6.9)	92.00	30.0 (±11.6)	24.5 (±11.6)	22.45	21.1 (±6.9)	16.4 (±6.3)	28.66	53.12
Young Adult	37.1 (±5.0)	23.0 (±4.0)	61.30	41.6 (±9.8)	34.0 (±9.6)	22.35	43.7 (±8.9)	29.3 (±7.8)	49.15	46.4 (±6.8)	40.7 (±6.7)	14.00	36.70
25–34	22.6 (±6.0)	13.4 (±3.1)	68.66	19.4 (±6.2)	14.1 (±5.5)	37.59	22.7 (±4.6)	14.4 (±3.7)	57.64	21.3 (±4.1)	15.8 (±3.7)	34.81	49.67
35–44	19.2 (±4.5)	8.4 (±3.4)	128.57	18.1 (±4.1)	12.0 (±3.5)	50.83	14.9 (±3.5)	7.8 (±2.6)	91.03	17.6 (±3.4)	13.1 (±3.1)	34.35	76.20
15–44	24.7 (±2.8)	13.6 (±2.2)	81.62	24.2 (±3.5)	17.6 (±3.2)	37.50	25.1 (±3.1)	16.3 (±2.7)	53.99	25.3 (±2.5)	20.2 (±2.3)	25.25	49.59

Notes: Underage are respondents ages 15–17 in Alberta, Manitoba, and Quebec, and ages 15–18 in the rest of Canada. Young adult are drinkers ages 18–24 in Alberta, Manitoba, and Quebec, and drinkers ages 19–24 in the rest of Canada.

All estimates (±95% CI) based on the weighted sample: 4+ and 5+ rates refer to proportion of sample in that age group reporting drinking 4+ or 5+ drinks per occasion at least monthly. † % Difference: (Rate 4+ − Rate 5+) × 100 / Rate 5+.

Sources: Adlaf, Begin, & Sawka (2005); Health Canada (n.d. a, n.d. b, n.d. c).

(alc5 or FIVEMN in CADUMS and 2004 CAS)? All estimates were based on the weighted sample and were adjusted for design effects.

NOTES

1 For example, Maker's Mark Whisky ad: "Your Bourbon has a great body and fine character. I wish the same could be said for my girlfriend."
2 Skyy Vodka ad: "Men are good for 2 things: Blocking the sun and pouring another drink" (image has a crotch shot of a man standing over a woman, who is lying down wearing a scanty bikini).
3 Wording of a campaign by New York City Department of Health & Mental Hygiene, depicting a bottle of Coca-Cola turning into fat as it is poured into a glass.

REFERENCES

Adlaf, E., Begin, P., & Sawka, E. (Eds.). (2005). *Canadian Addiction Survey (CAS): A national survey of Canadians' use of alcohol and other drugs; Prevalence of use and related harms: Detailed report.* Ottawa: Canadian Centre on Substance Abuse. Retrieved from www.ccsa.ca/ Resource%20Library/ccsa-004028-2005.pdf

Ahmad, N., Flight, F., Singh, V. A. S., Poole, N., & Dell, C. A. (2008). *Canadian Addiction Survey (CAS): Focus on gender.* Ottawa: Health Canada. Retrieved from http://publications.gc.ca/collections/collection_2009/sc-hc/H128-1-07-519E.pdf

Amaro, H., Blake, S. M., Schwartz, P. M., & Flinchbaugh, L. J. (2001). Developing theory-based substance abuse prevention programs for young adolescent girls. *Journal of Early Adolescence, 21*(3), 256–293.

Amaro, H., Fried, L., Cabral, H., & Zuckerman, B. (1990). Violence during pregnancy: The relationship to drug use among women and their partners. *American Journal of Public Health, 80*(5), 575–579.

Beller, S. (2013, April 1). *"Drunkorexia" is double trouble.* Retrieved from www.thefix.com/ content/drunkorexia-double-trouble91481

CASA. (2003). *The formative years: Pathways to substance abuse among girls and young women ages 8–22.* New York: National Centre on Addiction and Substance Abuse at Columbia University (CASA).

CCSA. (2012). *The Canadian Standards for Youth Substance Abuse Prevention: An Overview.* Ottawa: Canadian Centre on Substance Abuse.

Chen, W., Rosner, B., Hankinson, S., Graham, A., Colditz, G., & Willett, W. (2011). Moderate alcohol consumption during adult life, drinking patterns, and breast cancer risk. *JAMA, 306*(17), 1884–1890.

Crosariol, B. (2013, May 1). How you can sip your way to a skinnier figure with wine. *The Globe and Mail.*

Devereaux, D. (2003). *Study guide—deadly persuasion: The advertising of alcohol and tobacco.* Northampton, MA: Media Education Foundation.

Eliany, M., Giesbrecht, N., & Nelson, M. (Eds.). (1990). *National Alcohol and Other Drugs Survey (NADS): Highlights report*. Ottawa: Health and Welfare Canada. NADS data available from http://odesi1.scholarsportal.info/webview

Farhat, T., Iannotti, R., & Simons-Morton, B. (2010). Overweight, obesity, youth, and health-risk behaviors. *American Journal of Preventative Medicine, 38*(3), 258–267.

Fillmore, K. M., Golding, J. M., Leino, E. V., Motoyoshi, M., Shoemaker, C., Terry, H., . . . Ferrei, H. (1997). Patterns and trends in women's and men's drinking. In R. W. Wilsnack & S. C. Wilsnack (Eds.), *Gender and alcohol: Individual and social perspectives* (pp. 21–48). Piscataway, NJ: Rutgers University Center of Alcohol Studies.

Girls Action Foundation. (2010). *Amplify toolkit Montreal*. Quebec City: GAF. Retrieved from www.girlsactionfoundation.ca/en/amplify-toolkit-1.

Gladstone, J., Levy, M., Nulman, I., & Koren, G. (1997). Characteristics of pregnant women who engage in binge alcohol consumption. *Canadian Medical Association Journal, 156,* 789–794.

Greaves, L., & Poole, N. (2008). Bringing sex and gender into women's substance use treatment programs. *Substance Use & Misuse, 43*(9), 1271–1273.

Health Canada. (n.d. a). *Highlights report from the 2008 Canadian Alcohol and Drug Use Monitoring Survey (CADUMS)*. Retrieved from http://www.hc-sc.gc.ca/hc-ps/drugs-drogues/stat/_2008/summary-sommaire-eng.php#alc

Health Canada. (n.d. b). *Highlights report from the 2009 Canadian Alcohol and Drug Use Monitoring Survey (CADUMS)*. Retrieved from http://www.hc-sc.gc.ca/hc-ps/drugs-drogues/stat/_2009/summary-sommaire-eng.php

Health Canada. (n.d. c). *Highlights report from the 2010 Canadian Alcohol and Drug Use Monitoring Survey (CADUMS)*. Retrieved from http://www.hc-sc.gc.ca/hc-ps/drugs-drogues/stat/_2010/summary-sommaire-eng.php

Health Canada. (1995). *Canada's Alcohol and Other Drugs Survey (CADS), 1994*. Ottawa: Author. CADS data available for from http://odesi1.scholarsportal.info/webview

Hossfeld, B. (2008). Developing friendships and peer relationships: Building social support with the Girls Circle program. In C. W. LeCroy & J. E. Mann (Eds.), *Handbook of prevention and intervention programs for adolescent girls* (pp. 41–80). Hoboken, NJ: John Wiley & Sons Inc.

Johnston, A. D. (2011, November 21). Women are the new face of alcohol advertising. *Toronto Star*. Retrieved from www.thestar.com/atkinsonseries/atkinson2011/article/1090125--women-are-the-new-face-of-alcohol-advertising

Kilbourne, J. (1999). *Deadly persuasion: Why women and girls must fight the addictive power of advertising*. New York: Simon & Schuster.

LaBrie, J. W., Thompson, A. D., Huchting, K., Lac, A., & Buckley, K. (2007). A group motivational interviewing intervention reduces drinking and alcohol-related negative consequences in adjudicated college women. *Addictive Behaviors, 32*(11), 2549–2562.

LeCroy, C. W. (2008). Universal prevention for adolescent girls: The Go Grrrls program. In C. W. LeCroy & J. E. Mann (Eds.), *Handbook of prevention and intervention programs for adolescent girls* (pp. 11–40). Hoboken, NJ: John Wiley & Sons Inc.

Li, C. I., Chlebowski, R. T., Freiberg, M., Johnson, K. C., Kuller, L., Lane, D., . . . Prentice, R. (2010). Alcohol consumption and risk of postmenopausal breast cancer by subtype: The women's health initiative observational study. *Journal of the National Cancer Institute, 102*(18), 1422–1431.

Logan, T., Walker, R., Cole, J., & Leukefeld, C. (2002). Victimization and substance abuse among women: Contributing factors, interventions, and implications. *Review of General Psychology, 6*(4), 325–397.

Martin, S. L., Beaumont, J. L., & Kupper, L. L. (2003). Substance use before and during pregnancy: Links to intimate partner violence. *American Journal of Drug Alcohol Abuse, 29*(3), 599–617.

McCarty, C. A., Kosterman, R., Mason, W. A., McCauley, E., Hawkins, J. D., Herrenkohl, T. I., & Lengua, L. J. (2009). Longitudinal associations among depression, obesity, and alcohol use disorders in young adulthood. *General Hospital Psychiatry, 31*(5), 442–450.

McCreary Centre Society. (2010). *What a difference a year can make: Early alcohol and marijuana use among 16–18 year old BC students.* A report of the 2008 British Columbia Adolescent Health Survey. Vancouver: McCreary Centre Society.

Media Smarts. (n.d.). *Gender and alcohol—teaching backgrounder.* Retrieved from http://mediasmarts.ca/backgrounder/gender-and-alcohol-teaching-backgrounder

National Institute on Alcohol Abuse and Alcoholism. (2004, July). Alcohol—an important women's health issue. *Alcohol Alert, 62.* Retrieved from www.pubs.niaa.nih/gov/publications/aa62/aa62.htm.

Nolen-Hoeksema, S. (2004). Gender differences in risk factors and consequences for alcohol use and problems. *Clinical Psychology Review, 24*(8), 981–1010.

Poole, N., Urquhart, C., & Gonneau, G. (2010). *Girl-centred approaches to prevention, harm reduction, and treatment, gendering the national framework series* (Vol. 2). Vancouver: British Columbia Centre of Excellence for Women's Health.

Rehm, J., Baliunas, D., Brochu, S., Fischer, B., Gnam, W., Patra, J., . . . Tayler, B. (2006). *The costs of substance abuse in Canada 2002.* Ottawa: Canadian Centre on Substance Abuse.

Rose, G., Khaw, K., & Marmot, G. (2008). *Rose's strategy of preventative medicine.* Oxford: Oxford University Press.

Statistics Canada. (n.d.). *CANSIM Table 105-0501: Canadian Community Health Survey; Data on alcohol use from 2003 to 2010.* Data available from http://www5.statcan.gc.ca/cansim/a26?lang=eng&retrLang=eng&id=1050501&paSer=&pattern=&stByVal=2&p1=-1&p2=37&tabMode=dataTable&csid= Tables (custom age groupings ordered from Statistics Canada).

Statistics Canada. (2011). *CANSIM Table 105-0501: Health Canada indicator profile, annual estimates, by age group and sex, Canada, provinces, territories, health regions (2012 boundaries) and peer groups.* Tables on reported alcohol use for 2003, 2005, 2007/08, and 2009/10 based on custom age groupings purchased from Statistics Canada. Data on reported alcohol use based on standardized age grouping available from www5.statcan.gc.ca/cansim/a05?lang=eng&id=1050501

Stewart, S. H., & Brown, C. (2007). The relationship between disordered eating and substance use. In N. Poole & L. Greaves (Eds.), *Highs and lows: Canadian perspectives on women and substance use* (pp. 157–165). Toronto: Centre for Addiction and Mental Health.

Stigler, M. H., Neusel, E., & Perry, C. L. (2012). School-based programs to prevent and reduce alcohol use among youth. *Alcohol Research & Health, 34*(2), 157–162.

Tjepkema, M. (2004). Alcohol and illicit drug dependence. *Supplement to Health Reports: Vol. 15.* Cat. no. 82-003. Retrieved from http://www.statcan.gc.ca/pub/82-003-s/2004000/pdf/7447-eng.pdf

Walker, M., Al-Sahab, B., Islam, F., & Tamim, H. (2011). The epidemiology of alcohol utilization during pregnancy: An analysis of the Canadian Maternity Experiences Survey (MES). *BMC Pregnancy and Childbirth, 11*(1), 52.

6 Promoting the Mental Health of Immigrant Women by Transforming Community Physical Activity

Donna S. Lee, Wendy Frisby, and Pamela Ponic

Introduction

The World Health Organization (2001) has estimated that 20–25 percent of all people globally will experience mental health issues over their lifetimes and this has a significant negative impact, not only on the economy of societies, but also on the quality of life of individuals and their families. Women experience mental health issues, such as stress, depression, and anxiety, to a greater degree than men because of the adverse effects of inferior social status, the disproportionate burden of family caregiving, experiences of abuse and discrimination, and inequalities in educational and occupational opportunities (Morrow, 2007). For immigrant women, the migration process itself can lead to additional stress due to income and housing insecurities, cultural displacement, disruption of family relations and social supports, language barriers, and an unfamiliarity with how health and other services are provided (Khander & Koch, 2011; Vissandjee, Thurston, Apale, & Nahar, 2007).

There is growing evidence that participation in physical activity decreases depression, anxiety, and stress, suggesting that biomedical approaches are not the only treatment alternative (Bingham, 2009). The Victorian Health Promotion Foundation (VicHealth) in Australia has shown that community-based physical activity interventions are effective in promoting mental health as long as they include opportunities for community and social interaction, suggesting the importance of social and physical contributors to mental health promotion (Keleher & Armstrong, 2005). Yet physical activity and community engagement are seldom considered when mental health promotion interventions for women are being developed.

Thirty immigrant women who participated in our qualitative study confirmed that community physical activity participation had a significant positive impact on both their mental and physical health, although the pathways were neither linear nor uniform. The women primarily talked about health in terms of mental health, although they saw it as closely interconnected with their physical health. They also offered a number of suggestions for transforming how physical activity is currently offered at the community level to better meet their varied circumstances and mental health issues. In keeping with the transformational message of this book, rather than only describing the ways current health promotion programs and policies do not work for immigrant women, we advance a view of what might work and why, based on participant input. These findings provide a starting point for understanding the complex and contradictory connections between immigrant women's experiences with migration, mental health, and community physical activity, topics that are rarely considered in an integrative way in the literature or in health promotion policy and program development.

Migration and Women's Mental Health

Khander and Koch (2011) defined settlement as a health issue because although newcomers have lower rates of chronic disease and mental health conditions upon arrival in Canada, which is known as the "healthy immigrant effect," after settling many lose this advantage over time and their health problems sometimes exceed those of the Canadian-born population (Hyman & Jackson, 2010). Vissandjee et al. (2007) similarly argued that migration should be recognized as a social determinant of health. Migration can be voluntary or involuntary and there are a variety of factors driving decisions to relocate, including expectations about economic and educational opportunities, concerns about political changes, a desire for family reunification, and escaping persecution or environmental disasters (Vissandjee et al., 2007). Migration is a gendered process as immigrant women are more likely than men to be employed in informal sectors like domestic services and entertainment, which are often lower paying and subject to fewer regulations and human rights protection than other, male-dominated occupations (Kawar, 2004). Furthermore, despite having credentials in the same top four areas of post-secondary study, including (1) business, management, and public administration; (2) health; (3) parks and recreation; and (4) fitness, recent immigrant women are less likely than Canadian-born women with similar training to be employed in these fields (Chui, 2011). This disparity reflects the exclusion of recent immigrant women's voices and perspectives in planning and decision-making roles in organizations involved in health promotion program delivery. Discrimination based on race and having an accent rather than actual English language ability also compounds challenges to finding employment (Creese & Kambere, 2003).

Because most immigrant women enter Canada as dependants and are less likely than newcomer men to speak English or French fluently, they can encounter greater difficulties in securing employment and building social supports, and are therefore more prone to ill health (Khander & Koch, 2011). Previous research has shown that because the stress experienced throughout the migration and adaptation process can last for several years, marital and family relations can become strained, making newcomer women more vulnerable to abuse (Hyman, 2004). Vissandjee et al. (2007) argued that migration intersects with other social determinants of health such as gender, income, and social exclusion, yet when this is not taken into account, "it both reflects and perpetuates a culture of disadvantage that still persists for far too many women in Canada and around the world" (p. 222).

Like migration, mental health is gendered, in part because women have "historically been understood as located on the irrational or nature side of the nature/culture binary, [so] it is not surprising that in Western thinking, women more than men have come be to understood as mentally unstable" (Morrow, 2007, p. 356). Women are more likely than men to be diagnosed with depression and anxiety, to experience recurring depressive episodes, and to access traditional mental health care services, and this is sometimes attributed to hormonal imbalances or fragile psyches (Fullagar, 2008; Morrow, 2007). However, Dossa (2004) cautioned against medicalizing the effects of dislocation and social and economic exclusion through the use of mental health discourses that insinuate women cannot handle the stress of migration. Rather than individualizing the problem, it is important to consider how stressors are situated within the broader social and institutional conditions that immigrant women encounter. It is therefore important to consider how community physical activity is offered, along with how barriers to participation are tied to the social determinants of health, rather than assuming that immigrant women simply lack motivation or are uninterested in participating.

Community Physical Activity and Mental Health Promotion

By community physical activity, we are referring to settings where physical activities are offered by local governments through their recreation or leisure service departments, which also offer a range of other programs, including art, music, and competitive sport. The focus of our study was on programs like fitness, dance, swimming, yoga, and walking groups because women who are not currently participating often express the most interest in these types of physical activities (Frisby, 2011). We chose this setting because recreation departments usually have mandates for providing programs to all citizens, often at lower cost than in the private sector, and financial subsidies are sometimes available. However, these reduced program fees are often still too expensive for families living on low incomes (Taylor & Frisby, 2010).

While recreation departments in Canada typically position themselves as contributing to community health, few target immigrant groups specifically, despite rising immigration rates and the differential health effects of immigration. In addition, previous research has shown that immigrant women participate less in health-promoting forms of physical activity than immigrant men or native-born Canadians (Tremblay, Bryan, Perez, Ardern, & Katzmarzyk, 2006). This is likely tied to a number of factors such as unfamiliarity with the community recreation system in Canada, patriarchal norms that position women as unsuitable participants in organized physical activities in the public sphere, and a lack of time due to traditional gender-role responsibilities (Fullagar, 2008; Ponic, Nanjijuma, Pederson, Poole, & Scott, 2011). Moreover, most community physical activity programs target children, youth, and seniors rather than middle-aged adults, and many recreation departments are not well connected to other community organizations that offer health and immigration services (Frisby, 2011). As Yates, Hancock, and Hutchinson (2013) noted in their report on the health-recreation interface, the fields of community recreation, public health, primary care, chronic disease management, rehabilitation, and mental health could benefit significantly from improved interaction and integration with each other.

While the WHO (2001) acknowledged it is difficult to develop a single definition of mental health due to different cultural meanings, mental health is usually associated with feelings of subjective well-being, self-efficacy, autonomy, competence, and self-actualization of one's intellectual and emotional potential. Yet Fullagar (2008) argued that definitions of mental health that refer to reductionistic psychological factors often do not adequately take gendered relations of power into account. Following her qualitative study with women recovering from depression, Fullagar defined depression as "an intensification of emotional distress that arises from the performance of particular gender norms that regulate women's everyday lives" (p. 37). This definition illustrates that mental health is broader than the absence of clinically diagnosed mental disorders. The VicHealth framework built on a broader conceptualization by identifying three overarching determinants of mental health: social inclusion, freedom from violence and discrimination, and access to economic resources and participation (Keleher & Armstrong, 2005). Social inclusion referred to having opportunities for "social and community connections, stable and supportive environments, a variety of social and physical activities, access to networks and supportive relationships, and a valued social position" (ibid., p. 22). Freedom from violence, including gender-based violence, and discrimination entailed the valuing of diversity, physical security, opportunities for self-determination, and control over one's life. Finally, access to work and meaningful engagement, education, housing, and money were the factors contributing to economic resources and participation.

Immigrant Women's Health and Wellness Project

To obtain input directly from a population of women who may be experiencing declining mental health, 30 women who had recently immigrated to an urban area in western Canada were interviewed in their language of choice to obtain their perspectives on how their health had changed following migration, and what role community physical activity could play in facilitating their settlement. Study participants also completed a translated survey to provide background socio-demographic data. Inclusion criteria included women over the age of 18 who had migrated to Canada within the last five years who currently resided in the study community. Following the interviews, we arranged three meetings to share the findings and to discuss changes that would facilitate their participation in community physical activity. Translation and refreshments were provided and the meetings were held at convenient times so women with children could make child-care arrangements. Honoraria in the form of grocery vouchers were provided at interviews and meetings.

Study Participant Profile

A majority of interviewees were 30 to 59 years old, with one participant over 60. Participants originated from a number of different countries, including: Iran (13), China (7), Korea (2), the Philippines (2), the Czech Republic (1), France (1), Germany (1), India (1), Indonesia (1), and Mexico (1). They were recruited through multilingual notices posted at community recreation facilities, the multicultural society, a health authority, and the library. The women entered Canada through a variety of immigration categories, including: skilled workers (some were spousal applicants under this category) (18), family class (5), business class (2), live-in caregivers (2), investor class (1), and refugee class (1). This contrasts with Khander and Koch's (2011) findings that men are more likely to arrive in Toronto as skilled workers, whereas women were more likely to enter as dependants of skilled workers, family-class immigrants, or through the live-in caregiver program. The majority of women in our study had high levels of educational attainment, as 24 had completed a bachelor's or graduate degree prior to moving to Canada. All but seven participants migrated with dependent children. This diversity in the sample was intentional to avoid conflating experiences or views of individuals with a specific ethnic group (Meadows, Thurston, & Melton, 2001), and to more adequately reflect the diversity among recent immigrant women living in the community. It also helps illustrate the importance of considering how gender intersects with other social determinants of health.

Physical Activity Participation

In terms of physical activity participation, 18 of the 30 women had tried or were currently participating in community physical activity programs in Canada, 5 women had participated only in informal unorganized physical activities like walking or using fitness facilities in their apartment buildings, and 7 said they did not participate in any organized physical activity. Of these 7 women, 2 had enrolled their children in community physical activity programs and another 2 had visited community centres as part of their employment as caregivers.

Understandings of Health

The WHO (2001) report described mental health as a complex interaction between biological, psychological, and social factors that are deeply intertwined with one's physical health. The immigrant women in our study frequently referred to this connection between mental and physical health, as the following quotation from an Iranian woman who had been in Canada for three months illustrates: "If I just want to look at the one-dimensional, it's just physical. But, you come to understand that the health of mind and body together are important. When you have peace of body and mind, it means you are healthy." The majority of women had a holistic sense of well-being that was also tied to social and spiritual health, although a few associated health with the absence of chronic disease or adopting healthy lifestyles, such as not being overweight, eating and sleeping well, and being physically active.

For the seven women who reported good mental health after migration, a combination of two or more of the following factors were evident: they were partnered and the family migrated and stayed together; they or their partners held secure employment; they had previous experience living in Western nations or working in multinational companies; they had extended family living in Canada; and they were comfortable communicating in English. The remainder discussed declining mental health due to challenges adjusting to their new environment and spoke about feeling intimidated, being limited by their language abilities, and not knowing how to find information about their new community. Some women saw this as a personal failing rather than a problem with how community services are delivered. Emotional reactions to their new circumstances were diverse as some reported initial feelings of excitement and anticipation about the opportunities available, but when expectations were not met, positive emotions were replaced by feelings of despair, loneliness, and deep sadness.

Sources of Stress and Depression

The most common stressors were directly tied to the women's experiences with migration in relation to other social determinants of health, and included adjusting to a new society, financial insecurity, family separation, and social isolation. These four stressors were highly interrelated, as revealed in the following quotation from a woman from Iran who linked uncertainty with financial insecurity:

> I feel more stressed and it was even more before my husband got his job. Tension really changes everything and maybe even changes physical health, not maybe, it 100 percent changes it. Stress of what will happen tomorrow? Can you work or not? When can you finally work? What would happen to your child's education? But stress is the worst thing.

Another key source of stress was the lack of recognition of educational and professional qualifications, along with expensive ESL training not being recognized when the women applied for jobs. This was tied to financial insecurity because of exclusion from the job market, which compounded concerns about dwindling savings. The quotation below illustrates the impact this can have on making participation in health-promoting forms of physical activity a low priority. Many of the narratives were tied to ensuring that necessities were taken care of for other family members rather than for themselves, a typical gendered norm, and how the expenses and lack of information created additional barriers to participation.

> I know many people who are doing well financially. However, a newcomer family brought an amount of money and knows that they should spend this money for many things like children's educations, foods, rent of house, car, and etc. So in this case probably doing exercise would be the last priority. Since other things seem more fundamental and are primary needs.

Most of the women were not able to continue in the same types of careers they held prior to migration, and their partners, if they migrated together, also experienced difficulties entering the job market. While this is consistent with other studies (Man, 2004), it is important to recognize that not all women experienced economic exclusion. Two women were able to obtain the same type of employment within months of migrating to Canada and expressed high levels of job satisfaction. Another two women immigrated as live-in caregivers, so while their employment was more guaranteed, the work was highly gendered and not related to their education.

Financial insecurity resulted in family separation in some cases. Because male partners sometimes anticipated having difficulty obtaining work in Canada, some women migrated with their children in the hopes of providing them with more opportunities, while their partners remained in their country of origin to continue earning an income. Relocating with their children in tow with no social support contributed to these women's feelings of stress and depression. Not being valued because of changing roles, the loss of professional work status, and difficulties communicating in English also contributed to declining mental health.

For two women, their decision to migrate to Canada was in part precipitated by the dissolution of their marriages, while another divorced her husband one year after arrival, and a fourth was widowed months after she landed. Being newly single in a new country created a great deal of hardship for immigrant women who were underemployed and needed to care for children while concurrently negotiating a new legal and cultural system and coping with grief. Not only was social isolation linked to being temporarily or permanently separated from their partners, it was compounded when they encountered difficulty developing meaningful new relationships following migration. Community physical activity represented one non-traditional health setting that could contribute to reduced social isolation, although, as revealed in the next section, this did not always occur.

Role of Community Physical Activity in Promoting Women's Mental Health

Those with declining mental health are most likely to be sedentary, socially isolated, and disconnected from their community (Iwasaki, Coyle, & Shank, 2010). While there is growing evidence about the benefits of physical activity in preventing chronic diseases in culturally diverse populations (Caperchione, Kolt, & Mummery, 2009), less is known about the mechanisms that make it effective in promoting mental health. There is some research to suggest that participation under positive conditions can lead to improved mood, feeling better about oneself, relaxation, improved sleep, a heightened sense of belonging, and enjoyment (Bingham, 2009). Some immigrant women who had participated in community physical activity programs since coming to Canada confirmed this, even though relief was sometimes only temporary.

> The facilities that you have here to busy yourself with exercising have very good effect on mentality. I come here [to the community centre] every day to exercise and walk back home and it gives me good feelings at least for half of the day. Stresses may come back to me during a day again, but sport is so helpful for changing my morale.

While the WHO (2006, 2010) has acknowledged the positive link between physical activity and mental health in recent reports, inadequate attention has been given to intersections with gender, migration, and other social determinants of health.

As Fullagar (2008) argued, much can be learned about these intersections by unpacking power-knowledge relations to position women as the experts on their own lives. Hearing directly from immigrant women about the role community physical activity has on their mental health begins to shed light on the complexities and contradictions involved.

In our study, physical activity was often discussed as a mechanism for seeking social networks and intercultural connections while minimizing stress and anxiety to improve mental health. For women with families, their priority was ensuring their children could participate, so the women often put off their own participation indefinitely, even though many wanted to be positive and active role models for their children. This confirmed Fullagar's (2008) findings that pressures not to participate in leisure activities reinforces masculine-oriented subject positions of women as wives and mothers, as illustrated in the following comment from a woman from Iran about how physical activity became a diversion to cope with separation from a male partner:

> My loneliness is most likely because I had separated from my family suddenly, and also my husband was not here and my dependence to him is very much. But the thing that kept me was doing exercise. I tried to busy myself with doing exercise.

Fullagar (2008) found the most difficult issue for women in her study was feeling entitled to participate in activities because engaging in such self-care itself could become a source of stress and guilt. When these feelings were overcome or when women resisted traditional gender norms, new embodied habits were formed that were invigorating and tied to positive emotions (Fullagar, 2008). The following quotation from a woman who came to Canada from Mexico four years ago emphasizes this, but also speaks to the consequences of participating in less than ideal conditions, such as when physical activity instructors speak only in English:

> The first two years ... the first year was so frustrating, either for my English, for the weather, for my friends, for ... for everything.... I feel so lonely and my only companion was my family. And I need to open my mind to do ... you don't want to be depressed for months per year inside your house. You need to do something and that was when I start to join the fitness classes at the community centre. But it was so hard for me because I don't speak good English and the teacher used all these sophisticated words to do the movements.

Some of the women noted that they were "not really sporty," nor did they have any background in organized physical activity prior to migration. However, due to the stress encountered during and after migration, they sought out physical activities to relieve anxiety, boost morale, recharge their batteries, and release tension. According to Keleher and Armstrong (2005), combining physical activity with social interaction is key because solitary exercise alone does not reduce depression. To offset this, immigrants in a study by Stewart et al. (2008) attempted to build social networks with those outside their ethnic communities through participation in educational and health programs. The authors emphasized the need for service providers to be self-aware of discriminatory attitudes and to actively understand, empathize with, and support newcomers. Though few participants in our study spoke directly about discrimination, simply offering physical activity programs and assuming they will lead to increased social interaction was called into question when one woman, who moved to Canada from Korea three years ago, spoke about feeling like there was an "invisible wall" around her. Initially she sought out community physical activity programs to meet people, but she could not easily communicate with them and no one made an effort to befriend her, thus increasing her feelings of dislocation and isolation. When asked what she meant by an invisible wall, she explained:

> Ah ... the cashier or receptionist desk is very kind, but only kind. If I participate [in] some group, nobody knows me, and nobody talk to me. Maybe if someone talk to me and I will be nervous, so ... I can't contact them. I can't talk ... first time or second is ok, it's just about weather and small talk is okay, but the deep conversation is trouble for me.

Another interviewee from Germany also described the superficial and "othering" nature of some social interactions. She said that people asked her where she is from when they heard her accent, but that was usually where the conversation ended. Only one immigrant woman explicitly stated that she was able to develop lasting friendships, in this case with other immigrant women, through community physical activity programs: "I think that one of the most important things in my life is thanks to the recreation centres. Since I move here, I met my friends, my daughters are going there, I am volunteer there, I learn there." Social interaction was not a one-way process where newcomers were hoping that others would reach out to them. While there were few opportunities for the immigrant women to become physical activity instructors, one older woman from Iran taught yoga in her home and provided social support to her Canadian neighbours and newcomers, some of whom confided in her that they were suffering from depression.

I had some Canadian neighbours coming to my house and doing meditations together, but it was friendly and not for money. I had some other friends asking for yoga, I told them I perform yoga every day at 4 a.m. and anyone can join me. During the time I encountered some people who were really depressed and I was like a mother for them and helped them to pull themselves together.

Another woman from China said she provided social support to her immigrant friends by accompanying them to physical activity programs, but felt limited in how else to support them "because I am not [a] professional in this area; the only thing that I can do is to listen."

Other women said they sought out physical activity not to socialize primarily, but for their own health and time for themselves. To illustrate, an interviewee from China explained how daily life now required considerable mental focus and energy, for instance, to understand basic interactions with her neighbours or to process her two-and-a-half-hour English class, and how this made her feel mentally and physically exhausted by the end of the day. She explained that prior to migration, she was not regularly physically active because she felt healthy and didn't see a need for it. However, since immigrating, she consistently has less energy and sought out community physical activity as a way of coping.

I force myself to do it. Like last year, I'm choosing the class, like steps, 'cause it's included in the membership so I just use it. And like, three times a week the last year, I force to do it otherwise I don't feel like I'm healthy. I'm tired very easily.

She acknowledged that it seems contradictory to expend energy when she already feels tired, but offered this explanation: "I know when you exercise you are tired at that moment, but your energy still builds up after you relax." Thus, she intentionally increased her physical activity in order to "recharge her battery" and "have time for herself without her family" by participating in the $1 swimming session at the local swimming pool. She saw this as important to a balanced life when she stated: "You cannot, you know, always work like a machine. You have to get some entertainment for yourself." In this way she was transgressing traditional gender roles in her family by taking part in physical activity with the aim of keeping herself, as opposed to only others, healthy.

Becoming active was challenging when immigrant women were learning a new language, had other priorities, and when programs were too expensive, as the following comment from a woman from Iran illustrates:

When a newcomer comes here she/he stops doing many things. I mean she stops the activities that she used to do in Iran. The first thing is learning English and the second is finding a job. So she puts aside all the entertainments she once had. Firstly you think that this is not important, but it is. So, I think if you have these entertainments from the first days your mental pressure would be less and you can get familiar with the circumstances more easily. I think if they could have these classes with lower cost and conditions in which everyone can use them that would be so helpful.

Some women mentioned that they were quite active prior to migration, sometimes because fitness programs had been offered in their workplaces, as this woman from China explained:

I think the activity will help your health. That's true … because in China I worked in high-pressure environment, the company will supply opportunity to you to release this pressure. You can attend physical activity. That's a good way to release your pressure because practice this activity, practice this program, you can meet some person … during the exercise you can get to relax. That's true. I like.

Others, like some women of higher socio-economic status from Iran, had also been physically active prior to migration because there were a number of women-only options available in private membership-based facilities and pools. Some women did not want to participate in mixed-gender programs in Canada for religious and cultural reasons or because they felt less comfortable, and their participation levels had decreased.

The findings varied considerably, suggesting that simplistic solutions for all immigrant women are inappropriate. The complex links between migration, mental health, and physical activity were apparent because while community programs were seen as a setting for developing social networks or reducing feelings that contributed to stress, anxiety, and depression, trying to access programs sometimes become a source of stress when traditional gender roles were being transgressed or when social connections were not fostered. For a few newcomer women, the existing community physical activity programs worked fine, but the majority found them to be intimidating spaces because they were not familiar with how the programs were offered, few accommodations were made for non-English speakers, and opportunities for social interaction with others were limited.

Immigrant Women's Recommendations for Transforming Community Physical Activity

In keeping with the gender-transformative planning tools in this book, we see great value in engaging women about their mental health issues and ideas for improving health promotion programs. Study participants offered a number of key recommendations for health promotion policy and programming to better reach and engage immigrant women. The recommendations suggest ways that women can feel empowered to participate, instead of feeling alienated because of their newcomer status or being confined by traditional gender roles. Several of the recommendations address improving gender inequities, and point to how, in addressing these inequities, health promotion programming for newcomer women has the potential to be gender-transformative.

Promoting Immigrant Women's Leadership

A number of suggestions were provided to actively engage newcomer women in policy and program development. The women expressed interest in being consulted, in becoming volunteer hosts or participation "buddies," in conducting outreach to other newcomers in different languages, in leading physical activity programs, and being actively engaged in research in order to raise awareness about challenges faced by many immigrant women. Some of the newcomer women also expressed interest in teaching others about physical activities in their home countries. Opportunities for input and leadership can begin to transform practices toward balancing power relations and promoting social inclusion. Intentionally involving recent immigrant women in all aspects and levels of public service delivery can transform health promotion by recognizing their experiential knowledge and, for many, their professional skills and experience, as well as gaining a better understanding of how inequities translate into mechanisms of exclusion. There is potential to not only shed light on persistent gender-based inequities, but also on how different women are subject to inequities differentially based on intersecting social categories, such as immigrant status.

Understanding Multiple Barriers and Providing Suitable Options

Because of the financial insecurities that many newcomer women face, offering free or low-cost physical activities is essential. Although not all of the women in the study experienced downward socio-economic mobility, the only way many could participate was through the fee subsidy policy or by attending the few $1 drop-in sessions. In addition to cost, most of the women experienced multiple and compounding barriers to participation, including not feeling entitled to participate; difficulty communicating in English; lack of information about opportunities, child care, and transportation; a lack of skills; and a lack of available or suitable options.

Study participants provided a variety of suggestions that could be adopted by service providers to respond to these multiple barriers. For example, some immigrant women would like women-only programs for cultural and religious reasons or to learn with other women who were also beginners. Others suggested offering parallel adult programs at the same time as their children to address caregiving responsibilities. As well, others recommended that written and in-person information and program instruction should be available in languages that reflect those spoken in the community, which recognizes the diversity of many contemporary cities, acknowledges that learning a new language is a difficult and long-term process, and supports those who are learning dominant languages. A few participants also suggested that improving partnerships between recreation departments in local government and community organizations—such as multicultural societies, public health authorities, neighbourhood houses, women's shelters, and libraries—could help to pool resources and improve communications, policies, and programs. In this way, barriers could be tackled in a more integrative manner.

Attending to multiple and overlapping barriers to physical activity participation and providing suitable options to address them based on women's input destabilizes traditional top-down power relations. Doing so enables recent immigrant women to move beyond being passive observers to active participants and role models. As well, recognizing and addressing multiple and interrelated social and organizational barriers to participation counters discourses that blame the individual or culture for immigrant women's non-participation, and therefore begins to transgress inequities rooted in key determinants of health (Wallis & Kwok, 2008).

Intentionally Facilitating Social Interaction and Interculturalism

To preface this point, we are not suggesting a solidified gender norm that all immigrant women want to participate in physical activity as a social activity. In fact, a few interviewees explicitly stated that they exercise regularly for time for themselves and for their health, not to socialize. However, for most of the interviewees experiencing social isolation and a decline in mental health, they sought out physical activity opportunities in order to meet people and feel like they belong to the community. As discussed by Keleher and Armstrong (2005), the therapeutic effects of physical activity on mental health are garnered when it is offered in combination with social interaction. It is clear through interviews with recent immigrant women in our study that the types of social interactions are important.

Having opportunities to meet other women from both within and outside of their ethno-linguistic groups and develop meaningful relationships and friendships, rather than engaging in superficial conversations or doing physical activity in isolation, were seen as central to promoting mental health. Several interviewees indicated they did not want to stay only within their own ethno-linguistic group, but also wanted opportunities to meet local and other international people. Some suggested that they would like to be part of a newcomer support group that participates in physical activity together so they would not feel embarrassed by sometimes having limited language skills when asking questions or trying a new activity.

Opportunities that facilitate social interaction and friendships enable women to share knowledge and resources, provide mutual support to navigate a new system, work together and develop strength in numbers, and begin to advocate for themselves and others. Opportunities for mutual learning and meaningful social interaction will diversify Canada's physical culture and promote intercultural understanding to counter predominantly assimilationist approaches to community physical activity delivery, whereby newcomers are expected to adapt and fit into existing systems or approaches. For a population subgroup that is often left out of program planning circles, the potential to self-organize and voice their needs is an important step in gender-transformative health promotion that considers diversity within the category of "immigrant women."

Conclusion

As Vissandjee et al. (2007) argued, "[H]ealth policies and practices which are sensitive to both gender and the experience of migration will better pertain to women as Canadians in a globalizing world" (p. 221). As this chapter demonstrates, there is great diversity among immigrant women. Although practitioners work in environments that increasingly favour efficiency and maximum return on investment on health promotion interventions in terms of program reach and uptake, in order for gender-transformative health promotion to become realized, it is important to consider citizen engagement processes in the development and delivery of interventions (Taylor & Frisby, 2010).

Many of the recent immigrant women in this study were willing to contribute their skills, knowledge, and abilities to develop and implement public physical activity programs and policies. Their experiential knowledge of the multiple and compounding barriers faced in daily life enabled them to envision ways that programs and services can be developed to address or at least reduce these barriers.

Ultimately, gender-transformative health promotion encourages the social connection of women, which contributes to a sense of belonging, self-determination, and control over one's life (Keleher & Armstrong, 2005), not just in the realm of mental health or physical activity participation, but also for overall well-being.

ACKNOWLEDGEMENTS

We would like to thank all the newcomer women who participated in our study. We would also like to acknowledge the assistance of Parisa Faridi, Yalda Majidi, Liv Yoon, and Ying (Yamina) Zhang, who conducted and translated some of the interviews and provided interpretation at meetings.

REFERENCES

Bingham, P. B. (2009). *Physical activity for mental health: Literature review, minding our bodies.* Ottawa: Canadian Mental Health Association. Retrieved from www.mindingourbodies. ca/about_the_project/literature_reviews/physical_activity_ and_mental_health

Caperchione, C. M., Kolt, G. S., & Mummery, W. K. (2009). Physical activity in culturally and linguistically diverse migrant groups to Western society: A review of barriers, enablers, and experiences. *Sports Medicine, 39*(3), 167–177.

Chui, T. (2011). Immigrant women. *Women in Canada: A gender-based statistical report.* Catalogue no. 89-503-X. Ottawa: Statistics Canada. Retrieved from www.statcan.gc.ca/ pub/89-503-x/2010001/article/11528-eng.pdf

Creese, G., & Kambere, E. N. (2003). What colour is your English? *Canadian Review of Sociology & Anthropology, 40*(5), 565–573.

Dossa, P. (2004). *Politics and poetics of migration: Narratives of Iranian women from the diaspora.* Toronto: Canadian Scholars' Press Inc.

Frisby, W. (2011). Promising physical activity inclusion practices for Chinese immigrant women in Vancouver, Canada. *Quest, 63*(1), 135–147.

Fullagar, S. (2008). Leisure practices as counter-depressants: Emotional work and emotion-play within women's recovery from depression. *Leisure Sciences, 30* (1), 208–240.

Hyman, I. (2004). Setting the stage: Reviewing current knowledge on the health of Canadian immigrants. What is the evidence and where are the gaps? *Canadian Journal of Public Health, 9(3),* 14–8.

Hyman, I., & Jackson, B. (2010). The healthy immigrant effect: A temporary phenomenon? In N. Hamilton (Series Ed.), *Health Policy Research Bulletin: Migration Health Edition* (pp. 17–21). Health Canada. Retrieved from www.hc-sc.gc.ca/sr-sr/alt_formats/pdf/pubs/ hpr-rpms/bull/2010-health-sante-migr-eng.pdf

Iwasaki, I., Coyle, C. P., & Shank, J. W. (2010). Leisure as a context for active living, recovery, health, and life quality for persons with mental illness in a global context. *Health Promotion International, 25*(4), 483–494.

Kawar, M. (2004). Gender and migration: Why are women more vulnerable? In F. Reysoo & C. Verchur (Eds.), *Femmes en movement: Genre, migrations, et nouvelle divisions international du travail* (pp. 71–78). Berne: Commission Suisse pour l'UNESCO.

Keleher, H., & Armstrong, R. (2005). *Evidence-based mental health promotion resource.* Report for the Department of Human Services and VicHealth, Melbourne, Australia. Melbourne: Victoria Government Department of Human Services.

Khander, E., & Koch, A. (2011). *The global city: Newcomer health in Toronto.* Toronto Public Health and Access Alliance Multicultural Health and Service Community. Retrieved from www.toronto.ca/health/map/pdf/global_city/global_city.pdf

Man, G. (2004). Gender, work, and migration: Deskilling Chinese immigrant women in Canada. *Women's Studies International Forum, 27*(2), 135–148.

Meadows, L. M., Thurston, W. E., & Melton, C. (2001). Immigrant women's health. *Social Science & Medicine, 52*(9), 1451–1458. doi:10.1016/S0277-9536(00)00251-3

Morrow, M. (2007). Women's voices matter: Creating women-centered mental health policy. In M. Morrow, O. Hankivsky, & C. Varcoe (Eds.), *Women's health in Canada: Critical perspectives on theory and policy* (pp. 355–379). Toronto: University of Toronto Press Incorporated.

Ponic, P., Nanjijuma, R., Pederson, A, Poole, N., & Scott, J. (2011). *Physical activity for marginalized women in British Columbia: A discussion paper.* Vancouver: British Columbia Centre of Excellence for Women's Health. Retrieved from www.bccewh.bc.ca/publications-resources/default.htm

Stewart, M., Anderson, J., Beiser, M., Mwakarimba, E., Neufeld, A., Simich, L., & Spitzer, D. (2008). Multicultural meanings of social support among immigrants and refugees. *International Migration, 46*(3), 123–159.

Taylor, J., & Frisby, W. (2010). Addressing inadequate leisure access policies through citizen engagement. In H. Mair, S. M. Arai, & D. G. Reid (Eds.), *Decentring work: Critical perspectives on leisure, social policy, and human development* (pp. 30–45). Calgary: University of Calgary Press.

Tremblay, M. S., Bryan, S. N., Perez, C. E., Ardern, C. I., & Katzmarzyk, P. T. (2006). Physical activity and immigrant status: Evidence from the Canadian Community Health Survey. *Canadian Journal of Public Health, 97*(4), 277–282.

Vissandjee, B., Thurston, W., Apale, A., & Nahar, K. (2007). Women's health at the intersection of gender and the experience of international migration. In M. Morrow, O. Hankivsky, & C. Varcoe (Eds.), *Women's health in Canada: Critical perspectives on theory and policy* (pp. 221–243). Toronto: University of Toronto Press Incorporated.

Wallis, M. A., & Kwok, S. (2008). *Daily struggles: The deepening racialization and feminization of poverty in Canada.* Toronto: Canadian Scholars' Press Inc.

World Health Organization. (2001). *The world health report 2001—mental health: New understanding, new hope.* Retrieved from www.who.int/whr/2001/en/

World Health Organization. (2006). *A framework to monitor and evaluate implementation, WHO global strategy on diet, physical activity, and health.* Retrieved from www.who.int/dietphysicalactivity/M&E-ENG-09.pdf

World Health Organization. (2010). *Global recommendations on physical activity for health.* Retrieved from http://whqlibdoc.who.int/publications/2010/9789241599979_eng.pdf

Yates, B., Hancock, T., & Hutchinson, S. (2013). *Report on an "initial conversation" about the health-recreation interface.* Ottawa: Leisure Information Network.

7 Pioneering Women-Centred Heart Health Promotion

Ann Pederson, Mona Izadnegahdar,
Karin H. Humphries, and Lynne Young

Introduction

Ischemic heart disease (IHD) is the leading cause of mortality in both men and women in middle- and high-income countries (World Health Organization, 2011). The two most common manifestations of IHD are angina and acute myocardial infarction (AMI).[1] Although the overall incidence of AMI is lower in women, compared to their male counterparts, women are at a greater risk of death, re-hospitalization, and poorer physical and mental health following an AMI (Andrikopoulos et al., 2006; MacIntyre et al., 2001; Spertus, Jones, McDonell, Fan, & Fihn, 2002; Vaccarino, Parsons, Every, Barron, & Krumholz, 1999). Newer evidence also suggests that the nature of cardiovascular disease may be different in women than men, and that women are not consistently assessed for cardiovascular disease, nor treated to the same degree as men. Furthermore, research on temporal changes in ischemic heart disease by sex and gender has demonstrated that women have not benefited from the same declining hospitalization rates as men. Together, these findings highlight that greater attention is needed to prevent, diagnose, and manage heart disease in women across the entire spectrum of intervention levels.

Women have unique social, economic, psychosocial, and biological factors that put them at risk for heart disease (Fields, Savard, & Epstein, 1993; Wamala & Agren, 2002). Yet to date, heart health promotion, like cardiovascular research and clinical care, has tended to ignore women or apply a model of intervention derived from evidence based on men. Even large-scale multi-centre trials such as the Well-integrated Screening and Evaluation for Women Across the Nation (WISEWOMAN) program in the United States, arguably the most well-funded and evaluated cardiovascular health promotion project for women ever conducted, has not yet reported on how such programs explicitly engage with how sex and gender may affect women's risks for, experiences with, or outcomes for heart disease (Will, Farris, Sanders, Stockmyer, & Finkelstein, 2004; Will & Loo, 2008). Experts agree, however, that

> population-wide strategies are necessary to combat the pandemic of CVD in women, because individually tailored interventions alone are likely insufficient to maximally prevent and control CVD. Public policy as an intervention to reduce gender-based disparities in CVD preventive care and improve cardio-vascular outcomes among women must become an integral strategy to reduce the global burden of CVD. (Mosca et al., 2007, p. 1234)

This call to action unites us as epidemiologists, nurses, and social scientists committed to reducing the burden of cardiovascular disease—particularly IHD—in women.

Heart health promotion efforts need to be based on appropriate evidence, including evidence of what supports women to live in health-enhancing ways. Building on emerging evidence of sex and gender influences on women's heart health and the work of four demonstration projects conducted in British Columbia, Canada, this chapter promotes an approach to heart health promotion that is women-centred, gender-transformative, and culturally appropriate. This chapter particularly focuses on younger women (defined as age 55 or younger) as a key location for action because the evidence suggests they are particularly ill-served by current practices. The findings on heart health promotion advanced in this chapter support many of the principles articulated in the health promotion framework in Chapter 2 and illuminate that gender-transformative practice is not just something that happens to the women who participate in programs, but calls upon programmers (and those who fund and supervise them) to engage in new forms of practice and be agents of change themselves.

The Foundation for Action: Sex/Gendered Differences in Cardiac Risk Factors

Literature has consistently shown that, as compared to men, women have a greater risk of mortality and re-hospitalization following AMI. Such observed poorer outcomes in women with heart disease have been partly attributed to the fact that women are more likely to have co-morbid conditions, but also to be under-diagnosed and under-treated in comparison to men when presenting with AMI. Women are less likely than men to receive cardiac procedures such as coronary angiography and reperfusion therapies at the time of presenting with AMI and experience greater delays in starting therapy, even when they do receive them (Bangalore et al., 2012; Champney et al., 2009). Furthermore, women are less likely to receive evidence-based medications, such as lipid-lowering medication, upon discharge from hospital and are less likely to be referred to and attend cardiac rehabilitation programs (Bangalore et al., 2012; Jackson, 2005; Thomas et al., 1996). However, the observed differences in patients' clinical characteristics and treatment do not fully explain the observed sex gap in outcomes of AMI patients (Bangalore et al., 2012; Lawesson, Stenestrand, Lagerqvist, Wallentin, & Swahn, 2010; Vaccarino et al., 1999). This finding is particularly evident among younger adults who have the greatest sex gap in mortality following an AMI event (Vaccarino, Abramson, Veledar, & Weintraub, 2002).

To date, most of the research in this area has focused on older adults as women typically present with AMI at much older ages than men. Although the overall incidence of AMI among younger adults (55 years or younger) is lower, when it does occur, it can have significant clinical, psychological, and economic effects on women, their families, and society as a whole. The increasing prevalence of cardiac risk factors—such as diabetes, hypertension, obesity, and sedentary lifestyle—among younger adults in the general population has raised concerns about the imminent and growing risk of heart disease in this age group. Consequently, in 2010, the Heart and Stroke Foundation of Canada identified younger adults, particularly women, as a vulnerable and at-risk population for heart disease (Heart and Stroke Foundation, 2010).

In addition to traditional cardiac risk factors, socio-economic and psychosocial factors also play important roles in the development and outcome of heart disease in women. Women's average lower education and income level, coupled with their higher prevalence of depression, stress, anxiety, and poorer social support, can be barriers to making healthy lifestyle choices to prevent heart disease and/or accessing care and cardiac prevention programs following a heart disease diagnosis, which subsequently could lead to poorer outcomes. For instance, a mixed methods research program exploring lone mothers' risk for cardiovascular disease suggested that lone mothers were more likely than partnered mothers to live in low socio-economic circumstances, and to have increased behavioural and clinical risks for, and presence of, CVD than their married counterparts (Young, Cunningham, & Buist, 2005; Young, James, & Cunningham, 2004). Lone mothers in both American and Canadian quantitative studies were more likely to be smokers and, in the U.S. study (Young, Cunningham, & Buist, 2005), lone mothers were more likely to be non-white. In the qualitative study within this program of research, results suggested that lone mothers lacked the resources and power to effect change in their heart health behaviours (Wharf-Higgins, Young, Naylor, & Cunningham, 2006).

Sex Differences in Cardiac Risk Profile

Beginning in the 1940s, the Framingham Heart Study identified age, sex, smoking, high blood pressure, high blood cholesterol, and diabetes as major cardiac risk factors, and this led to the development of the Framingham Risk Score for cardiovascular disease (Wilson et al., 1998). A more recent global case-control study of risk factors for AMI, the INTERHEART study, extended these early findings and identified nine modifiable risk factors, which collectively were shown to explain more than 90 percent of the population-attributable risk for AMI in both men and women, suggesting that the risk of AMI could be reduced by more than 90 percent if all these nine risk factors were eliminated (Anand et al., 2008). These modifiable risk factors include smoking, hypertension, abnormal lipids, diabetes, abdominal obesity, high-risk diet, psychosocial factors, lack of physical activity, and excessive alcohol intake (Yusuf et al., 2004). Anand et al. (2008) found, however, that the strength of the association of the risk factors for AMI varied by age, including current smoking, lipid abnormalities, diabetes, and hypertension, which had a greater impact among younger than older women, and smoking, lipids abnormalities, hypertension, and abdominal obesity, which had a greater impact in younger men, compared to older men.

Among younger patients with AMI, smoking is the most prevalent cardiac risk factor in both women and men, with more than two-thirds of patients being either former or current smokers (Champney et al., 2009; Lawesson et al., 2010; Sozzi et al., 2007). Furthermore, based on the Framingham Heart Study, Kannel, McGee, and Castelli (1984) found that among young adults (35–44 years) smoking was associated with a threefold increase in risk of developing CAD.

One of the earlier studies of sex differences in risk profile and outcomes of younger adults revealed that younger women were more likely to have a history of diabetes, hypertension, and prior stroke, but were less likely to have hypercholesterolemia or be current smokers (Vaccarino et al., 1999). More recent studies stratified their analysis of sex differences in cardiac risk factors and co-morbidities by both age and AMI type (STEMI and NSTEMI).[2] Similarly, their findings revealed that, regardless of the type of AMI, younger women have a greater burden of risk factors, with a higher prevalence of diabetes, obesity, heart failure, stroke, renal insufficiency, and chronic obstructive pulmonary disease (Champney et al., 2009).

Trends in Cardiac Risk Factors

The 2010 Heart and Stroke Foundation of Canada's annual report, titled *A Perfect Storm*, highlights the rising trends in the prevalence of several cardiac risk factors, including hypertension, obesity, and diabetes, in the general population, particularly among Canadians younger than 50 years of age (Heart and Stroke Foundation, 2010; Lee et al., 2009). Overall, among adults 35–49 years, hypertension (regardless of being on anti-hypertensive treatment) increased from 5.6 percent to 13.2 percent, diabetes from 1.6 percent to 2.6 percent, and obesity from 13.5 percent to 16.2 percent between the years 1994 and 2005.

Given the association of obesity with other cardiac risk factors, including diabetes and hypertension (Mokdad et al., 2003), reports of the rising prevalence of obesity among young adults during the recent decade are worrisome. Based on the most recent available data in Canada and the United States, obesity—defined as a body mass index (BMI) greater than or equal to 30 kg/m2—has been reported to be present in more than one-third of young American men and women between the ages of 40–59 years (Ogden, Carroll, Kit, & Flegal, 2012) and in approximately 23 percent of young Canadian men and 17 percent of young women between the ages of 35–54 (Statistics Canada, 2011).

It is expected that these obesity trends among young adults in the general population would be reflected in the risk profile of young patients presenting with AMI; however, only a few studies have assessed the temporal changes in risk factors of young adults with AMI in recent years. Similar to earlier reports of a deteriorating cardiac risk profile among all adult patients in recent decades (Goldberg et al., 2004), the Worcester Heart Study also demonstrated a worsening cardiac risk profile among younger patients presenting with their first AMI event, including increasing trends in diabetes and hypertension (McManus et al., 2011). Furthermore, a recent study, based on four nationwide French registries, indicated that the proportion of patients less than 60 years of age, particularly women, who present with smoking and/or obesity as their sole risk factors at the time of their hospitalization for STEMI, continuously increased between the years 1995 to 2010 (Puymirat et al., 2012). Based on this study, approximately 45 percent of young French women and 40 percent of young men presented with smoking and/or obesity as their only risk factors. Together, these trends suggest that more and more younger adults, including women, are at risk for AMI than previously recognized.

Summary

Women, particularly those younger than 55 years of age, are more likely to present with cardiac risk factors and co-morbidities at the time of presenting for an AMI and are also at a greater risk of death following their cardiac event. The reasons for the observed higher short-term mortality following AMI in younger women compared to younger men are not fully understood. The sex differences in cardiac risk profile, use of evidence-based therapies (such as lipid-lowering medication) at the time of discharge, or timely use of reperfusion therapies (i.e., percutaneous coronary intervention [PCI] or thrombolysis) following an AMI, do not fully explain the excess risk of mortality in women. In sum, the face of heart disease is changing with emerging at-risk populations such as younger women. Given the recent unfavourable trends in cardiac risk factors and AMI hospitalization rates, and the overall poorer outcomes of younger women following events such as AMI, there is an urgent need to develop evidence-informed heart health promotion initiatives that are effective for women.

Sex/Gender Influences on the Pathway to Cardiovascular Disease

To translate these complex and multiple epidemiological data and observations of clinical trends to inform new health promotion strategies, it is helpful to conceptualize the pathway to cardiovascular disease. Keleher, MacDougall, and Murphy (2007), in their text on health promotion, present a diagram of the pathways to cardiovascular disease and diabetes that integrates a multi-level understanding of the determinants of health and links it to an action framework.

This framework illustrates the complex pathways to the development of cardiovascular disease and diabetes, as well as the wide array of interventions that may contribute to reducing the risk of developing either or both of these conditions. Specifically, this framework identifies a range from "upstream" to "midstream" to "downstream" factors that contribute to CVD and diabetes. These range, in turn, as per the Dahlgren and Whitehead framework (Dahlgren & Whitehead, 1991), from distal material factors such as housing, racism and discrimination, and poverty, and social structural conditions through psychosocial mediating factors to more immediate health-related practices such as smoking, alcohol use, physical activity, weight control, and healthful eating. (Age, genetics, and sex are understood to be immutable individual characteristics in this framework.) Interventions to prevent cardiovascular disease and diabetes range in turn from those at the macro or population level to those at the community and organizational (meso) level through to those that immediately affect the individual and are closely linked to health services. Accordingly, interventions to prevent CVD and diabetes range from reducing social inequities through public policies to addressing parenting skills and creating social networks to ensuring the availability of appropriate and acceptable health care.

Notably, this framework identifies gender inequity as both a macro- and meso-determinant of health, and hence it starts with the understanding that women's health is grounded in the context of their lives—in the social, economic, educational, and political context in which they live, work, and socialize (Reid, Pederson, & Dupéré, 2012). That is, women's health is a product of gendered social systems that shape their opportunities for health and their exposure to health-damaging agents, conditions, and environments (Keleher, 2004). Social norms about the roles women play in the household, in the workplace, and in the community contribute to women's economic security, as well as their access to resources and information—and, in turn,

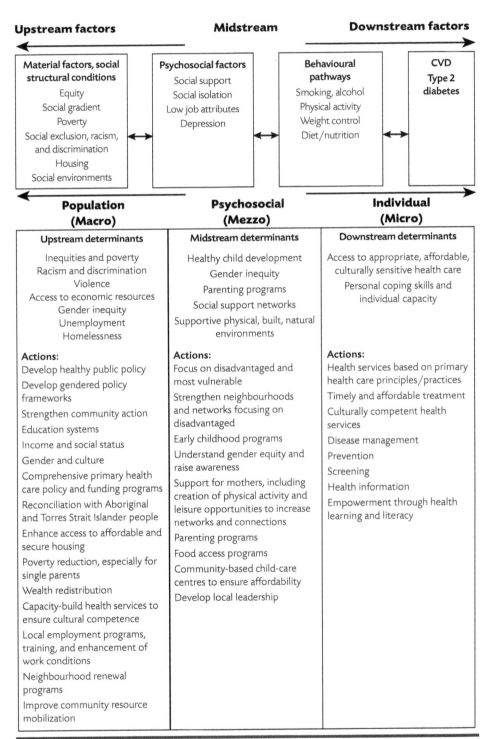

Upstream factors   **Midstream**   **Downstream factors**

Material factors, social structural conditions	Psychosocial factors	Behavioural pathways	CVD
Equity	Social support	Smoking, alcohol	Type 2 diabetes
Social gradient	Social isolation	Physical activity	
Poverty	Low job attributes	Weight control	
Social exclusion, racism, and discrimination	Depression	Diet/nutrition	
Housing			
Social environments			

Population (Macro)	**Psychosocial (Mezzo)**	**Individual (Micro)**
Upstream determinants	**Midstream determinants**	**Downstream determinants**
Inequities and poverty	Healthy child development	Access to appropriate, affordable, culturally sensitive health care
Racism and discrimination	Gender inequity	
Violence	Parenting programs	Personal coping skills and individual capacity
Access to economic resources	Social support networks	
Gender inequity	Supportive physical, built, natural environments	
Unemployment		
Homelessness		
Actions:	**Actions:**	**Actions:**
Develop healthy public policy	Focus on disadvantaged and most vulnerable	Health services based on primary health care principles/practices
Develop gendered policy frameworks	Strengthen neighbourhoods and networks focusing on disadvantaged	Timely and affordable treatment
Strengthen community action	Early childhood programs	Culturally competent health services
Education systems	Understand gender equity and raise awareness	Disease management
Income and social status	Support for mothers, including creation of physical activity and leisure opportunities to increase networks and connections	Prevention
Gender and culture		Screening
Comprehensive primary health care policy and funding programs	Parenting programs	Health information
Reconciliation with Aboriginal and Torres Strait Islander people	Food access programs	Empowerment through health learning and literacy
Enhance access to affordable and secure housing	Community-based child-care centres to ensure affordability	
Poverty reduction, especially for single parents	Develop local leadership	
Wealth redistribution		
Capacity-build health services to ensure cultural competence		
Local employment programs, training, and enhancement of work conditions		
Neighbourhood renewal programs		
Improve community resource mobilization		

FIGURE 7.1: Pathways for CVD-Diabetes: Determinants and Interventions

Source: Adapted from Keleher, MacDougall, & Murphy (2007).

their health (Wamala & Agren, 2002). The central assumption of this approach is that empowering individual women to increase control over their health through activities such as health education and the promotion of health literacy must be accompanied by efforts to address the structural constraints that limit women's health, including gender-based assumptions and practices that limit women economically, socially, and politically (Keleher, 2010).

This pathway to cardiovascular disease and diabetes links to the framework outlined in Chapter 2 in some specific ways. First, it is consistent with the overarching path that the framework illustrates in the way that it documents in detail the journey from structural determinants through psychosocial and behavioural factors to health outcomes, though it does not comment on potential social or economic outcomes that may also arise. Second, it illustrates how the health and other systems of care or services play a role in the development of disease. In addition, the pathway is explicit that gender inequity contributes to poor health. However, in contrast to the framework, this pathway positions equity as an input into the pathway to health or illness rather than as a potential outcome. Hence, where the framework differs from this model is that it positions health promotion interventions—particularly those that embrace action on gender inequities—as a resource to potentially change this pathway.

An Exploration of Heart Health Promotion for Women in British Columbia

As noted, a program of heart health promotion at the BC Women's Hospital & Health Centre was prompted by *Women's Heart Health: An Evidence Review* (Greaves, Humphries, & Hemsing, 2008). Consistent with the existing literature, the review identified the importance of engaging in primary prevention to improve women's heart health in British Columbia, paying particular attention to reducing smoking, increasing physical activity, improving nutrition, and enhancing weight management. The report argued, however, that interventions in these areas needed to be conducted in ways that acknowledge how gender and diversity shape differences in risk among men and women, and among subgroups of women. Moreover, the review authors argued that actions at the individual level needed to be complemented by policy changes and improved access to health care services.

The authors proposed that a number of factors be considered when developing interventions to promote women's heart health and prevent cardiovascular disease. These suggestions included recognizing and incorporating changes in women's health through the life course within programs; addressing health literacy to support women modifying their risk factors for cardiovascular disease; improving social support and addressing psychosocial factors that are both a contributor to and affected by cardiovascular disease in women; and developing tailored, women-centred interventions related to diet, physical activity, and smoking. The review also identified a number of women at greater risk for developing cardiovascular disease in the province, based on epidemiological and population trends, including older women, low-income women, Aboriginal women, South Asian women, and women with mental illnesses and/or addictions. Given their findings, the authors suggested that both broad, population-based interventions and more targeted, tailored programs directed at these high-risk groups be offered. Moreover, they commented that there was not a proven universal intervention that can be applied to all women and that, instead, programs need to be tailored to women and subpopulations of women.

Project Background

Building on that evidence review, a project team at BC Women's Hospital & Health Centre and the British Columbia Centre of Excellence for Women's Health, in partnership with Fraser Health, initiated a heart health promotion project to explore the potential of tailoring programs to women, including low-income and Aboriginal women. A follow-up literature review was commissioned to identify the core elements that should comprise heart health promotion interventions for women. The reviewers looked specifically for interventions that focused on changing cardiovascular risk by addressing clinical, behavioural, socio-cultural, and/or economic risk factors in adult women (Context, 2010). In summing up their findings, the reviewers observed that there is

> a complex mass of evidence existing around primary prevention activities for heart disease targeted towards women. The results of this update do not point us in one clear direction for intervening but provide multiple starting points for consideration and a host of effective, "better practices" across the range of risk areas. (p. 1)

Interventions ranged from programs aimed primarily at individual risk factor reduction to those that worked simultaneously to influence the system, the community, and individual behaviour, such as the U.S. Office of Women's Health initiative, Improving, Enhancing, and Evaluating Outcomes of Comprehensive Heart Health Care Programs for High Risk Women (Foody, Villabalanca, Giardina, Gill, & Taylor, 2010). The reviewers noted promising high-level, process-oriented approaches that are likely to be valuable in primary prevention activities to promote women's heart health. These include

- aiming to concurrently have influence across the system, community/institution, and individual, thereby creating the supportive environments and structures necessary to facilitate individual change;
- linking or partnering the clinical environment with the community;
- integrating multidisciplinary clinical involvement (i.e., through collaboratives, referrals);
- designing and delivering activities within the context of women's lives, readiness for change, and unique barriers through the use of participatory approaches that involve women in identifying problems and solutions and delivering activities;
- connecting women to their immediate environment and community (or capitalizing on existing connections, where they exist);
- identifying and overcoming access barriers;
- integrating peer facilitators where possible;
- aiming to improve awareness and health literacy prior to promoting behaviour change;
- creating social support for behaviour change;
- creating ethnoculturally relevant approaches, materials, and resources; and
- allowing sufficient time for changes to occur.

However, the authors concluded that there was a dearth of information about interventions that were developed, implemented, or evaluated using a gender lens. This updated review became the starting point for a set of small demonstration projects in two health authorities in British Columbia, Canada, conducted between 2010 and 2012. The remainder of this chapter offers reflections on the elements of women-specific interventions to promote heart health in the demonstration projects.

Four Demonstration Projects

A total of four projects were undertaken, two in Vancouver at two community-based sites in the east side of the city, and two in Surrey at a community health centre offering supports to pregnant women and mothers dealing with substance use and/or violence and abuse. The first program in Vancouver was undertaken at the RayCam Community Centre (www.raycam.org/) in the downtown area of Strathcona; the second was conducted in partnership with the Pacific Association of First Nations Women (http://pafnw.ca/) and held at the Aboriginal Mother Centre (www.aboriginalmothercentre.ca/). The two programs in Surrey were conducted at the Maxxine Wright Community Health Centre (MWCHC; www.atira.bc.ca/maxxine-wright-community-health-centre), a unique facility providing health, housing, and social care to pregnant and mothering women affected by both violence and substance use. The women in all four programs were variously marginalized by income, racialization, ethnicity, substance use, violence and trauma, experiences of residential schooling, and/or the neighbourhood they resided in, so they were at increased risk for developing cardiovascular disease over their lifetimes.

While each project was distinct and there are detailed project reports describing the setting, participants, program activities, and outcomes for each project, they also shared common elements, which are the focus of this discussion. Across all the project sites, the project teams provided a series of educational sessions, clinical assessments, and psychosocial supports to some 60 women. Women in the programs were linked to community services; provided with healthful meals; invited to learn new skills such as gardening, meal planning, and stress management; and supported in managing relationship challenges, navigating housing issues, and exploring their identities as indigenous women when appropriate.

Consistent with the emerging literature on gender and health promotion (Reid et al., 2012), these projects paid explicit attention to issues of women's safety, their roles as family caregivers and mothers, and gendered opportunities and barriers for engaging in heart health promotion as they worked with women to try to change health-related practices such as tobacco use, physical activity, and healthful eating. In keeping with the principles described above, efforts were made across the continuum of health promotion action. These included working with women to support them in identifying and defining their own heart health priorities, to involve women in partnerships that would sustain them in promoting their health, and to engage community stakeholders beyond health authority personnel in enhancing the health of women. Moreover, activities extended beyond addressing the traditional risk factors for cardiovascular disease—tobacco use, physical activity, and diet—by including social support, community engagement, and empowerment within relationships as explicit program goals.

The experiences of the women, health care service providers, and program leadership were documented, and the processes of each program described for their impact on the women themselves, as well as service providers (Chopova, Penaloza, & Shrestha, 2013; Ziabakhsh, Prodan-Bhalla, Middagh, King, & Jinkerson-Brass, 2013). The evaluation reports—both qualitative and quantitative—indicate that participation and engagement with the two project sites was high among both staff and target group participants. Heart health was not an obvious priority for the women and staff in any of the settings, yet the primary prevention approach enabled women and the program staff to come together in new ways to learn about heart health, to build community, to raise awareness of the women's risks for heart disease, and to work on reducing those risks. Despite the complexity of the women's everyday lives and the challenges faced by living on low incomes, mothering, and histories of violence and/or substance use, the women were interested in being healthier and in supporting their families to be as well.

All project sites focused on enhancing women's health literacy and skills develop-ment while working to reduce their barriers to access to heart-healthy food, increase their access to physical activity, reduce the stress in their lives, and reduce their use of tobacco. By being embedded in communities, program staff at all sites were able to link women to community resources such as community recreation facilities, community gardens, food banks, and community kitchens; to secure discounts on services; to facilitate participation in community structures; and to link women to health and social services.

None of the approaches adopted by these demonstration projects is a recipe for women-specific heart health promotion, yet all four project sites developed programming tailored to their context and clientele. Project sites were careful to ensure that basics such as the provision of meals and child-minding were part of the fabric of their program offerings when appropriate. Program participants and staff all operated on principles of trust, communication, and respect. For example, because the Maxxine Wright Community Health Clinic explicitly takes a stance of harm reduction toward substance use and is engaged in creating a safe, welcoming space for women with experiences of violence, the principles of safety, communica-tion, and relationship were core elements of the programming at MWCHC. These same principles were generated through the processes undertaken in Strathcona, for example, when the nurse practitioners (NPs) engaged community members in a photographic journey to explore and illustrate the meaning of heart health as part of the project development. Whereas at MWCHC the heart health program was integrated into an existing drop-in program, the NPs worked with community members in Strathcona to develop a program model that would work in a broader community-wide context, and the program at the Aboriginal Mother Centre was aimed at developing leadership among women in the community to help support other women in improving their heart health profile.

Much of the women-centred nature of these programs rests deep in the details of program delivery and staff competencies. Project teams agreed that their pro-jects shared common themes with respect to issues facing the women as they tried to manage their heart health, including mothering, safety, poverty, housing, and racialization because they were members of visible minority groups. Among the ways that the program staff addressed these issues were the following:

- trauma-informed services (i.e., harm reduction approach, client-led smoking cessation, attention to physical and emotional safety)

- provision of supports regarding the social determinants of health (e.g., lei-sure-access pass funding, help with housing, access to healthy food)
- provision of child-minding to enable the women to attend the session and know their children were safe and cared for
- negotiating women-only time at local recreation facilities or accompanying women to such facilities (addressing issues of safety and comfort)
- managing partners during program time (e.g., creating boundaries about when and where men were able to be on the premises)
- enhancing skills in mothering through teaching, modelling, and practising
- teaching relationship skills (e.g., offering a course on relationships to the women at MWCHC who had histories of difficult relationships)
- providing women with opportunities for social engagement and support through group educational sessions as well as individual appointments
- embracing elements of First Nations health and spirituality as facets of health promotion, particularly incorporating elements of ceremony, teaching, and storytelling as ways of learning and validating experiences
- adapting educational resources to the specific group of women participating in the program
- transforming the client–provider relationship such that the providers participated in the program activities as women themselves, not as professionals who stood apart from the other women

Thus the core of these initiatives was not limited to heart health education offered in a traditional format, but rather as a way of offering health information, skills development, and support that recognized the complexity of these women's lives and explicitly took context, relationship, language, culture, and identity into consideration.

Women were provided with information and education on the risk factors for heart disease; screened for heart health risk factors; taught the importance of and strategies for eating healthfully and engaging in more physical activity; managing stress; and supported in tobacco cessation efforts. But each of these traditional risk factor–reduction activities was undertaken in ways that supported women's health literacy, started with women's priorities for change, recognized the constraints on their lives, and supported them in their progress. The women were also linked into community support systems for housing, recreation, grocery shopping, and employment to the extent possible.

The impact of these demonstration programs was measurable only in the short term. The evaluations recorded reductions in smoking, increases in physical activity, reductions in stress levels, increased interest in heart-healthy cooking, and improvements in knowledge about heart health. Program staff experienced the building of communities, the sharing of stories, and the development of women as mothers. They provided women with links to community services, helped them solve problems with housing and income assistance, and, in some cases, provided them with shelter and safety. Each of these things is a small piece of the heart health puzzle.

It was challenging for these health promotion projects to tackle existing sex differences and gender inequities at a systemic level. Nevertheless, by actively approaching heart health through the lens of empowerment and by working on the determinants of health and not just on a small set of risk behaviours, the demonstration projects embraced important elements of gender-informed practice. Specifically, offering gender-responsive heart health promotion required the program staff (which included nurse practitioners and other advanced practice nurses, community nutritionists, and other public health professionals) to work in ways that challenged their roles as experts with knowledge to impart to uninformed "patients," calling upon them instead to become actively engaged with the program participants, to share leadership and program development, to be flexible in how programming was conducted, and to be willing to divulge of themselves and their experiences as women if they expected the women to share of themselves in the process of learning about heart health.

Conclusion:
Transforming Heart Health Promotion for Women

Emerging evidence confirms that younger women would benefit from greater attention to the prevention of cardiovascular disease, particularly through increased physical activity and reduction in smoking. As well, particular groups of women, including lone mothers, who are at disproportionate risk for developing cardiovascular disease, need supports to improve their cardiovascular risk profile and likelihood of surviving an acute MI. As the pathways for CVD-diabetes illustrated, however, the behavioural pathway to cardiovascular disease and diabetes is embedded in and linked to psychosocial and material factors that will not be affected by increased knowledge of healthful eating and smoking cessation. Enhancements in the social and economic conditions of women's lives are also essential in reducing women's risk for CVD. Ideally, actions need to be taken across multiple levels of the pathway to disease, but particularly vulnerable groups of women will require appropriately tailored interventions. The demonstration projects involved women in various communities who are understood to be vulnerable to cardiovascular health problems.

The literature and demonstration projects described in this chapter suggest that it is valuable to work with women in ways that respect their knowledge, capacity for change, and cultural and spiritual practices, and foster self-care and mutual aid. Through the provision of women-only spaces and the discussion of the ways that social norms, relationships, and responsibilities constrain some women's ability to live healthfully, these programs had positive effects on both the women who attended them and the providers who offered them.

The projects undertaken in British Columbia go some way to articulating how gender-responsive health promotion is more than health promotion with women. Indeed, the question of how our work was different from just "good" health promotion practice challenged us repeatedly throughout the years we worked on these projects. We concluded that the essence of what makes our work distinctive is our attention to women in context. This means that rather than trying to find general practices that work for all women all of the time, we are willing, as health promoters, to work with particular women in their unique circumstances. Moreover, we recognized the so-called "risk behaviours" as coping strategies that women develop to manage complex lives and that sometimes we have to work on the material and structural factors before we can address substance use or healthful eating.

The gender-transformative framework positions health promotion interventions as a mechanism for potentially transforming women's health, but as a high-level framework, it cannot provide details on how programs and interventions actually transform women's lives. This chapter suggests that health services that are women-centred, community-based, culturally safe, and participatory can be a site for promoting healthier living conditions, as well as addressing the more immediate health behaviours that contribute to cardiovascular disease.

NOTES

1   Angina refers to chest pain or discomfort that occurs when an area of the heart is deprived of oxygen. It is typically described as a crushing or squeezing sensation in the chest and may radiate to the jaw, shoulders, arm, or back. Acute myocardial infarction occurs when blood flow to a part of the heart is blocked for a long enough time that part of the heart muscle is damaged or dies.

2   The definition of AMI was modified in 2000 to distinguish between the two subtypes of AMI: ST-elevation MI (STEMI) and Non-ST elevation MI (NSTEMI) (Alpert, Thygesen, Antman, & Bassand, 2000). In general, STEMI patients have higher in-hospital mortality rates and are more likely to be younger and male compared to NSTEMI patients.

REFERENCES

Alpert, J. S., Thygesen, K., Antman, E., & Bassand, J. P. (2000). Myocardial infarction redefined—a consensus document of the Joint European Society of Cardiology/American College of Cardiology Committee for the redefinition of myocardial infarction. [Practice guideline]. *Journal of the American College of Cardiology, 36*(3), 959–969.

Anand, S. S., Islam, S., Rosengren, A., Franzosi, M. G., Steyn, K., Yusufali, A. H., ... Yusuf, S. (2008). Risk factors for myocardial infarction in women and men: Insights from the INTERHEART study [Comparative study multicentre study research support, non-U.S. government]. *European Heart Journal, 29*(7), 932–940. doi:10.1093/eurheartj/ehn018

Andrikopoulos, G. K., Tzeisa, S. E., Pipilis, A. G., Richter, D. J., Kappos, K. G., Stefanadis, C. I., ... Chimonas, E. T. (2006). Younger age potentiates post myocardial infarction survival disadvantage of women. *International Journal of Cardiology, 108*(3), 320–325.

Bangalore, S., Fonarow, G. C., Peterson, E. D., Hellkamp, A. S., Hernandez, A. F., Laskey, W., ... Bhatt, D. L. (2012). Age and gender differences in quality of care and outcomes for patients with ST-segment elevation myocardial infarction. *The American Journal of Medicine, 125*(10), 1000–1009. doi:10.1016/j.amjmed.2011.11.016

Champney, K. P., Frederick, P. D., Bueno, H., Parashar, S., Foody, J., Merz, C. N., ... Vaccarino, V. (2009). The joint contribution of sex, age, and type of myocardial infarction on hospital mortality following acute myocardial infarction [Multicentre study research support, National Institutes of Health, extramural]. *Heart, 95*(11), 895–899. doi:10.1136/hrt.2008.155804

Chopova, D., Penaloza, D., & Shrestha, H. (2013). *Women's heart health second demonstration project: My wellness at Maxxine Wright.* Surrey, BC: Maxxine Wright Community Health Centre.

Context Research. (2010). *Women's heart health evidence update for primary prevention strategies, activities, and programs.* Vancouver: Primary Prevention of Heart Disease in Women Project, BC Women's Hospital and British Columbia Centre of Excellence for Women's Health.

Dahlgren, G., & Whitehead, M. (1991). Policies and strategies to promote social equity in health. Stockholm: Institute of Future Studies.

Fields, S. K., Savard, M. A., & Epstein, K. R. (1993). The female patient. In P. S. Douglas (Ed.), *Cardiovascular health and disease in women* (pp. 3–21). Philadelphia: W. B. Saunders.

Foody, J. M., Villabalanca, A. C., Giardina, E. G., Gill, S., & Taylor, A. L. (2010). The Office of Women's Health initiative to improve women's heart health: Program description, site characteristics, and lessons learned. *Journal of Women's Health, 19*(3), 507–516.

Goldberg, R. J., Spencer, F. A., Yarzebski, J., Lessard, D., Gore, J. M., Alpert, J. S., & Dalen, J. E. (2004). *A 25-year perspective into the changing landscape of patients hospitalized with acute myocardial infarction (the Worcester Heart Attack Study)* [Research support, U.S. Government, Public Health Service]. *The American Journal of Cardiology, 94*(11), 1373–1378. doi:10.1016/j.amjcard.2004.07.142

Greaves, L., Humphries, K. H., & Hemsing, N. (2008). *Women's heart health: An evidence review.* Vancouver: Provincial Health Services Authority, BC Women's Hospital and Health Centre.

Heart and Stroke Foundation. (2010). *A perfect storm of heart disease looming on our horizon.* 2010 Heart and Stroke Foundation annual report on Canadians' health. N.p.: Author.

Jackson, L. (2005). Getting the most out of cardiac rehabilitation: A review of referral and adherence predictors. *Heart, 91*, 10–14.

Kannel, W. B., McGee, D. L., & Castelli, W. P. (1984). Latest perspectives on cigarette smoking and cardiovascular disease: The Framingham Study. *Journal of Cardiopulmonary Rehabilitation, 4,* 267–277.

Keleher, H. (2004). Why build a health promotion evidence base about gender? *Health Promotion International, 19*(3), 277–279.

Keleher, H. (2010). Gender norms and empowerment: "What works" to increase equity for women and girls. In G. Sen & P. Östlin (Eds.), *Gender equity in health: The shifting frontiers of evidence and action* (pp. 161–183). New York: Routledge.

Keleher, H., MacDougall, C., & Murphy, B. (Eds.). (2007). *Understanding health promotion.* Melbourne: Oxford University Press.

Lawesson, S. S., Stenestrand, U., Lagerqvist, B., Wallentin, L., & Swahn, E. (2010). Gender perspective on risk factors, coronary lesions, and long-term outcome in young patients with ST-elevation myocardial infarction [Multicentre study research support, non-U.S. government]. *Heart, 96*(6), 453–459. doi:10.1136/hrt.2009.175463

Lee, D. S., Chiu, M., Manuel, D. G., Tu, K., Wang, X., Austin, P. C., ... Tu, J. V. (2009). Trends in risk factors for cardiovascular disease in Canada: Temporal, socio-demographic, and geographic factors. *CMAJ, 181*(3/4), E55–66.

MacIntyre, K., Stewart, S., Capewell, S., Chalmers, J. W., Pell, J. P., Boyd, J., ... McMurray, J. J. (2001). Gender and survival: A population-based study of 201,114 men and women following a first acute myocardial infarction [Research support, non-U.S. governmentt]. *Journal of the American College of Cardiology, 38*(3), 729–735.

McManus, D. D., Piacentine, S. M., Lessard, D., Gore, J. M., Yarzebski, J., Spencer, F. A., & Goldberg, R. J. (2011). Thirty-year (1975 to 2005) trends in the incidence rates, clinical features, treatment practices, and short-term outcomes of patients <55 years of age hospitalized with an initial acute myocardial infarction [Comparative study research support, National Institutes of Health, extramural]. *The American Journal of Cardiology, 108*(4), 477–482. doi:10.1016/j.amjcard.2011.03.074

Mokdad, A. H., Ford, E. S., Bowman, B. A., Dietz, W. H., Vinicor, F., Bales, V. S., & Marks, J. S. (2003). Prevalence of obesity, diabetes, and obesity-related health risk factors, 2001. *JAMA, 289*(1), 76–79.

Mosca, L., Banka, C. L., Benjamin, E. J., Berra, K., Bushnell, C., Dolor, R. J., ... Wenger, N. K. (2007). Evidence-based guidelines for cardiovascular disease prevention in women: 2007 update. *Journal of the American College of Cardiology, 49*(11), 1230–1251.

Ogden, C. L., Carroll, M. D., Kit, B. K., & Flegal, K. M. (2012). Prevalence of obesity in the United States, 2009–2010. *National Center for Health Statistics Data Brief* (82), 1–8.

Puymirat, E., Simon, T., Steg, P. G., Schiele, F., Gueret, P., Blanchard, D., ... Danchin, N. (2012). Association of changes in clinical characteristics and management with improvement in survival among patients with ST-elevation myocardial infarction. [Research support, non-U.S. government]. *JAMA, 308*(10), 998–1006. doi:10.1001/2012.jama.11348

Reid, C., Pederson, A., & Dupéré, S. (2012). Addressing diversity and inequities in health promotion: The implications of intersectional theory. In I. Rootman, S. Dupéré, A.

Pederson, & M. O'Neill (Eds.), *Health promotion in Canada: Critical perspectives on practice* (3rd ed., pp. 54–66). Toronto: Canadian Scholars' Press Inc.

Sozzi, F. B., Danzi, G. B., Foco, L., Ferlini, M., Tubaro, M., Galli, M., … Mannucci, P. M. (2007). Myocardial infarction in the young: A sex-based comparison [Comparative study]. *Coronary Artery Disease, 18*(6), 429–431. doi:10.1097/MCA.0b013e3282583bfc

Spertus, J. A., Jones, P., McDonell, M., Fan, V., & Fihn, S. D. (2002). Health status predicts long-term outcome in outpatients with coronary disease. *Circulation, 106*(1), 43–49.

Statistics Canada. (2011). *Overweight and obese adults (self-reported), 2011.* Retrieved from www.statcan.gc.ca/pub/82-625-x/2012001/article/11664-eng.htm

Thomas, R. J., Miller, N. H., Lamendola, C., Berra, K., Hedbäck, B., Durstine, J. L., & Haskell, W. (1996). National survey on gender differences in cardiac rehabilitation programs: Patient characteristics and enrollment patterns. *Journal of Cardiopulmonary Rehabilitation and Prevention, 16*(6), 402–412.

Vaccarino, V., Abramson, J. L., Veledar, E., & Weintraub, W. S. (2002). Sex differences in hospital mortality after coronary artery bypass surgery: Evidence for a higher mortality in younger women. *Circulation, 105*(10), 1176–1181.

Vaccarino, V., Parsons, L., Every, N. R., Barron, H. V., & Krumholz, H. M. (1999). Sex-based differences in early mortality after myocardial infarction [Original articles]. *New England Journal of Medicine, 341*(14), 217–225.

Wamala, S., & Agren, G. (2002). Gender inequity and public health: Getting down to real issues. *European Journal of Public Health, 12,* 163–165.

Wharf-Higgins, J., Young, L. E., Naylor, P. J., & Cunningham, S. (2006). Out of the mainstream: Low-income lone mothers' life experiences and perspectives on heart health. *Health Promotion Practice, 7*(2), 221–233.

Will, J. C., Farris, R. P., Sanders, C. G., Stockmyer, C. K., & Finkelstein, E. A. (2004). Health promotion interventions for disadvantaged women: Overview of the WISEWOMAN projects. *Journal of Women's Health, 13*(5), 484–502.

Will, J. C., & Loo, R. K. (2008). The WISEWOMAN program: Reflection and forecast. *Preventing Chronic Disease, 5*(2), 1–9.

Wilson, P. W., D'Agostino, R. B., Levy, D., Belanger, A. M., Silbershatz, H., & Kannel, W. B. (1998). Prediction of coronary heart disease using risk factor categories. *Circulation, 97*(18), 1837–1847.

World Health Organization. (2011). *The top 10 causes of death.* Retrieved from www.who.int/mediacentre/factsheets/fs310/en/index.html

Young, L. E., Cunningham, S., & Buist, D. (2005). Lone mothers are at higher risk for cardiovascular disease compared to partnered mothers. Data from the National Health and Nutrition Examination Survey III (NHANES III). *Health Care for Women International, 26*(7), 604–621.

Young, L. E., James, A., & Cunningham, S. (2004). Lone motherhood and risk for cardiovascular disease: The National Population Health Survey, 1998–99. *Canadian Journal of Public Health, 95*(5), 329–335.

Yusuf, S., Hawken, S., Ounpuu, S., Dans, T., Avezum, A., Lanas, F., … Lisheng, L. (2004). Effect of potentially modifiable risk factors associated with myocardial infarction in 52 countries (the INTERHEART study): Case-control study [Comparative study multicentre study research support, non–U.S. government]. *Lancet, 364*(9438), 937–952. doi:10.1016/S0140-6736(04)17018-9

Ziabakhsh, S., Prodan-Bhalla, N., Middagh, D., King, C., & Jinkerson-Brass, S. (2013). Women's heart health demonstration project: Seven sisters healthy heart project (unpublished). Vancouver: Provincial Health Services Authority.

8 Housing, Violence, and Women's Health: Addressing the Social Determinants of Health in Health Promotion

Pamela Ponic and Jill Atkey

Introduction

Housing instabilities are gendered, reflecting both social and health inequities (Bryant, 2009; Shaw, 2004) as evidenced by the degree to which socially marginalized groups, including women who have been abused, experience housing challenges. Shapcott (2008) succinctly describes the ongoing housing instability and homelessness crisis in Canada, highlighting that it is particularly acute for women and children living in poverty and First Nations peoples. This calls for action because housing is a known determinant of health (Dunn, Hayes, Hulchanski, Hwang, & Potvin, 2006; World Health Organization, 2008); the Ottawa Charter for Health Promotion identifies shelter as a primary prerequisite for health (World Health Organization, 1986); and housing instabilities and related health inequities are rectifiable through targeted interventions and policies (Dunn, 2004; Groton, 2013; Shaw, 2004). Bringing a gender lens to such interventions is essential to addressing the specific contexts and needs of women.

The purpose of this chapter is to bring attention to the importance of fostering health promotion interventions that explicitly address the social determinants of health—such as housing—and the utility of doing so through a gender lens. We begin by discussing literature that provides an overview of gendered housing patterns and the role of intimate partner violence (IPV); housing and related social determinants of health; and housing/health interventions from a gendered perspective. We then describe a study that brought a gender-transformative lens to studying and taking action to address the barriers to housing for women in the context of IPV. Shedding Light on the Barriers to Housing for Women Fleeing Violence was a feminist participatory action research (FPAR) project that sought to understand the barriers to housing and related health effects. By examining how housing inter-acted with other social determinants, this project aimed to initiate actions toward improving housing for women in a way that was comprehensive, systemic, and gender-transformative. Finally, we make the argument that health promoters need to attend to the social determinants of health from a gendered perspective because dominant approaches tend to be structured around male-centred norms that often fail to serve women or address disparities in women's social and health outcomes.

Housing, Gender, and Violence against Women

Analysis of census data illustrates the gendered nature of housing patterns in the Canadian context. The Canada Mortgage and Housing Corporation (CMHC) measures acceptable housing in terms of: (1) affordability—shelter costs are less than 30 percent of the before-tax household income; (2) suitability—dwellings have enough bedrooms per person as defined by National Occupancy Standards; and (3) adequacy—dwellings are not requiring major repairs (Canada Mortgage and Housing Corporation, 2012a). If housing fails to meet any one of these three criteria or if a household has to spend 30 percent or more of its pre-tax income to pay the median rent in their local market, the household is said to be in core housing need. According to 2006 Canadian Census data, women were more likely than men to be in core housing need, with lone female parents (27.9 percent) and women living alone (24.8 percent) having the highest rates of need (ibid.). Female-led lone-parent households had double the incidence of core housing need compared to male-led lone-parent households (at 30.2 percent and 15.2 percent respectively). These num-bers jump dramatically when looking solely at renter households, with 45.7 percent of female-led lone-parent households and 27.6 percent of male-led lone-parent households in core housing need (Canada Mortgage and Housing Corporation, 2012b). Aboriginal women were more than twice as likely to live in core housing need as non-Aboriginal women, and 46 percent of Aboriginal women living in lone-parent households lived in core housing need. Lone-parent households (of which 81 percent are led by women) in core housing need had lower levels of income and education and higher levels of unemployment and shelter cost-to-income ratio, indicating links between gender, Aboriginal status, socio-economic resources, and housing need (ibid.).

A growing body of literature suggests that intimate partner violence (IPV) is the primary cause of women's housing instability and homelessness (Miller & DuMont, 2000; Weber-Sikich, 2008; Wesley & Wright, 2005). IPV is defined as repeated physical, sexual, and/or emotional abuse by an intimate partner in the context of coercive control (Tjaden & Thoennes, 2000). Analysis of data from the California

Women's Health Survey showed that women who experienced IPV within the previous year were four times more likely to report housing instability than women who had not experienced IPV, with housing instability measured by move frequency, difficulty in paying the rent or mortgage, or being without housing (Pavao, Alvarez, Baumrind, Induni, & Kimerling, 2007). In Baker, Cook, and Norris's (2003) sample of 110 women who left IPV, 38 percent reported becoming homeless after separation and 25 percent reported having to relocate in the first year due to financial problems or continued harassment. Australian researchers found that women's housing instability increased after they left a violent partner, and that a lack of secure housing tenure contributed to women feeling unsafe after leaving (Champion et al., 2009). In a nationwide Canadian study, women who moved two to six times in the year after leaving IPV had lower incomes, were more likely to live in unaffordable housing, and experienced greater levels of violence than those who moved once or not at all (Ponic et al., 2011). Barata and Stewart (2010) found that women leaving IPV face discrimination from private-market landlords. Housing instability can force women to return to an abusive partner and contributes to the difficulty in leaving the relationship (Melbin, Sullivan, & Cain, 2003; Taylor-Butts, 2007).

Housing and Interconnected Social Determinants of Health

Housing is widely acknowledged as a social determinant of health (Mikkonen & Raphael, 2010; World Health Organization, 2008). Research shows that the health effects of inappropriate and unstable housing include respiratory illnesses caused by mould, mites, lead, and asbestos (Hwang, Martin, Tolomiczenko, & Hulchanski, 2003; Jacobs, Wilson, Dixon, Smith, & Evens, 2009) and compromised child development (Cooper, 2004). Unaffordable housing can result in psychological strain and social disconnection (Dunn, 2002), while also limiting access to other health-promoting resources such as nutritious food or recreation because high proportions of income are used to cover housing-related costs (Kirkpatrick & Tarasuk, 2007).

A complex policy web contributes to conditions that impact poor housing options in combination with other health determinants (Wilkinson & Pickett, 2009; World Health Organization, 2008). Bryant (2008) describes how policies that reduce availability of adequate financial resources and acceptable housing options can compromise health-promoting early life development, food security, and access to education and recreation. Such limits, in turn, foster social exclusion, which further contributes to poor health outcomes (Bryant, 2008). Importantly, gender is an underlying factor that influences the ways in which such determinants disproportionately impact women and their health, as the evidence on housing in the context of violence illustrates (Benoit, Shumka, & Vallance, 2010; Bryant, 2009; Spitzer, 2005).

Housing and Health Promotion for Women

Housing interventions can promote health and well-being (Pevalin, Taylor, & Todd, 2008; Thomson, Thomas, Sellstrom, & Petticrew, 2009), particularly for people with mental health and substance use issues and those with other stigmatized health concerns such as HIV/AIDS (Kyle & Dunn, 2008; Leaver, Garagh, & Dunn, 2007). In fact, researchers suggest that not only is the provision of affordable social housing a key to health promotion and disease prevention, it is also solid economic policy given its connections to other determinants of health (Bryant, 2008; Dunn et al., 2006). The primary housing interventions for women leaving IPV are safe homes, transition houses (i.e., shelters), and second-stage housing, all of which seek to provide safe, short-term housing options. While this is an important strategy to help women leave abusive partners, its efficacy is limited. Ponic et al. (2011) found that only 16 percent of women in a Canadian sample used transition house services in the one-year period after leaving IPV. These programs often have policies or norms that exclude or alienate women with male teenaged children, women of colour, immigrant women, women using substances, or those with mental health issues, which may account for low levels of uptake (Baker, Holditich Niolon, & Oliphant, 2009; Barron, 2005; BC Society of Transition Houses, 2011). Such barriers are highly problematic because transition house–type services are typically the gateway to other services and, at times, longer-term housing options.

Housing First is a housing intervention first conceptualized in New York in the mid-1990; its core premise is that providing homeless people with stable housing is primary and can be a base from which related health and social services are accessed (The Homeless Hub, 2013). This approach seeks to eliminate barriers in traditional approaches to housing provision. For example, access is not contingent upon residents accessing specific services, having psychological treatment, or abstaining from drugs or alcohol. Early evaluations of the Housing First model show promising results in promoting stable housing and reducing harms associated with substance use and mental health issues (Groton, 2013). The Mental Health Commission of Canada recently concluded a three-year national study testing the efficacy of the Housing First model in five Canadian cities (Hwang, Stergiopoules, O'Campo, & Gozdzik, 2012). The interim reports from the study articulate key successes of the Housing First model, from the improvement in individual lives and cost savings to interventions and cross-ministry approaches (Mental Health Commission of Canada, 2012).

Housing First studies and interventions are primarily gender-blind in their conceptualization, so we know little of the efficacy of the approach for women in general, and for women leaving IPV specifically (Klowdawsky, 2009). The only known study examining housing interventions from a gender perspective suggests that men and women experience housing interventions differently, with women revealing more complex outcomes, in part related to trauma (Rich & Clark, 2005). The focus on street-entrenched homelessness fails to recognize that the experience of homelessness is gendered, whereby homeless men are more likely than women to be enumerated by absolute homeless counts. Women are under-represented in homeless counts and comprise a significant share of the hidden homeless because of safety and protective mechanisms, so they couch surf or enter into relationships to gain access to shelter (Bopp et al., 2007; Paradis, Bandy, Cummings Diaz, Athumani, & Pereira, 2012; Regional Steering Committee on Homelessness, 2012). Where women are served, the approach does not intentionally or comprehensively take IPV into account despite evidence suggesting it is the primary cause of women's homelessness and housing instability. The critiques of both women-specific and non-gendered housing interventions point to the need for housing interventions and research that bring a gender lens and that support women's health and social outcomes.

The Shedding Light Project

The Shedding Light project was initiated by a research partnership between two provincial umbrella agencies—the BC Non-Profit Housing Association (www.bcnpha.ca) and the BC Society of Transition Houses (www.bcsth.ca). Both agencies have a mandate to support non-profit housing options for vulnerable populations. The partnership grew out of the recognition that women leaving violent relationships face considerable challenges in obtaining long-term, acceptable, and affordable housing and an interest in systematically documenting the BC-specific barriers. The project had two research questions: (1) What are the barriers to long-term housing for women leaving violent relationships across BC? and (2) How do the barriers impact women's health? As the description of our process will outline, we used the "engage, analyze, review, and identify" steps outlined in the planning tool that accompanies the framework (see Chapter 11) to answer these questions and take actions toward addressing them.

Shedding Light was guided by FPAR methodology and Photovoice methods. FPAR blends feminist theories with participatory action research methodology (Frisby, Maguire, & Reid, 2009). It centres on women's diverse experiences through varied and creative forms of representation, challenges patriarchy, and accounts for intersecting oppressions along lines such as race, class, age, and sexual orientation; fosters women's participation and inclusion in all aspects of the research process; and generates evidence toward action and social change (Lykes & Coquillon, 2006; Maguire, 2001; Reid & Frisby, 2008). Photovoice is a method that is well aligned with FPAR and has its roots in women's health and social justice issues (Wang, 1999).

The goal of Photovoice is to provide space for women's empowerment through creative and collaborative photo-taking and analysis, including in the context of violence against women (Frohmann, 2005). In Photovoice, participants take photos to illustrate their experiences, engage in photo-elicitation interviews to give meaning to the pictures, and work in groups to discuss common themes and potential actions (Hergenrather, Rhodes, Cowan, Bardhoshi, & Pula, 2009). Photos provide rich material for high-impact knowledge-translation activities (Packard, 2008), an important feature when action and social change are goals of the project.

The project took place in four communities across British Columbia that were deliberately chosen by a provincial advisory committee to reflect the diverse social, economic, and geographical contexts of BC. In each community, we created local advisory committees and hired a community-based researcher. Our recruitment strategy sought to include a diverse range of women by conducting outreach at multiple sites beyond women-serving agencies that focused on women against violence. Forty-five women participated in the six-month data collection and analysis process. They ranged in age from 19 to 66 years old, and all but four were single. Most had children, yet less than half of those who identified as mothers had full-time custody of their children. Mean annual income was $13,846. Twelve of the 45 (26.7 percent) identified as Aboriginal whereas the Canadian Aboriginal female population is less than 4 percent of the total population. These demographics show diversity in the group of participants, while also mirroring the profile of women living in core housing need in CMHC statistics.

The entire research team collaboratively created an Ethics and Safety Protocol that was guided by a trauma-informed lens (Ponic & Jategaonkar, 2011; Poole & Greaves, 2012) and prioritized women's safety and autonomy throughout the project. Participants engaged in a five-step research process that unfolded over six months:

1. An initial group meeting to review ethical and safety protocols, discuss women's involvement and concerns, and train participants in taking photos safely and for research purposes.
2. One-to-one meetings between a community-based researcher and participant to review protocols, conduct a structured demographic interview, and provide cameras.
3. Participant photo-taking.
4. Photo-elicitation interviews to provide a narrative explaining the photos.
5. A final group meeting during which the research team provided initial analysis for participants to confirm and extend. Participants also shared select photos with one another and collaboratively brainstormed actions and outcomes.

This process produced a data set of 547 photographs and 42 transcripts from interviews and group meetings. The research team further analyzed the data and identified the following findings.

Women's Barriers to Housing after Leaving a Violent Relationship

The 45 women in the Shedding Light project reported a complex set of interrelated barriers to housing, which together exacerbated the health effects of violence:

- poverty
- unsafe and unacceptable housing options
- persistent patterns of discrimination
- health effects of violence

Poverty

All 45 women reported experiences of poverty, including a lack of income and resources to meet basic needs and lack of opportunity to find meaningful employment. Some women described lifelong experiences of poverty, whereas others became impoverished after leaving a violent relationship. Experiences of poverty were heightened for women who had custody of their children and the expenses associated with providing adequate food, clothing, and shelter for them, as indicated by this woman:

> Again, it's a money issue. These pants are my son's, my eldest son's pants, and as you can see, they're tattered, torn. Do you pay the rent or do buy your kid a couple of pair of jeans to go to school in? Then you don't have food.

The causes of women's poverty were multi-faceted. Many women described financial abuse from ex-partners that at times continued long after they had left the relationship. Unaffordable or unavailable child-minding, communication, and transportation, along with post-abuse health issues, compromised women's ability to secure or maintain employment. Over half of the women in this study were receiving government social or disability assistance, which in British Columbia is inadequate to cover basic needs, including shelter (Atkey & Siggner, 2008). For those who were employed, many worked at jobs for minimum wage or just above. One women described earning "$10 per hour, 40 hours per week from two jobs, gross income $1,600 per month." In a context where the average monthly rent in communities with populations higher than 10,000 in BC is nearly $900 (Canada

Mortgage and Housing Corporation, 2012c), housing is thus unaffordable for most of the women in the study. Women managed these financial constraints by using food banks and free clothing stores, getting food from dumpsters, feeding their children before themselves, and turning off the heat.

Unacceptable and Unsafe Housing

In the context of poverty, participants reported living in housing that was unacceptable (i.e., unaffordable, unsuitable, and inadequate) and unsafe. Nearly all the women in this study were living in unaffordable housing, paying more than 30 percent of their income—and some as high as 70 percent—on housing costs. High costs also resulted in women with children living in unsuitable housing because they could not afford a place with an appropriate number of bedrooms per person. This woman describes her five-year-old son's room:

> These pictures show my son's room, in the closet.... He can't use the whole closet because his bed is in there and we only have room for the one dresser. When we first moved in, his crib was in the closet too.

The majority of participants lived in private market housing because public or non-profit housing did not exist in their communities or waiting lists were years long. Dependency on private market rentals is problematic because their condition goes largely unregulated. Participants described renting inadequate homes that were dirty, mouldy, full of asbestos, uninsulated, and without working appliances and plumbing. One single mother recalls:

> We were actually getting really, really sick. And as soon as we turn the heat on I started smelling mould, and I found that there was a lot of mould underneath the housing and in the walls. I talked to my landlord, but they didn't want to do anything about it.

These issues were without remedy because landlords were often left unaccountable when they disregarded the Residential Tenancy Act as tenants are responsible for managing the time-consuming complaints processes.

The unacceptable housing that participants described was also often unsafe. One woman described her tub falling through the floor into her kitchen and others lived near known gang houses. Violence, threats, and harassment by landlords who took advantage of women's vulnerable situations and dependency on housing were also prevalent, as one woman described: "One time the landlord suggested I screw him for rent."

Persistent Patterns of Re-victimization

Participants reported persistent patterns of re-victimization in the forms of continued harassment from ex-partners, gaps in policies and services, and discrimination by landlords, all of which acted as barriers to housing and healing. Many women, particularly those in tenuous custody relationships with ex-partners, experienced being stalked, deprived of joint finances, and denied access to their children. Some participants reported being caught in long-term legal battles and had lost custody of their children because they did not have adequate resources to pay for housing. One woman said that she "applied for ... low income housing [BC Housing], but they said if you don't have the kids 50/50 time you can't use the facility.... But I can't get custody if I don't have the housing." There were similar policy paradoxes in employment, child care, education, and income assistance systems.

Many women experienced discrimination on the basis of race, source of income, and family status in the private market. Some landlords explicitly stated that they would not rent to people on social assistance and others refused to rent to families with children. One Aboriginal woman described repeatedly being denied apartments because of her skin colour:

> My colour, my skin and all that: that's a roadblock right away. We've already had that experience here. The man would phone and say "Yes, the apartment's open." We'd go see it and he looks at me: "Oh, it's not available anymore."

For most women, their experiences of ongoing abuse and discrimination came at the hands of men, which this woman describes:

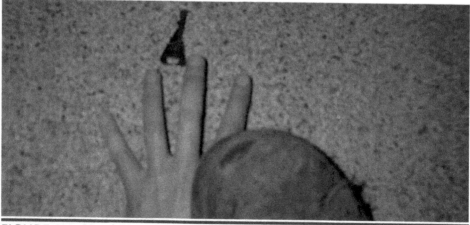

FIGURE 8.1: Hand/Key
Source: Authors.

This photo represents … men in my life that have either not protected me or interfered in the housing—either the partners I've had, the landlords I've had that have interfered with my safety and caused me to come to harm.

Health Effects of Violence

The mental and physical health effects of violence are well demonstrated in the literature, including depression, post-traumatic stress disorder, chronic pain, and respiratory issues (Campbell, 2002). Participant reports illustrated that lack of housing and poor health had a mutually reinforcing relationship in that the health effects of violence were a barrier to housing, and that the unsafe and unacceptable housing options that women were able to access exacerbated their poor health.

Mental health issues and a sense of powerlessness were identified as women's most pervasive issue as they tried to regain control over their lives. One woman said that "sometimes there are walls and you don't know how to get past them.… You become really hard. It's like hearts of stone sometimes, especially when you come out of abuse situations or there's just all these barriers … it's hard."

Some women spoke of being depressed, suicidal, lost, or overwhelmed during the transition period after leaving a violent situation. Mental health concerns were worsened during the transition period as women were forced to navigate complex systems, discrimination, poverty, and other persistent barriers in an effort to obtain stable housing and income.

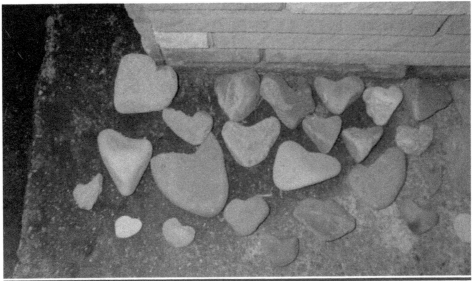

FIGURE 8.2: Hearts/Wall

Source: Authors.

Physical health issues were also a barrier to housing. Many women experienced chronic pain as a result of physical abuse, which limited their employability and therefore adequate income. They also found it challenging to secure housing that accommodated their physical disabilities. For example, one community lacked apartment buildings with elevators, forcing a participant with chronic hip and knee pain to walk up and down stairs for laundry and groceries, thus worsening her pain. Lack of accessible housing options contributed to women's isolation because of the physical difficulties associated with leaving the house. Inadequate housing also impaired the health of many women and children, which in turn increased their housing instability:

> We had to move out because there was asbestos in the walls. My son was getting really sick—he was on two inhalers. My baby was getting bleeding noses every night—so were all of us—but hers were worst.

The overall lack of resources also limited women's ability to access other health-promoting resources, including healthy food and recreation.

Barriers to Housing as Systemic and Interconnected
In summary, these four sets of barriers are systemic and interconnected as illustrated by the collective experiences of the 45 women in this study. Violence left them in poverty and unable to afford acceptable and safe housing. Landlord abuse and discrimination, as well as gaps between policy systems, failed to support adequate levels of income and housing stability. The health effects of violence heightened women's financial instabilities, and the unacceptable and unsafe housing that they were able to access on limited income further compromised their health. The women spoke of these barriers as a cycle that felt nearly impossible to break and at times sent them back to abusive partners.

Knowledge Translation Strategies: Policy Change and Public Awareness
Shedding Light was initiated to garner evidence to inform actions toward improved housing for women who have been abused. The research team, provincial and local advisory committees, and participants identified two key actions: (1) influence changes in policy and practice, and (2) increase public awareness. The knowledge translation strategies that we developed are described in Box 8.1.

Conclusion: Women, Violence, and Housing: From Gender-Blind to Gender-Transformative
The Shedding Light findings contribute to the growing body of literature that illustrate women's housing instability in the context of IPV (Pavao et al., 2007; Ponic et

BOX 8.1: **KNOWLEDGE TRANSLATION STRATEGIES**

1. *Surviving Not Thriving: The Systemic Barriers to Housing for Women Leaving Violent Relationships* (Ponic & Jategaonkar, 2010) is an advocacy report directed toward public, non-profit, and private sectors. It provides a succinct summary of project findings and 25 recommendations that address the four systemic and interconnected barriers. Examples of the gender-specific recommendations are:

- Use a gender and violence lens in the development of anti-poverty policy and programming.
- Develop a national housing strategy that pays attention to the needs of women leaving violence and the provision of family housing.
- Create a women's advocate position within senior levels of provincial government that would be responsible for upholding the legal and safety rights of women who have experienced violence. (pp. 4–5)

2. *The Surviving Not Thriving Tool Kit: A DVD and Facilitator's Guide to the Barriers to Housing for Women Leaving Violence* (BC Non-profit Housing Association, 2012) was designed to educate and build awareness. It includes a nine-minute DVD and a facilitator's guide that supports planning and facilitation of community events adaptable for various settings and audiences. The DVD utilizes the project photographs to tell a collective story of women's experiences accessing housing after leaving IPV. The facilitator's guide includes gender-specific activities that help participants

- distinguish between individual and systemic barriers to housing;
- understand the policy web that contributes to the production of gendered housing patterns and the role of intimate partner violence; and
- identify actions that can be taken to address housing issues for women.

al., 2011). The links between violence against women, housing, and health—along with poverty, policy gaps, and patterns of discrimination—clearly illustrate how gender underpins women's experiences of the social determinants of health. The finding that the housing-health relationship is mutually reinforcing (Jategaonkar & Ponic, 2011) highlights the need for health promoters to work toward breaking these cycles. In fact, recent research illustrates that heightened levels of housing instability have as great an impact on negative mental and physical health outcomes as severity of violence (Rollins et al., 2012). What's more, Greene, Chambers, Masinde, and O'Brien-Teengs (2012) illustrate how race and immigration status

further contributed to these cycles for immigrant mothers with HIV. The disproportionate number of Aboriginal women who participated in Shedding Light mirror
Canadian housing statistics (Canadian Mortgage and Housing Corporation, 2012a,
2012b) and warrant further specific attention to the ways in which colonialism
contributes to patterns of violence, housing instability, poverty, and poor health.

Yet housing policy, programming, and research remain primarily gender-blind
(Gabriel, 2008; Saugeres, 2009). The Shedding Light project is an example of how
a gender-transformative lens can be applied to housing research and interventions.
To do so, we sought to enact FPAR and Photovoice principles that align with
the gender-transformative health promotion principles outlined in this book. For
example, the project was women-centred and action-oriented in that our underlying
and ambitious goal was to contribute to the transformation of patriarchal power
relations to improve women's housing conditions, reduce the incidence of violence
against women, and promote their health. We brought an intersectional lens to the
recruitment of participants in an effort to reflect a range of experiences across various
systems of oppression, including race. Our team applied a trauma-informed lens to
promote women's safety and autonomy in light of the violence and trauma they had
experienced. Photovoice provided women with an empowering method to illustrate
their experiences creatively and have them be seen and heard. And, finally, our
analysis of findings was integrative in order to illustrate the ways in which barriers
were interconnected and therefore required responses across systems and sectors.

We also applied steps identified in the planning tool. First we engaged with
women, community organizations, researchers, and practitioners to identify the
gender-specific research questions and plan a safe and meaningful research process.
Second, we analyzed the evidence generated through the project in light of existing
literature and demographics through a gender and diversity lens. Third, we reviewed
existing housing practices and related health and social service interventions to
highlight gaps and discriminatory policies. And fourth, we identified ways in which
these gendered gaps and discriminatory policies could be rectified, and devised two
knowledge translation strategies to help address them.

As the gender-transformative health promotion for women framework (see
Chapter 1) highlights, the social determinants of health are a central factor in producing women's health and social outcomes. Given the health promotion mandate
to create supportive environments for health (World Health Organization, 1986),
housing and related social determinants should be well within the purview of health
promotion. However, the tendency in health promotion is to focus on individual
behaviours rather than structural inequities. In instances when structural factors or
social determinants are taken into account in health promotion, they tend to be

conceptualized more as the social contexts of individual behaviours rather than sites of health promotion in and of themselves.

We see that addressing housing and related social determinants is crucial health promotion work in light of the overwhelming evidence on the degree to which social inequities perpetuate health inequities (Raphael, 2009; Spitzer, 2005; Wilkinson & Pickett, 2009). In fact, the core health promotion philosophies of equity and empowerment may well serve housing interventions to become more accessible for marginalized populations.

Bringing a gender-transformative lens is crucial to this work because of the ways in which all social determinants of health are gendered and contribute to negative health outcomes for women. Certainly health promoters must address issues of violence against women and women's housing instability to be gender-transformative.

REFERENCES

Atkey, J., & Siggner, R. (2008). *Still left behind: A comparison of living costs and income assistance in British Columbia.* Vancouver: Social Planning and Research Council of BC.

Baker, C. K., Cook, S. L., & Norris, F. H. (2003). Domestic violence and housing problems: A contextual analysis of women's help-seeking, received informal support, and formal system response. *Violence Against Women, 9*(7), 754–783.

Baker, C. K., Holditch Niolon, P., & Oliphant, H. (2009). A descriptive analysis of transitional housing programs for survivors of intimate partner violence in the United States. *Violence Against Women, 15*(4), 460–481.

Barata, P. C., & Stewart, D. E. (2010). Searching for housing as a battered woman: Does discrimination affect reported availability of a rental unit? *Psychology of Women Quarterly, 34*(1), 43–55.

Barron, J. (2005). Multiple challenges in services for women experiencing domestic violence. *Housing, Care, and Support, 8*(1), 11–15.

BC Non-profit Housing Association. (2012). *Surviving not thriving tool kit: A DVD and facilitator's guide to the barriers to housing for women leaving violence.* Vancouver: BC Non-profit Housing Association and BC Society of Transition Houses.

BC Society of Transition Houses. (2011). *Reducing barriers to services and supports for substance use and mental wellness concerns among women fleeing violence.* Vancouver: Author.

Benoit, C., Shumka, L., & Vallance, K. (2010). *Violence as a determinant of girls' and women's health: Research brief.* Vancouver: Women's Health Research Network.

Bopp, J., van Bruggen, R., Elliott, S., Fuller, L., Hache, M., Hrenchuk, C., ... McNaughton, G. (2007). *You just blink and it can happen: A study of women's homelessness North of 60.* Yellowknife, NWT: Four Worlds Centre for Development Learning, Qulliit Nunavut Status of Women Council, YWCA Yellowknife, Yellowknife Women's Society, Yukon Status of Women's Council.

Bryant, T. (2008). Housing and health: More than bricks and mortar. In D. Raphael (Ed.), *Social determinants of health: Canadian perspectives* (pp. 235–249). Toronto: Canadian Scholars' Press Inc.

Bryant, T. (2009). Housing and income as social determinants of women's health in Canadian cities. *Women's Health and Urban Life, 8*(2), 1–20.

Campbell, J. (2002). Health consequences of intimate partner violence. *The Lancet, 359*(9314), 1331–1336.

Canada Mortgage and Housing Corporation. (2012a). *Housing conditions of girls and women.* 2006 Housing Census Series: Issue 19. Ottawa: Author.

Canada Mortgage and Housing Corporation. (2012b). *Housing conditions of lone-parent-led households.* 2006 Housing Census Series: Issue 19. Ottawa: Author.

Canada Mortgage and Housing Corporation. (2012c). *Rental market report: British Columbia highlights.* Housing Market Information, Spring 2012. Ottawa: Author.

Champion, T., Gander, C., Camacho Duarte, O., Phibbs, P., Crabtree, L., & Kirkby, M. (2009). *The impact of housing on the lives of women and children: Post domestic violence crisis accommodation.* Sydney: NSW Women's Refuge Movement Resource Centre and University of Western Sydney.

Cooper, M. (2004). Housing affordability: A children's issue. In D. Hulchanski & M. Shapcott (Eds.), *Finding room: Options for a Canadian rental housing strategy* (pp. 89–114). Toronto: CUCS Press.

Dunn, J. R. (2002). Housing and inequalities in health: A study of socioeconomic dimensions of housing and self reported health from a survey of Vancouver residents. *Journal of Epidemiology and Community Health, 56*(9), 671–681.

Dunn, J. R. (2004). Housing and population health—research framework. Ottawa: Canadian Mortgage and Housing Corporation.

Dunn, J. R., Hayes, M. V., Hulchanski, J. D., Hwang, S. W., & Potvin, L. (2006). Housing as a socio-economic determinant of health. *Canadian Journal of Public Health, 97*(3), 11–15.

Frisby, W., Maguire, P., & Reid, C. (2009). The "f" word has everything to do with it: How feminist theories inform action research. *Action Research, 7*(1), 13–29.

Frohmann, L. (2005). The framing safety project: Photographs and narratives by battered women. *Violence Against Women, 11*(11), 1396–1419.

Gabriel, M. (2008). Savvy investors and domestic goddesses? New challenges for feminist housing research. *Housing, Theory, and Society, 25*(3), 191–201.

Greene, S., Chambers, L., Masinde, K., & O'Brien-Teengs, D. (2012). A housing is not a home: The housing experiences of African and Caribbean mothers living with HIV. *Housing Studies, 28*(1), 116–134.

Groton, D. (2013). Are housing first programs effective? A research note. *Journal of Sociology and Social Welfare, 40*(1), 51–63.

Hergenrather, K. C., Rhodes, S. D., Cowan, C. A., Bardhoshi, G., & Pula, S. (2009). Photovoice as community-based participatory research: A qualitative review. *American Journal of Health Behaviour, 33*(6), 686–698.

The Homeless Hub. (2013). Retrieved from www.homelesshub.ca/topics/housing-first-209.aspx

Hwang, S., Martin, R., Tolomiczenko, G., & Hulchanski, J. (2003). The relationship between housing conditions and health status of rooming house residents in Toronto. *Canadian Journal of Public Health, 94*(6), 436–440.

Hwang, S., Stergiopoulos, V., O'Campo, P., & Gozdzik, A. (2012). Ending homelessness among people with mental illness: The At Home/Chez Soi randomized trial of a Housing First intervention in Toronto. *BMC Public Health, 12,* 787–803.

Jacobs, D., Wilson, J., Dixon, S., Smith, J., & Evens, A. (2009). The relationship of housing and population health: A 30-year retrospective analysis. *Environmental Health Perspectives, 117*(4), 597–604.

Jategaonkar, N., & Ponic, P. (2011). Unsafe and unacceptable housing: Health and policy implications for women leaving violent relationships. *Women's Health and Urban Life, Special issue on women's health and public policy, 10*(1), 32–58.

Kirkpatrick, S., & Tarasuk, V. (2007). Adequacy of food spending is related to housing expenditures among lower-income Canadian households. *Public Health Nutrition, 10*(12), 1464–1473.

Klodawsky, F. (2009). Rights to the city: Thinking social justice for chronically homeless women. In D. Hulchanski, P. Campsie, S. Chau, S. Hwang, & E. Paradis (Eds.), *Finding home: Policy options for addressing homelessness in Canada* (Chapter 4.4) [E-book]. Toronto: Cities Centre, University of Toronto. Retrieved from www.homelesshub.ca/FindingHome

Kyle, T., & Dunn, J. (2008). Effects of housing circumstances on health, quality of life, and healthcare use for people with severe mental illness: A review. *Health and Social Care in the Community, 16*(1), 1–15.

Leaver, C., Gargh, G., Dunn, J., & Hwang, S. (2007). The effects of housing status on health-related outcomes in people living with HIV: A systematic review of literature. *AIDS Behavior, 11*(Supp. #6), S85–S100.

Lykes, M. B., & Coquillon, E. (2006). Participatory and action research and feminisms: Towards transformative praxis. In S. Hesse-Biber (Ed.), *Handbook of feminist research: Theory and praxis* (pp. 297–326). Thousand Oaks, CA: Sage Publications.

Maguire, P. (2001). Uneven ground: Feminisms and action research. In P. Reason & H. Bradbury (Eds.), *Handbook of action research: Participative inquiry and practice* (pp. 59–69). London: Sage Publications.

Melbin, A., Sullivan, C. M., & Cain, D. (2003). Transitional supportive housing programs: Battered women's perspectives and recommendations. *Affilia, 18*(4), 445–460.

Mental Health Commission of Canada. (2012). *At home/Chez soi.* Interim report. Ottawa: Author.

Mikkonen, J., & Raphael, D. (2010). *Social determinants of health: The Canadian facts.* Toronto: York University School of Health Policy and Management.

Miller, K. L., & DuMont, J. (2000). Countless abused women: Homeless and inadequately housed. *Canadian Woman Studies, 20*(3), 115–122.

Packard, J. (2008) "I'm gonna show you what it's really like out here": The power and limitation of participatory visual methods. *Visual Studies, 23*(1), 63–77.

Paradis, E., Bardy, S., Cummings Diaz, P., Athumani, F., & Pereira, I. (2012). *We're not asking, we're telling: An inventory of practices promoting the dignity, autonomy, and self-determination of women and families facing homelessness.* Toronto: The Canadian Homelessness Research Network Press.

Pavao, J., Alvarez, J., Baumrind, N., Induni, M., & Kimerling, R. (2007). Intimate partner violence and housing instability. *American Journal of Preventative Medicine, 32*(2), 143–146.

Pevalin, D., Taylor, M, & Todd, J. (2008). The dynamics of unhealthy housing in the UK: A panel data analysis. *Housing Studies, 23*(5), 679–695.

Ponic, P., & Jategaonkar, J. (2010). *Surviving not thriving: The systemic barriers to housing for women leaving violent relationships.* Vancouver: BC Non-profit Housing Association.

Ponic, P., & Jategaonkar, N. (2011). Balancing safety and action: Ethical protocols for Photovoice research with women who have experienced violence. *Arts and Health: An International Journal for Research, Policy, and Practice, 4*(3), 189–202.

Ponic, P., Varcoe, C., Davies, L., Ford-Gilboe, M., Wuest, J., & Hammerton, J. (2011). Leaving ≠ Moving: Housing patterns of women who have left an abusive partner. *Violence Against Women, 17*(12), 1576–1600.

Poole, N., & Greaves, L. (Eds.). (2012). *Becoming trauma-informed.* Toronto: Centre for Addiction and Mental Health.

Raphael, D. (Ed.). (2009). *Social determinants of health: Canadian perspectives.* Toronto: Canadian Scholars' Press Inc.

Regional Steering Committee on Homelessness. (2012). *One step forward: Results of the 2011 Metro Vancouver homeless count.* Vancouver: Metro Vancouver.

Reid, C., & Frisby, W. (2008). Continuing the journey: Articulating dimensions of feminist participatory action research. In P. Reason & H. Bradbury (Eds.), *Handbook of action research: Participative inquiry and practice* (2nd ed., pp. 93–105). London: Sage Publications.

Rich, A. R., & Clark, C. (2005). Gender differences in response to homelessness services. *Evaluation and Program Planning, 28*(1), 69–81.

Rollins, C., Glass, N., Perrin, N., Billhardt, A., Barnes, J., Hansen, G., & Bloom, T. (2012). Housing instability is as strong a predictor of poor health outcomes as level of danger in an abusive relationship. Findings from the SHARE study. *Journal of Interpersonal Violence, 27*(4), 623–643.

Saugeres, L. (2009). "We do get stereotyped": Gender, housing, work, and social disadvantage. *Housing, Theory, and Society, 26*(3), 193–209.

Shapcott, M. (2008). Housing. In D. Raphael (Ed.), *Social determinants of health: Canadian perspectives* (pp. 221–234). Toronto: Canadian Scholars' Press Inc.

Shaw, M. (2004). Housing and public health. *Annual Review of Public Health, 25,* 397–418.

Spitzer, D. (2005). Engendering health disparities. *Canadian Journal of Public Health, 96*(2), S78–S96.

Taylor-Butts, A. (2007). Canada's shelters for abused women, 2005/2006. *Juristat: Canadian Centre for Justice Statistics, 27*(4), 1–20.

Tjaden, P., & Thoennes, N. (2000). *Full report of the prevalence, incidence, and consequences of violence against women.* Washington, DC: National Institute of Justice.

Thomson, H., Thomas, S., Sellstrom, E., & Petticrew, M. (2009). The health impacts of housing improvement: A systematic review of intervention studies from 1987 to 2007. *American Journal of Public Health, 99*(S3), S681–S692.

Wang, C. (1999). Photovoice: A participatory action research strategy applied to women's health. *Journal of Women's Health, 8*(2), 185–192.

Weber-Sikich, K. (2008). Global female homelessness: A multi-faceted problem. *Gender Issues, 25,* 147–156.

Wesely, J., & Wright, J. (2005). The pertinence of partners: Examining intersections between women's homelessness and their adult relationships. *American Behavioral Scientist, 48*(8), 1082–1101.

Wilkinson, R., & Pickett, K. (2009). *The spirit level: Why greater equality makes societies stronger.* New York: Bloomsbury Press.

World Health Organization. (1986). *The Ottawa Charter for health promotion.* Ottawa: Author.

World Health Organization. (2008). *Closing the gap in a generation: Health equity through action on the social determinants of health.* Geneva: Author.

9 Illuminating Gender-Transformative Mental Health Promotion in the Workplace

Paola Ardiles, Kathy GermAnn, and Farah Mawani

> Mental health can flourish in environments that are safe,
> just and equitable, and that foster quality connections.
>
> —Canadian Institute for Health Information,
> *Improving the Health of Canadians: Exploring Positive Mental Health*

Introduction

A multiplicity of factors influence our mental well-being, from the complex inter-action of our cells and the environment, to the broad social and political structures that govern our societies. But gender is a key determinant of mental well-being. And a highly influential environment for women and men, bearing on their mental well-being, is the workplace, where so many of us spend a third to half of our waking lives. Despite this, current conceptualizations of workplace "mental health" (which typically focus on mental illness) and the dominant discourse on workplace health promotion tend to neglect gender and mental well-being. In particular, these views overlook the power of relationships in the workplace to influence mental well-being.

In this chapter, we articulate an approach based on a positive articulation of mental health and briefly describe principles of mental health promotion. Next, we critically examine the interaction of gender, social support, and the relational dynamics through which mental well-being can be co-generated in the workplace. Finally, drawing from existing literature and case scenarios, we identify a basic set of key elements, principles, and practices upon which to build gender-transformative health promotion for the workplace, an important location for health promotion where relatively little action on gender has taken place.

166

Mental Well-being and Mental Health Promotion

Mental well-being is the capacity to "feel, think and act in ways that enhance our ability to enjoy life and deal with the challenges we face" (Centre for Health Promotion, University of Toronto, 1997, cited in Joubert & Raeburn, 1998, p. 15) and recognize its multiple dimensions: emotional, relational/social, spiritual, and intellectual (Epp, 1998). Individuals may experience mental well-being in different ways, but examples of commonly identified experiences include having quality connections with others; having choice, autonomy, and a sense of competence; feeling vital and full of energy; feeling happy; having a sense of meaning and purpose in one's life; enjoying one's life; and having a sense that one is living a life worth living (Canadian Institute for Health Information, 2009; Diener, 2000; Russell, 1930/1996; Ryan & Deci, 2001; Ryff & Singer, 1998).

Reflecting a multi-level determinants of health framework, mental well-being is generated through the dynamic interaction of individuals, groups, and the opportunities and influences in their environments (Epp, 1998), including living and working conditions. Mental health promotion, therefore, aims to promote mental well-being through a range of strategies implemented at multiple levels. Key principles of mental health promotion include

- a positive conceptualization of mental health (mental well-being);
- approaches that emphasize meaningful engagement and participation, and that foster empowerment;
- a focus on building upon existing strengths and assets;
- collaborative actions on the determinants of mental well-being at multiple levels; and
- tailored and culturally appropriate actions (GermAnn & Ardiles, 2009, p. 26).

However, within these broad conceptualizations of mental health promotion in the literature there are gaps to fill relevant to the interaction of gender, social support, and the relational dynamics that can co-generate mental well-being in the workplace.

Gender: A Key Determinant of Mental Well-being

As mental well-being has been recognized as a key resource for population well-being and the social and economic prosperity of society (Barry, 2009), there is a critical need to better integrate considerations of gender in developing mental health promotion strategies, programs, and policies. Although gender is often mentioned as a key determinant of mental health, issues related to gender roles, gender relations, and gendered social structures have largely been ignored or minimized in the major mental health promotion evidence reviews, as well as in government policies and in mental health promotion practice across diverse settings.

Complicating this picture, much of the research on mental health promotion in the workplace has approached mental health from a deficit perspective that emphasizes the burden of illness (e.g., ranging from mild to severe mental disorders), economic cost of illness (e.g., loss of productivity), or on the risk factors for illness (e.g., workplace stressors) (Standing Senate Committee on Social Affairs Science and Technology, 2006). Again, gender is often a neglected factor in workplace mental health initiatives even though it is recognized that workplaces are gendered—for example, in workforce characteristics, leadership practices, and sex discriminatory practices (Armstrong, 2009).

Using the framework for gender-transformative health promotion as a catalyst for our analysis, we advance a new approach that not only acknowledges gender as a key determinant of mental health in the workplace, but also identifies the need to employ a strength-based perspective to create healthy and vibrant workplaces where women have the opportunity to flourish. To do this, we have reviewed literature on social support, and integrated an innovative exploration into relational dynamics to promote mental well-being for women in the workplace.

A Gendered Approach to Mental Health Promotion in the Workplace

Workplace environments affect mental well-being but exemplify and, in many cases, reify stereotypical masculine traits in social relationships within them (Fletcher, 1998), and result in different experiences of social support for men and women. They occupy the majority of waking time for working-age adults; can involve intense psychological, intellectual, and/or physical demands; and are key social environments across the adult lifespan (Ray & Bergeron, 2007). In addition, the dynamic relationship between individual employees, workplaces, and their broader socio-political context can affect mental well-being.

Social Support

Social support is a key social determinant within workplace environments, affecting the human relationships that impact mental well-being. Social support can involve formal and/or informal sources/relationships. Formal support refers to organizational support (Simich, Mawani, Wu, & Noor, 2004), including that provided by governments, health and social services, and workplaces. Informal support refers to relationships among individuals within social networks, including those between family members, friends, neighbours, colleagues, and so forth. Peer support, the relationship between peers, is currently at the forefront of international literature, policy, and programming because of its unique contribution to mental well-being. Though much of the focus on peer support is about people with lived experience of mental health issues/illnesses (O'Hagan, Cyr, McKee, & Priest, 2010), it is an important concept for workplace mental health promotion, as workplace relationships are often primarily peer relationships involving shared goals and shared experience.

Social support affects mental well-being in two ways: structurally and functionally. Structural support refers to the existence and quantity of social relationships and the interconnectedness of a person's social network. Functional support refers to the ways in which support can be informational, instrumental, emotional, and affirmational, and clearly implies that the existence and quantity of social relationships alone are not sufficient to promote mental well-being. Informational support is the provision of information, advice, and guidance (Cohen & Wills, 1985) to meet particular needs, and instrumental support is "help, aid, or assistance with tangible needs" (Berkman & Glass, 2000, p. 145) such as job tasks or common objectives. Emotional support refers to love, care, sympathy, empathy, and appreciation, and affirmational support is validation and constructive feedback, based on shared experience, a central component of peer support that affects mental well-being (Berkman & Glass, 2000).

Social support is transactional, involving giving and receiving (Berkman & Glass, 2000). This reciprocity is key to building relationships and generating well-being. This is particularly true of relationships between peers in workplace settings. A gender analysis of social support reveals that men and women need and offer different types of support, give and receive different levels of social support, and seek support in different ways (Heaney & Israel, 1997). Research highlights that women foster more intimate peer relationships, seek more social support during periods of stress, and provide more frequent and effective social support than men (Kawachi & Berkman, 2001). Research has found associations between lower perceived adequacy of social support and increased psychological distress, depressive symptoms, and anxiety (ibid.). A growing body of evidence has found associations between peer support and improvements in quality of life (Miyamoto & Sono, 2012, O'Hagan et al., 2010).

Receiving support has been found to increase self-esteem (Turner, Lloyd, & Roszell, 1999), and belonging (Kawachi & Berkman, 2001), and giving support has shown a stronger association to well-being than receiving support (Bracke, Christiaens, & Verhaeghe, 2008). How women and men experience social support creates a differential impact on their health (Kawachi & Berkman, 2001) as women tend to have more intimate peer relationships than men and may be more negatively impacted by the suffering of those close to them (ibid.). Women are also more likely to be in relationships where they give more support than they receive, and this can have a detrimental effect on their mental well-being, particularly for those with low financial or other resources.

Gender intersects with other factors to affect social support and mental health. For example, in a Canadian study of social support among immigrants and refugees, Somali refugees described experiencing distress due to their inability to give social support when their own needs for support were so great (Simich et al., 2004). They longed to be part of a community of reciprocal relationships, where they could give as well as receive support, seeing this as vital to their cultural identities (ibid.). Social support is a fundamental and gendered determinant of mental and physical health and a foundation of health promotion practice.

Relational Dynamics and Organizational Analysis

Insights from relational cultural theory (RCT) (Jordan, Kaplan, Baker Miller, Stiver, & Surrey, 1991; Jordan, Walker, & Hartling, 2004) are particularly informative for our purposes. In contrast to models of human growth and development, which emphasize separation and individuation, RCT posits that human growth occurs in connection—that is, through "growth-fostering interactions" with others (Baker Miller & Stiver, 1997, p. 22). These interactions generate outcomes that are highly resonant with the notions of mental well-being and flourishing. However, most workplaces are not "structured to attend to, let alone foster mutuality and relational bonding" (Jordan, 1991, p. 94) as an emphasis on productivity is deemed to be enhanced by competition and individualism.

Fletcher's work (1998, 2007) has significant potential to inform a gender-transformational approach to mental health promotion in the workplace as she draws attention to how workplaces are gendered, exemplifying stereotypical masculine traits while devaluing or ignoring feminine ones. Re-examining these gendered assumptions to include perspectives that have previously been discounted or ignored, however, can stimulate new ways of thinking about organizing workplace settings. Enacting relational skills and adopting a relational stance is one way in which women "do gender" in the workplace and in society at large (Fletcher, 2007) in keeping with their gender socialization. However, most organizations are modelled on masculine models where independence, individualism, and toughness are perceived as "ideal," while relational skills and practices (e.g., fostering empathy, mutual empowerment, and caring) are perceived as implying weakness and powerlessness.

Fletcher (2007) describes a way of working in organizations that stems from a relational belief system, and envisions how organizations might be different if they embraced three strengths associated with connection and affiliation: vulnerability, empathy, and empowerment. Vulnerability, viewed not as a personal failure but rather as an inevitable part of human interdependence, becomes a way of building rapport and equalizing or humanizing working relationships so they can be strengthened and it opens people to learning and growth. Empathy enables responsiveness to the feelings and expressions of others and helps people develop broader understandings of one another. Finally, empowering, from Fletcher's perspective, is about gaining satisfaction from participating in the development of others.

Kahn's work on holding environments, relational systems, and patterns of caregiving in organizations illuminates the importance of relational practices such as those identified by Fletcher (Kahn, 1993, 1998, 2001, 2005). Kahn (1993) mapped patterns of caregiving among social workers that provide insight into how mental well-being can be promoted in workplace relationships. In essence, when the one who is caring for "the other" makes herself accessible and attends to the other in ways that help her feel understood, heard, valued, joined, and cared for, feelings of being connected, which are so important for mental well-being, are generated.

In order to understand relational dynamics that generate well-being in the workplace, GermAnn (2006) conducted an ethnographic study of a rural hospital and long-term care facility—reputed to be a "great place to work" and one that delivered exemplary care to patients and residents—in order to identify relational dynamics and organizational practices that produced mental well-being. Staff and managers in this facility described "well-being" in terms of an affective experience based on global appraisals of one's life (feeling successful and that one is "doing okay"; feeling happy with oneself and one's work) and more specific feelings of being accepted for who one is and that one is "making a difference" (ibid.). Without exception, interviewees said that working in this facility contributed to their well-being and described numerous ways in which this occurred. Four patterns of relating with co-workers and patients/residents that produced well-being were identified. These included the following:

- *Creating a comfort zone:* People made themselves open and available to one another, signalling their receptiveness to being with and helping each other.
- *Caring for each other:* In the giving and receiving of care, those receiving care came to feel accepted for who they are and those who cared for them came to feel that they were making a difference in other people's lives.
- *Carrying each other:* Grounded in a comfort zone in which the giving and receiving of care flowed unimpeded, workers were able to compensate for one another. Feeling safe and accepted, they could be vulnerable—they could say,

"I don't know," "I'm not fully functioning today—help me." This pattern of interacting was crucial in terms of working together effectively to produce good outcomes for patient and resident care.

- *Learning with and from each other:* Being able to learn from each other was another important vehicle for feeling included, of fitting in, while being honoured for who one is and what one does.

Further examination revealed an abundance of caring relationships that combined, constituting a caring relational landscape—"a dynamic matrix of mutually affirming and supportive patterns of relating characterized by the enactment of a genuine concern for the well-being of others" (GermAnn, 2006, p. 139). This matrix of caring relationships had been nurtured and sustained over many years, revealing that the caring relational landscape was created and sustained by the active and consistent enactment of two core sets of principles. The first emphasized service and working together as a team, with a strong focus on patient/family-centred care. The second core principle was "treating people well," which included respecting, supporting, and enjoying one another and demonstrating positive regard. The caring nature of the organizational relational landscape was sustained through the respectful navigation of differences, tensions, and conflict; vigilant monitoring of the landscape and, when necessary, the containment of degenerative dynamics. In other words, relational work was valued and visible and therefore sustained. GermAnn's work demonstrates that there are some workplaces in which relational practices are clearly important, visible, and actively nurtured and sustained. This requires a high degree of relational competence, which Surrey (1991) defines as "the interest and capacity to stay emotionally present with, to enlarge or deepen the relational context to create enough space for both or all people to express themselves and allow possible conflict, tension, and creative resolution" (p. 167).

Social Support, Relational Practices, and Workplace Mental Health Promotion

Both the social support and relational dynamics evidence illuminate the need to critically reconsider the notion of "mental health" in the workplace from a gendered point of view. A gender-transformative approach, at least in part, is one that emphasizes social support and relational dynamics as a seedbed for the co-generation of mental well-being in the workplace. Women's (and men's) social support and relational skills can be leveraged to promote mental well-being in the workplace and, importantly, make social support and relational practices visible and valued at an organizational level. There is a need for visible and committed enactment of espoused values that promote the development of relational competencies such as service and treating people well, combined with vigilant monitoring and interventions to identify and forestall degenerative relational dynamics in a workplace environment. This is particularly important when considering that gender and power interact across various social environments.

Power and its distribution in workplace environments are critically important. Baker Miller (1986) asserted that "the greater the development of each individual, the more able, more effective, and less needy of limiting or restricting others she or he will be" (p. 116). A shift to this mindset would require significant reconfiguration of ideas about and practices pertaining to power and leading in organizational settings. In such a paradigm, others can be viewed as a potential source of learning regardless of where that other person is in the organizational hierarchy, and power in the workplace can be viewed as fluid and a positive contribution to growth-fostering interactions that support mental well-being.

A multi-level framework for gender-transformative mental health promotion in the workplace includes roles for women, men, the organization, and the broader society. At the individual level, strategies may focus on building resilience and empowerment skills, especially among women, as well as promoting psychological and social well-being. There is also a need to look at what happens between women and other individuals and groups—to nurture and sustain interactions and relationships that are positive and generative. At an organizational level, other types of actions may be oriented toward the creation of supportive environments such as building gender-sensitive relational competence at all levels, recognizing the importance of taking time to build positive relationships, and promoting participation in decision making or engagement in the workplace. At a broader societal level, strategies may address the gendered structural determinants of mental health, and reduce health and social inequities that affect women and men through more equitable access to economic resources, equitable employment, and educational opportunities. Within all these levels, it is critical to acknowledge complexity when taking into account the diversity of women and men in the workplace.

In summary, creating a healthy work environment that will promote mental health requires ways to shift power from power-over, to power-with. Attention needs to be given to what happens between women and men and individuals in different roles, and social support and positive relationships need to be fostered among individuals, groups, and teams in an organization. Organizations need to embrace the importance of building social inclusion and relational competence—the ability to develop mutually trusting and respectful (i.e., positive) organizational relationships—to navigate conflict and tensions, and maintain a supportive and inclusive relational environment in the workplace to accomplish the organization's work and to protect and promote mental well-being.

Key Elements of a Gender-Transformative Workplace Mental Health Promotion

Determining the key elements of a gender-transformative approach to workplace mental health promotion requires drawing from women's lives and experiences in order to re-vision organizational life and the promotion of mental well-being in the workplace in ways that will benefit managers, employees, and the organization as a whole. A gender-transformative approach offers an opportunity to expand an understanding of organizing and how mental well-being can be protected and promoted in workplace settings to benefit both women and men. While this is a preliminary list, a gender-transformative mental health promotion approach in workplaces would include the following:

- A focus on mental well-being for women and men—that is, the capacity to feel, think, and act in ways that enhance our ability to enjoy life and deal with challenges, to develop a sense of inclusion and belonging, to have meaning in life and feel that one is living a life worth living
- A strengths-based approach that acknowledges the importance of social support, social inclusion, and relational dynamics as core strengths that produce mental well-being, and that honours women's roles in the workplace
- An emphasis on the relational landscape of the workplace with particular attention to the gendered elements of social support and the relational dynamics through which mental well-being is co-produced
- Making gendered versions of relational work both visible and valued as an integral aspect of the accomplishment of the organization's work and the co-generation of mental well-being
- An awareness of the gendered distribution of power and a reconceptualization of the effective use of power in the workplace, shifting from the dominant power-over approach to greater enactment of power-with and the fluid shifting of power according to expertise and nee
- Attention to enacting gender- and culturally relevant policies and practices throughout the organization to respond to the interaction of factors affecting women's mental health in the workplace
- Multiple levels of action and understanding of how gender affects mental well-being

Conclusion

Applying a gender lens to promote mental well-being is greatly needed, not only to integrate gender considerations into mental health programs, policies, and practices across diverse settings, but, more importantly, to create gender-transformative health promotion for women and men that makes traditional feminine strengths visible and respected in the generation of mental well-being and enhances women's status in the process. We are not there yet. More research and application to practice and policy is needed to inform gender-transformative workplace mental health promotion in general and in varied workplace settings. Individuals, teams, organizations, and society at large all have a role to play, and can share the responsibility of creating transformative workplace environments for both women and men. In transforming our relationships in the workplace, we can also support the transformation of families, communities, and society at large to promote health and well-being for all.

REFERENCES

Armstrong, P. (2009). Ancillary workers: Forgotten women in health care. In P. Armstrong & J. Deadman (Eds.), *Women's health: Intersections of policy, research, and practice* (pp. 175–186). Toronto: Women's Press.

Baker Miller, J. (1986). *Toward a new psychology of women* (2nd ed.). Boston: Beacon Press.

Baker Miller, J., & Stiver, I. P. (1997). *The healing connection: How women form relationships in therapy and in life.* Boston: Beacon Press.

Barry, M. M. (2009). Addressing the determinants of positive mental health: Concepts, evidence, and practice. *International Journal of Mental Health Promotion, 11*(3), 4–17.

Berkman, L. F., & Glass, T. (2000). Social integration, networks, and health. In L. F. Berkman & I. Kawachi (Eds.), *Social epidemiology* (pp. 137–173). New York: Oxford University Press.

Bracke, P., Christiaens, W., & Verhaeghe, M. (2008). Self-esteem, self-efficacy, and the balance of peer support among persons with chronic mental health problems. *Journal of Applied Social Psychology, 38*(2), 436–459.

Canadian Institute for Health Information. (2009). *Improving the health of Canadians: Exploring positive mental health.* Ottawa: Author.

Centre for Health Promotion, University of Toronto. (1997). *Proceedings from the International Workshop on Mental Health Promotion,* Toronto.

Cohen, S., & Wills, T. A. (1985). Stress, social support, and the buffering hypothesis. *Psychological Bulletin, 98*(2), 310–357.

Diener, E. (2000). Subjective well-being: The science of happiness and a proposal for a national index. *American Psychologist, 55*(1), 34–43.

Epp, J. (1998). *Mental health for Canadians: Striking a balance.* Ottawa: Government of Canada.

Fletcher, J. K. (1998). Relational practice: A feminist reconstruction of work. *Journal of Management Inquiry, 7*(2), 163–186.

Fletcher, J. K. (2007). Leadership, power, and positive relationships. In J. Dutton & B. R. Ragins (Eds.), *Exploring positive relationships at work: Building a theoretical and research foundation* (pp. 347–372). Mahwah, NJ: Lawrence Erlbaum and Associates.

GermAnn, K. (2006). Caring matters: Working, relating, and well-being in a caregiving organization (Unpublished doctoral dissertation). University of Alberta, Edmonton.

GermAnn, K., & Ardiles, P. (2009). *Toward flourishing for all: Mental health promotion and mental illness prevention policy background paper.* Retrieved from http://www.bemhsus.ca/toward-flourishing-for-all

Heaney, C. A., & Israel, B. A. (1997). Social support and social networks. In K. Glanz, B. Rimer, & F. Lewis (Eds.), *Health behavior and health education: Theory, research, and practice* (2nd ed., pp. 179–205). San Francisco: Jossey-Bass.

Kawachi, I., & Berkman, L. F. (2001). Social ties and mental health. *Journal of Urban Health, 78*(3), 458–467.

Jordan, J. (1991). The meaning of mutuality. In J. V. Jordan, A. G. Kaplan, J. Baker Miller, I. Stiver, & J. Surrey (Eds.), *Women's growth in connection: Writings from the Stone Center* (pp. 81–96). New York: Guilford Press.

Jordan, J. V., Kaplan, A. G., Baker Miller, J., Stiver, I. P., & Surrey, J. L (1991). *Women's growth in connection: Writings from the Stone Center.* New York: Guilford Press.

Jordan, J. V., Walker, M., & Hartling, L. M. (2004). *The complexity of connection: Writings from the Stone Center's Jean Baker Miller Training Institute.* New York: The Guilford Press.

Joubert, N., & Raeburn, J. (1998). Mental health promotion: People, power and passion. *International Journal of Mental Health Promotion,* Inaugural Issue, 15–22.

Kahn, W. A. (1993). Caring for the caregivers: Patterns of organizational caregiving. *Administrative Science Quarterly, 38*(4), 539–563.

Kahn, W. A. (1998). Relational systems at work. *Research on Organizational Behavior, 20,* 39–76.

Kahn, W. A. (2001). Holding environments at work. *The Journal of Applied Behavioral Science, 37*(3), 260–279.

Kahn, W. A. (2005). *Holding fast: The struggle to create resilient caregiving organizations.* New York: Brunner-Routledge.

Miyamoto, Y., & Sono, T. (2012). Lessons from peer support among individuals with mental health difficulties: A review of the literature. *Clinical Practice and Epidemiology in Mental Health, 8,* 22–29.

O'Hagan, M., Cyr, C., McKee, H., & Priest, R. (2010). *Making the case for peer support: Report to the Mental Health Peer Support Project Committee of the Mental Health Commission of Canada.* Ottawa: Mental Health Commission of Canada.

Ray, B., & Bergeron, J. (2007). Geographies of ethnocultural diversity in a second-tier city. *Our Diverse Cities, 4,* 91–94.

Russell, B. (1996). *The conquest of happiness.* New York: W. W. Norton & Co. (Original work published 1930.)

Ryan, R. M., & Deci, E. L. (2001). On happiness and human potential: A review of research on hedonic and eudaimonic well-being. *Annual Review of Psychology, 52*(1), 141–166.

Ryff, C. D., & Singer, B. (1998). The contours of positive human health. *Psychological Inquiry, 9*(1), 1–28.

Simich, L., Mawani, F., Wu, F., & Noor, A. (2004). *Meanings of social support, coping, and help-seeking strategies among immigrants and refugees in Toronto.* Toronto: University of Toronto Press.

Standing Senate Committee on Social Affairs Science and Technology. (2006). *Out of the shadow at last: Transforming mental health, mental illness, and addiction services in Canada.* Ottawa: Parliament of Canada.

Surrey, J. L. (1991). Relationship in empowerment. In J. V. Jordan, A. G. Kaplan, J. Baker Miller, I. Stiver, & J. Surrey (Eds.), *Women's growth in connection: Writings from the Stone Center* (pp. 162–180). New York: Guilford Press.

Turner, R. J., Lloyd, D. A., & Roszell, P. (1999). Personal resources and the social distribution of depression. *American Journal of Community Psychology, 27*(5), 643–672.

10 Rethinking Preconception and Maternal Health:
A Prime Opportunity for Gender-Transformative Health Promotion

Lauren Bialystok, Lorraine Greaves, and Nancy Poole

Introduction

For decades, prenatal health has been the target of public health campaigns and one of the most visible subjects of health promotion. These efforts have been exemplars of some of the most gender-exploitative types of health promotion: shaming, blaming, and fetus-centric, they reinforce the view that maternal health is subordinate to fetal health and women are entirely responsible for their children's well-being (Wade, 2011; Wise, 2008). For example, the now ubiquitous admonitions to quit smoking and drinking during pregnancy show little regard for the woman's lifelong health, nor any sensitivity to the circumstances of her substance use; not surprisingly, tobacco and alcohol cessation efforts are often abandoned postpartum, resulting in rates of relapse as high as 90 percent once the fetus is no longer a motivator or a reference point for medical treatment (Fleming, Lund, Wilton, Landry, & Scheets, 2008; Greaves et al., 2011). Only recently have critiques of such approaches begun to generate more women-centred, supportive prenatal health promotion interventions (Greaves & Poole, 2005).

Even so, the reach of prenatal health promotion is drastically limited. From the standpoint of both women's and children's health, our current practices are failing. The high rate of unplanned pregnancy (about 50 percent) and the continuing barriers to accessing complete and timely prenatal care mean that many of the outcomes it is intended to prevent, such as low birth weight, are still very common (Finer & Henshaw, 2006). For example, the percentage of preterm babies in the United States rose from 9.4 percent in 1981 to 12.3 percent in 2003, and those with low birth weight from 6.8 percent in 1981 to 7.9 percent in 2003 (Martin et al., 2006). There are varied reasons for these trends, including infertility treatments; rising maternal age; tobacco, drug, and alcohol use; obesity; and chronic disease (Ohlsson & Shah, 2008). Because of the acute and lifelong health costs associated with preterm birth and low birth weight, there is growing recognition that care for the health of mothers and children cannot be confined to the period between conception and birth. Instead, we need to think about the "preconception" or "inter-conception" period as a critical opportunity for health promotion. Preconception care is not only a way of improving maternal and child health, but also of practising gender-transformative health promotion, which facilitates reproductive autonomy and contributes to women's overall well-being.

The term "preconception care" has been used in North America since the 1980s to describe child-bearing-related health care for women before they become pregnant. It was first associated with the care provided to women who had already experienced adverse pregnancy outcomes (Chamberlain, 1980), but shortly came to be recommended for all women (Institute of Medicine, Committee to Study the Prevention of Low Birth Weight, 1985). Despite this history, there is no uniform definition or universal recognition of preconception care (Curtis, Abelman, Schulkin, Williams, & Fassett, 2006). While a smattering of guidelines and documents have brought the concept to life in several Canadian jurisdictions, there is no consistent set of national guidelines for this important component of well-woman care (Bialystok, Greaves, & Poole, 2013).

Conceptualizing Preconception Care

The degree of variation in both the practice and theory of preconception care may not be surprising as there is no agreed-upon definition to anchor the literature or guide its practice. The definitions of preconception care seem to fall into two main categories, illustrating different concepts of health and the relationship between mothers and children.

First, there are definitions that define preconception care as an extension of prenatal care whose primary purpose is to produce healthy, full-term babies. This approach is supported by evidence that factors such as poor maternal nutrition, substance use, and chronic disease can negatively affect a fetus even prior to conception, and that other health hazards (such as sexually transmitted infections) cannot always be treated in a timely fashion during pregnancy (Atrash, Jack, & Johnson, 2008). One study found that in the three months prior to conception or before women realized they were pregnant, 15.8 percent of women in Canada used tobacco and 62.4 percent drank alcohol (Public Health Agency of Canada, 2009). Many women have diabetes, hypertension, and other chronic conditions that can negatively affect a pregnancy and can be treated prior to conception (Atrash, Jack,

& Johnson, 2008; Bombard, Robbins, Dietz, & Valderrama, 2013). Based on this evidence, it is often deemed prudent for women and their partners to engage in healthier behaviours even before becoming pregnant, so that the full length of the pregnancy is conducive to fetal health. Men are often invoked in these definitions in their role as future fathers, since sperm fitness and partner health are important determinants of pregnancy achievement and perinatal outcomes. The Centers for Disease Control in the United States defines preconception care this way:

> [Preconception care is] a set of interventions that aim to identify and modify biomedical, behavioural, and social risks to a woman's health or pregnancy outcome through prevention and management, emphasizing those factors that must be acted on before conception or early in pregnancy to have maximal impact. (quoted in Posner, Johnson, Parker, Atrash, & Biermann, 2006, p. S198)

In a similar vein, some define preconception care simply as "the identification of those conditions that could affect a future pregnancy or fetus and that may be amenable to intervention" (Morgan, Hawks, Zinberg, & Schulkin, 2006, p. S59). Operating in these definitions is an assumption that health promotion consists of providing information, which any would-be parents who care about their future children's health will effortlessly convert into action. Women in particular are construed as unencumbered agents who can and will do anything to secure their children's health; those who fail to do so are simply insufficiently informed or, worse, "bad mothers." This message is consistent with the prenatal care messages that invoke babies' interests to provoke women into changing their behaviour during pregnancy. These types of prenatal messages quickly stigmatize women who are unable to stop drinking, smoking, or using other substances during pregnancy, and may deter them from seeking treatment by implying that changing is a simple choice (Greaves & Poole, 2005; Poole & Isaac, 2001). As Wise (2008) observes, this approach "has helped to generate a tragically counterproductive public rage at childbearing women, often minority women, who fall into one of these high-risk behavioural groupings" (p. S15). Preconception care messages that extend the logic of conventional prenatal care approaches are likely to be gender-regressive, not to mention ineffective. The emphasis on the mother's individual responsibility for changing herself, as well as the exclusive focus on fetal and infant health, has been criticized for being anti-woman, hetero-normative, and "pronatalist" (Moos, 2010; Wade, 2011).

In contrast to these views of preconception, there is a second category of definitions that emphasizes the woman's health and the importance of incorporating reproductive health and planning into routine care. This approach carefully avoids treating the woman as simply a vessel for a future baby and instead recognizes her as an autonomous reproductive agent:

> Preconception care is not something new being added to the already overburdened primary care provider, but a part of routine primary care for women of reproductive age, and much of preconception care merely involves the provider reframing his or her thinking, counselling, and decisions in light of the reproductive plans and sexual and contraceptive practices of the patient. (Atrash, Jack, & Johnson, 2008, p. 586)

This definition makes no mention of pregnancy outcomes or fetal health specifically, but acknowledges that fertile women, including lesbians, need comprehensive health care that takes into account their reproductive plans and capacities. Women may choose not to become pregnant or be at very low risk of pregnancy but still require care that supports the health of their whole bodies. Atrash et al. (2008) also note that "for women who do not desire pregnancy, a preconception care program can reduce personal health risks and the risk of an unwanted pregnancy" (p. S261). Furthermore, unlike most definitions of the first type, this category does not assume that women have a stable (male) partner who will father her future children or that all men are potential biological fathers.

As Moos (2010) argues, preconception care should benefit the woman's health first and, should she become pregnant, "the benefits are expanded" (p. 263). Clearly this is the approach that is most aligned with the principle of gender-transformative health promotion for women. In the remainder of this chapter, we will outline existing efforts to mainstream preconception health, address the challenges involved, and point to positive examples of preconception health promotion that incorporate the principles of the gender-transformative health promotion framework.

The Current Context of Preconception in Canada

Canada does not have current national guidelines regarding preconception care, although there have been several efforts at a variety of levels to standardize and promote preconception health. Some of these efforts reprise the shaming tendencies of most prenatal health promotion, but overall there are encouraging signs of woman-centredness. At the national level, the Society of Obstetricians and Gynaecologists of Canada (SOGC) does not have a clinical practice guideline for preconception care, but it published *Healthy Beginnings*, a book that covers preconception to postpartum. The Public Health Agency of Canada (PHAC) published preconception guidelines in 2000 in a resource that advocates that "preconception care and education be incorporated into school curricula and the workplace, delivered through the media, and offered through community-based agencies" (Public Health Agency of Canada, 2000). It takes a diversity-sensitive, non-judgmental approach to family planning and preconception care, detailing the risks of smoking in particular while acknowledging that "women who are contemplating pregnancy and smoke are caught in a very real dilemma" (ibid.). The document also provides specific guidelines for health care providers on preconception screening. However, it is not evident that the SOGC or PHAC recommendations have been taken up in any systematic way.

Several preconception initiatives have taken place at the provincial level. Best Start Resource Centre released a trio of reports in 2009 on preconception health in Ontario following surveys of physicians, public health units, and the public (Best Start Resource Centre, 2009a, 2009b, 2009c). It found that most public health units (88 percent) had implemented at least one preconception initiative in the past five years (Best Start Resource Centre, 2009b). The initiatives broke down into: 75 percent resource distribution, 53 percent resource development, 47 percent information sessions, 47 percent awareness campaigns, 44 percent media strategies, 44 percent displays, 22 percent research, and 28 percent others (Best Start Resource Centre, 2009b). However, the report did not specify the criteria used to assess whether an initiative was directed at preconception and how the respondents understood the research question. The survey of family physicians found that 78.4 percent claimed to deliver preconception care at least weekly, and only 1.6 percent never provided it (Best Start Resource Centre, 2009a). Conversely, 58 percent of women and men surveyed in the same series claimed their health care provider had not brought up the topic of preconception health (Best Start Resource Centre, 2009c). There appears to be a lack of clarity and communication between family physicians and the public about what preconception care consists of and why it is necessary.

The images and words chosen in these campaigns show attentiveness to shared responsibility for health and a desire to avoid hetero-normativity, and attempt to address the needs of particular subgroups of Canadian women, such as Aboriginal women, in a culturally appropriate way. For example, the brochure for men includes information about paternal health as it influences conception and fetal health, and also encourages men to consider whether they are ready to become fathers (Best Start Resource Centre, 2012). Compared to health promotion campaigns that have saddled women with all the biological and social responsibility of parenthood, this constitutes an improvement. While lesbian mothers are never mentioned directly, at least one picture in one campaign features two women who appear to be a couple.

Preconception interventions have also been undertaken in other provinces, but evaluation of their effects is not available. Overall these efforts are disparate, inconsistent, and informed to a great extent by guidelines for prenatal health promotion and the first type of definition of preconception health. In short, Canada does not yet have a coordinated national mandate to promote preconception health, nor a unified vision of what this means. National preconception guidelines exist in the United States, where the Centers for Disease Control (CDC) released a comprehensive report on preconception health and care in 2006 that detailed 10 recommendations that everyone in the health care sector can refer to (Johnson et al., 2006; Lu, 2007). Since the publication of the CDC guidelines, a number of federally funded efforts have resulted in preconception programs in specific cities, targeting populations who are most vulnerable to poor maternal and newborn outcomes and least likely to have access to prenatal care (Thompson, Peck, & Brandert, 2008). Although the CDC's definition of preconception is relatively narrow, it has enabled some gender-transformative practices to emerge at the grassroots level. Several of these interventions are reviewed in the final section of this chapter.

Challenges of Creating Effective Health Promotion for Preconception

There is little evidence available on the impact of preconception health campaigns to date. All the Canadian efforts described have centred on awareness-raising and the distribution of information in the form of public posters/brochures, websites, and recommendations to physicians. The effectiveness of such interventions is difficult to evaluate because they do not track particular individuals over time, nor can they control for any other factors that may influence one's knowledge of and receptiveness to preconception health. Such brochures and websites rely on the individual reading the information to process it and initiate personal change. As has been identified in Motivational Interviewing practice, providing individuals with clear instructions does not necessarily empower them to improve their health (Rollnick, Miller, & Butler, 2008). This may be especially true for those who are marginalized and have less control over their circumstances, including women with low income, Aboriginals, young mothers, women in abusive relationships, recent immigrants, and non-English or non-French speakers (Harelick, Viola, & Tahara, 2011; Roberts & Pies, 2011). In fact, although some groups of people may benefit from health promotion based in awareness-raising, this approach may actually exacerbate the inequality between women who have the best reproductive outcomes and those who have the worst, condemning women in certain groups to further exclusion. When the realities of poverty, racism, violence against women, and addictions and mental health are taken into account, there is an urgent need to find creative ways of improving reproductive and perinatal health within the constraints of complex forms of deprivation and disadvantage. Women who have the time, money, social capital, and background health to respond to new information may incorporate changes such as taking a folic acid supplement relatively effortlessly, while women who are isolated and disempowered could find this a very real challenge.

In the case of improving preconception health, as in other health issues, the individual ability to effect change is also tied to a greater or lesser extent to the availability of appropriate health and social services. Preconception health requires preconception care. As long as health promotion takes the form of campaigns without corresponding enhancements in service and accessibility, the recommendations are unlikely to be heeded consistently. Preconception care needs to be embedded in well-woman care, rather than added as a separate encounter with the health system or divorced from women's health entirely. Women are not very likely to schedule and undergo tests for sexually transmitted infections and hypertension prior to conception, much less to spontaneously quit drinking and smoking. But if discussions of these issues are part of an ongoing care program with all the requisite non-judgmental supports, initiatives to incorporate elements of preconception health are more likely to be integrated into women's life plans. Preconception health promotion, then, is not only the domain of obstetricians and health promotion agencies, but of family physicians, nurses, midwives, and other care providers who treat women throughout their reproductive years (Bialystok, Greaves, & Poole, 2013; Carl & Hill, 2009; Files, David, & Frey, 2008). The provision of women-centred care and the promotion of preconception health are inseparable.

Another related challenge in the effective delivery of preconception health care is to distinguish it appropriately from other forms of care, such as prenatal, contraceptive, and perinatal, without losing the important continuity between these stages in a woman's reproductive life cycle. The correct balance is difficult to achieve, but imperative if we are to avoid confounding women's various needs. If the focus is too heavily on health prior to conception, there is the risk of treating women as persistently "pre-pregnant," even if they have no plans to conceive. Yet if the focus is too heavily on contraception and sexual health, important opportunities for conception-related health promotion may be missed. In practice such matters are often addressed all at once, especially if women are not able to see a family doctor regularly.

In light of these challenges to the effective and appropriate promotion of preconception health, several conclusions emerge. First, the awareness-building approaches that have formed most of the organized preconception interventions to date are at best a small component of a larger task. Health promotion techniques that offload responsibility onto individuals by calling for behavioural changes are most likely to be effective with those who are already privileged, healthy, literate, and well informed, and these are the individuals who arguably need it the least. Second, health care professionals and policy-makers are integral to the coordinated implementation of preconception care because individuals must have somewhere to turn when they are ready to address health needs prior to pregnancy. Health promotion and health care need to be equally accessible and mutually reinforcing. Third, while it is crucial to start with a conceptual understanding of preconception that differentiates it from prenatal and contraceptive care, the exact components and priorities within preconception care must be tailored to the needs of individual women and groups of women. Interventions will be most successful if they are to some extent top-down (in the form of, for example, national guidelines and provincial resources) as well as bottom-up, located in particular communities and developed with an awareness of specific circumstances (Prochaska, Mauriello, Dyment, & Gökbayrak, 2011).

The principles of gender-transformative health promotion are perfect guidelines to responding to these challenges. In particular, preconception health is best enabled by approaches that are culturally sensitive, adaptive, tailored, harm reduction–oriented, integrative, equity-oriented, intersectional, and strengths-based. Encouraging examples of these approaches are already underway.

Promising Practices: Improving Preconception Health and Empowering Women

The CDC preconception guidelines and associated resources have enabled a variety of programs in the United States to promote preconception health in locally relevant ways. Some of the highlights of these efforts are reported in a special issue of *American Journal of Health Promotion*. Selected examples are grouped here according to the gender-transformative principles they most exemplify.

Culturally Safe and Relevant

Cultural relevance is paramount both in the content of health promotion messages and in their delivery mechanisms. In Oregon, a preconception health program is attending to the needs of Latinas, this time by experimenting with the health promotion medium. *Amor y Salud* (Love and Health) is the title of a preconception health campaign that used the popular Spanish radio soap opera (*radionovela*) format to deliver preconception messages to Latina women (Dixon-Gray Mobley, McFarlane, & Rosenberg, 2013). Instead of stacking pamphlets in doctors' offices, this program used familiar communication devices to convey important health information in the women's own language. Women were able to access *Amor y Salud* through radio, Facebook, and MySpace (Dixon-Gray et al., 2013). Although there were impediments to the systematic evaluation of the intervention, the researchers concluded that it is possible to design culturally specific, community-informed, low-cost preconception messages that will reach a large population; for about $31,000, the *radionovela* episodes were played on the radio over 2,000 times, and the Facebook page was viewed 11,000 times (Dixon-Gray et al., 2013).

Adaptive and Tailored

While the need for individualized, patient-centred care is well recognized and has been shown to be effective in providing preconception care to vulnerable women (Biermann, Dunlop, Brady, Dubin, & Brann, 2006), there are numerous obstacles to providing all women with preconception care that is sufficiently tailored, timely, and meaningful. Increasingly, health information technology is being devised to meet these types of gaps in the health care system and to enhance health promotion. In order to meet the needs of more women, a team of preconception researchers have designed a technology-based "virtual patient advocate" (VPA), known as "Gabby," to help screen and advise women on preconception health (Gardiner et al., 2013). The technology allows women to move at their own pace through different stages of assessment, health education, and creation of a "My Health to-Do List," by clicking on the answers that best represent their response to the VPA, as in a real conversation. The information and order of questions is not fixed but rather tailored to the user based on her input. "Gabby" is a computer-generated image of a woman (focus groups helped researchers to determine her appearance and name) who "emulates the face-to-face conversational behavior of an empathic clinician, including nonverbal communicative behavior such as gaze, posture, and hand gestures" (Gardiner et al., 2013, p. eS12). Evaluation of the Gabby approach suggests that health information technology has the potential to not only boost women's knowledge about preconception risks, but also to appropriately scaffold action plans that result in positive changes to their health.

Harm Reduction–Oriented

Researchers and health care providers working with highly vulnerable women repeatedly find that their intended messages about preconception are dwarfed by more urgent needs (Handler et al., 2013). In light of the overlapping health and social needs of marginalized women, it is unrealistic to expect all preconception programs to achieve the kinds of improvements that depend on multiple support systems. Hence the primary goal of preconception health promotion is sometimes to reduce the harms that are most amenable to improvement and clear the way for more thorough treatment of others. For example, in one intervention directed at American Indian women of the Northern Plains who have a higher risk of having a child with fetal alcohol spectrum disorder, the goal was to reduce binge drinking and/or to improve contraception so that binge drinkers would be less likely to conceive (Hanson, Miller, Winberg, & Elliott, 2013). The rationale was that preconception care in a highly vulnerable population must begin with better contraception, which can buy time for health issues to be addressed before conception becomes a factor. The intervention did not have an impact on binge drinking levels, but it was successful in the goal of delaying pregnancy; participants were using contraception more consistently within three months of the start of the program (Hanson et al., 2013).

Integrative

Harm reduction in this context can also mean pausing reproductive health interventions temporarily in order to help women secure more fundamental (or what they perceive to be more fundamental) needs. Integrative health promotion recognizes that health is inseparable from necessities such as personal safety, stable housing, and employment, without which improvements in preconception health are unlikely to materialize. In one program piloted in Chicago for African-American women with a history of low birth weight and infant mortality, women in the program mostly perceived themselves to be healthy and could not find time in their stressful lives for preventative medicine, despite having high rates of hypertension, acute infections, and other health problems (Handler et al., 2013). They were in a constant need of triaging, and program staff found that "participants, even if fully intent on keeping an appointment, frequently changed their plans at the last minute to respond to other pressing needs" (Handler et al., 2013, p. eS28). The program provided both a physician and case managers for each participant to develop individual needs assessments and integrate social and medical services. The results confirmed that preconception programs cannot impose a view of which needs are most critical for a certain population or for individual women. As the authors explain, "[Interconception care] should not be thought of so much as a prescription, but rather as a complex process of matching interventions and services to meet women's unique needs" (Handler et al., 2013, p. eS30). An integrative approach therefore must be paired with adaptive, women-centred approaches based upon listening to women rather than imposing priorities or health messages on them. Over time, the expected improvements will be apparent not only in perinatal health outcomes but also in women's social stability and overall empowerment.

Equity-Oriented, Intersectional

Several other studies have found that the effectiveness of preconception health promotion is hampered by the impacts of racism, which has a particularly detrimental effect on health and is of course highly correlated with other forms of oppression (Hogan et al., 2013). For example, African-American women have less access to prenatal care than white women, have higher rates of infant mortality, and are almost twice as likely to have preterm births (Handler et al., 2013; Hogan et al., 2013). These inequities are then compounded by the intersection of race and poverty, "resulting in the disproportionate burden of having to care for high-need children in an environment that is already resource poor" (Hogan et al., 2013, p. eS40). When racialized women access medical services, stereotypes and latent prejudices can affect the quality of care they receive. Gender-transformative health promotion must attend to how women's experiences are affected by racism and other forms of discrimination. Such correlations may be especially salient in the context of preconception health promotion because of stereotypes about women's reproductive habits and family structure in different racial and ethnic communities. In order to qualify as gender-transformative, health promotion efforts must listen to women's individuals needs and work with them to define personal and familial goals rather than making assumptions on the basis of race or other factors.

Strengths-Based

Because it is difficult both on the health system and on individual women to address preconception care in designated medical visits, some health practitioners have found ways to build on existing opportunities to reach women when they access other services. This "piggybacking" is a more efficient and woman-centred way to promote preconception health among some of the neediest women.

A prime example of this strategy is a program that added individualized preconception risk assessment and brief counselling to a mandatory nutrition class for poor women receiving a government-funded nutritional supplement (Special Supplemental Nutrition Program for Women, Infants, and Children, or WIC). Wait times at WIC clinics are notoriously long, a fact that was creatively converted into an opportunity for additional service provision in the Georgia program. The results were very promising: "Nearly all of the participants, 148 (98.7%), reported that the reproductive health risk assessment and counseling received during the encounter was important to them" (Dunlop, Dretler, Badal, & Logue, 2013, p. S63). The effectiveness of bundling services was enhanced by the individualized, woman-centred approach taken by the preconception counsellors. The participants were highly responsive to the face-to-face interaction and tailored provision of information (Dunlop et al., 2013). For women who are regularly stigmatized and underserved, this unexpected attention was not only effective, but empowering. As one participant explained, "I feel like I'm important, like I matter, even though

I'm using WIC and some people, they talk bad about the people that use WIC or use public assistance. But it's good to know you have a voice" (Participant W099) (Dunlop et al., 2013, p. S64).

Other studies have confirmed that piggybacking on existing opportunities, even by adding brief interventions, can measurably improve knowledge of preconception risks and health care. One study found that brief targeted interventions at publicly funded primary care clinics produced "a significant increase in knowledge related to preconception health from baseline to 3 to 6 months post-encounter, including recognition of the importance of folic acid supplementation, seeking medical care for chronic conditions, and review of medication" (Dunlop, Logue, Thorne, & Badal, 2013, p. S50).

However, obstacles such as rigid billing codes, even in publically paid health care systems, can prevent this type of additive counselling or integrated care. For example, some medical practitioners in Canada restrict health visits to "one issue" to confine the range of the visit and expand their billing purview, practices that counter the development of this woman-centred integrative approach. Health promoters need to move beyond distributing pamphlets and do a better job of meeting women where they are by building on the strengths of women themselves, reframing existing resources, and maximizing opportunities for service integration.

Conclusion

Although the health care system and population in the United States have their own characteristics, some lessons from the American context may be applicable elsewhere. In the United States some preconception programs have yielded positive outcomes by employing principles of gender-transformative health promotion and building on best practices derived from other forms of health care. The existence of national guidelines and associated funding has also been critical in enabling this progress, and would presumably have the same effects in Canada and other countries. In order to address serious concerns about perinatal outcomes, and to do so without stigmatizing and shaming women, coordinated efforts at a variety of levels are needed. Health promoters can play a critical role by developing and insisting on preconception interventions that are responsive to women's complex needs, not to decontextualized notions of individual responsibility.

REFERENCES

Adams, E. K., Kenney, G. M., & Galactionova, K. (2013). Preventive and reproductive health services for women: The role of California's family planning waiver. *American Journal of Health Promotion, 27*(Supp. 3), eS1–eS10.

Atrash, H., Jack, B. W., & Johnson, K. (2008). Preconception care: A 2008 update. *Current Opinion in Obstetrics and Gynaecology, 20*(6), 581–589.

Atrash, H., Jack, B. W., Johnsen, K., Coonrod, D. V., Moos, H.-K., Stubblefield, R. C., Damus, K., & Reddy, U. M. (2008) Where is the "W"oman in MCH? *American Journal of Obstetrics and Gynecology, 199*(6), S259–S265.

Best Start Resource Centre. (2009a). *Preconception health: Awareness and behaviours in Ontario.* Toronto: Author.

Best Start Resource Centre. (2009b). *Preconception health: Physician practices in Ontario.* Toronto: Author.

Best Start Resource Centre. (2009c). *Preconception health: Public health initiatives in Ontario.* Toronto: Author.

Best Start Resource Centre. (2012). *How to build a healthy baby: Men's information.* Toronto: Health Nexus.

Bialystok, L., Greaves, L., & Poole, N. (2013). Preconception care: A call for national guidelines. *Canadian Family Physician, 59,* e435–e437.

Biermann, J., Dunlop, A., Brady, C., Dubin, C., & Brann, A. (2006). Promising practices in preconception care for women at risk for poor health and pregnancy outcomes. *Maternal and Child Health Journal, 10*(Supp. 5), S21–S28.

Bombard, J. M., Robbins, C. L., Dietz, P. M., & Valderrama, A. L. (2013). Preconception care: The perfect opportunity for health care providers to advise lifestyle changes for hypertensive women. *American Journal of Health Promotion, 27*(Supp. 3), S43–S49.

Carl, J., & Hill, D. A. (2009). Preconception counseling: Make it part of the annual exam. *Journal of Family Practice, 58*(6), 307–314.

Chamberlain, G. (1980). The prepregnancy clinic. *British Medical Journal, 281*(6232), 29–30.

Curtis, M., Abelman, S., Schulkin, J., Williams, J., & Fassett, E. (2006). Do we practice what we preach? A review of actual clinical practice with regards to preconception care guidelines. *Maternal and Child Health Journal, 10*(1), 53–58.

Dixon-Gray, L. A., Mobley, A., McFarlane, J. M., & Rosenberg, K. D. (2013). *Amor y Salud* (Love and Health): A preconception health campaign for second-generation Latinas in Oregon. *American Journal of Health Promotion, 27*(Supp. 3), S74–S76.

Dunlop, A. L., Dretler, A. W., Badal, H. J., & Logue, K. M. (2013). Acceptability and potential impact of brief preconception health risk assessment and counseling in the WIC setting. *American Journal of Health Promotion, 27*(Supp. 3), S58–S65.

Dunlop, A. L., Logue, K. M., Thorne, C., & Badal, H. J. (2013). Change in women's knowledge of general and personal preconception health risks following targeted brief counseling in publicly funded primary care settings. *American Journal of Health Promotion, 27*(Supp. 3), S50–S57.

Files, J. A., David, P. S., & Frey, K. A. (2008). The patient-centered medical home and preconception care: An opportunity for internists. *Journal of General Internal Medicine, 23*(9), 1518–1520.

Finer, L. B., & Henshaw, S. K. (2006). Disparities in rates of unintended pregnancy in the United States, 1994 and 2001. *Perspectives on Sexual and Reproductive Health, 38*(2), 90–96.

Fleming, M. F., Lund, M. R., Wilton, G., Landry, M., & Scheets, D. (2008). The healthy mom's study: The efficacy of brief alcohol intervention in postpartum women. *Alcoholism: Clinical & Experimental Research, 32*(9), 1600–1606.

Gardiner, P., Hempstead, M. B., Ring, L., Bickmore, T., Yinusa-Nyahkoon, L., Tran, H., ... Jack, B. (2013). Reaching women through health information technology: The Gabby preconception care system. *American Journal of Health Promotion, 27*(Supp. 3), eS11–eS20.

Greaves, L., & Poole, N. (2005). Victimized or validated? Responses to substance-using pregnant women. *Canadian Women's Studies Journal, 24*(1), 87–92.

Greaves, L., Poole, N., Okoli, C. T. C., Hemsing, N., Qu, A., Bialystok, L., & O'Leary, R. (2011). *Expecting to quit: A best practices review of smoking cessation interventions for pregnant and postpartum girls and women* (2nd ed.). Vancouver: British Columbia Centre of Excellence for Women's Health and Health Canada.

Handler, A., Rankin, K., Peacock, N., Townsell, S., McGlynn, A., & Issel, M. (2013). The implementation of interconception care in two community health settings: Lessons learned. *American Journal of Health Promotion, 27*(Supp. 3), eS21–eS31.

Hanson, J. D., Miller, A. L., Winberg, A., & Elliott, A. J. (2013). Prevention of alcohol-exposed pregnancies among nonpregnant American Indian women. *American Journal of Health Promotion, 27*(Supp. 3), S66–S73.

Harelick, L., Viola, D., & Tahara, D. (2011). Preconception health of low socioeconomic status women: Assessing knowledge and behaviors. *Women's Health Issues, 21*(4), 272–276.

Hogan, V. K., Culhane, J. F., Crews, K. J., Mwaria, C. B., Rowley, D. L., Levenstein, L., & Mullings, L. P. (2013). The impact of social disadvantage on preconception health, illness, and well-being: An intersectional analysis. *American Journal of Health Promotion, 27*(Supp. 3), eS33–eS42.

Institute of Medicine, Committee to Study the Prevention of Low Birth Weight. (1985). *Preventing low birth weight.* Washington, DC: National Academy Press.

Johnson, K., Posner, S. F., Biermann, J., Cordero, J. F., Atrash, H. K., Parker, C. S., ... & Curtis, M. G. (2006). *Recommendations to improve preconception health and health care: A report of the CDC/ATSDR Preconception Care Work Group and the Selected Panel on Preconception Care.* Atlanta: Morbidity and Mortality Weekly Report, Centres of Disease Control and Prevention.

Lu, M. C. (2007). Recommendations for preconception care. *American Family Physician, 76*(3), 397–400.

Martin, J. A., Hamilton, B. E., Sutton, P. D., Ventura, S. A., Menacker, F., & Kirmeyer, S. (2006). *Births: Final data for 2004: National vital statistics reports.* Hyattsville, MD: National Center for Health Statistics.

Moos, M.-K. (2010). *What are the challenges and knowledge gaps for implementing preconception health?* Paper presented at the 1st European Congress Preconception Care and Preconception Health, Brussels.

Morgan, M. A., Hawks, D., Zinberg, S., & Schulkin, J. (2006). What obstetrician-gyne-cologists think of preconception care. *Maternal and Child Health Journal, 10*(S1): S59–S65.

Ohlsson, A., & Shah, P. (2008). *Determinants and prevention of low birth weight: A synopsis of the evidence.* Edmonton: Institute of Health Economics.

Poole, N., & Isaac, B. (2001). *Apprehensions: Barriers to treatment for substance-using mothers.* Vancouver: British Columbia Centre of Excellence for Women's Health.

Posner, S., Johnson, K., Parker, C., Atrash, H., & Biermann, J. (2006). The national summit on preconception care: A summary of concepts and recommendations. *Maternal and Child Health Journal, 10*(Supp. 5), S199–S207.

Prochaska, J. M., Mauriello, L., Dyment, S., & Gökbayrak, S. (2011). Designing a health behavior change program for dissemination to underserved pregnant women. *Public Health Nursing, 28*(6), 548–555.

Public Health Agency of Canada. (2000). *Preconception care, family-centred maternity, and newborn care: National guidelines.* Ottawa: Author.

Public Health Agency of Canada. (2009). *What mothers say: The Canadian maternity experiences survey.* Ottawa: Author.

Roberts, S. C. M., & Pies, C. (2011). Complex calculations: How drug use during pregnancy becomes a barrier to prenatal care. *Maternal and Child Health Journal, 15*(3), 333–341.

Rollnick, S., Miller, W. R., & Butler, C. C. (2008). *Motivational interviewing in health care.* New York: Guilford Press.

Thompson, B. K., Peck, M., & Brandert, K. T. (2008). Integrating preconception health into public health practice: A tale of three cities. *Journal of Women's Health, 17*(5), 723–727.

Wade, L. (2011). Pre-conception care: Good for babies, bad for women? *The Society Pages.* Retrieved from http://thesocietypages.org/socimages/2011/02/03/pre-conception-care-good-for-babies-bad-for-women.

Wise, P. H. (2008). Transforming preconceptional, prenatal, and interconceptional care into a comprehensive commitment to women's health. *Women's Health Issues, 18*(6), S13–S18.

PART 3

11 Provoking Gender-Transformative Health Promotion

Nancy Poole, Judie Bopp, and Lorraine Greaves

Introduction: The Challenge

Gender-transformative health promotion provokes us to engage with broad concepts of health, social determinants of health, health promotion, gender, and individual and system change. This engagement involves consideration of past approaches to health promotion, analysis of current data and context, applying additional lenses, and imagining forward to ways of working differently. Collective reflective and action-oriented processes are called for.

As described in Chapter 1, in developing the gender-transformative health promotion framework, we led wide engagement and exchange processes. Key informants engaged with our research team through telephone interviews, face-to-face consultations, web meetings, and e-survey mechanisms that helped us to revise and expand the framework. At the same time as engaging with the framework concepts, participants in the consultation processes stressed the importance of making the application of the framework practical for all those prepared to implement gender-transformative health promotion. Indeed, a key suggestion from an early consultation (Melbourne, Australia, in April 2012) was to solicit more input on the usability, applicability, and feasibility of the framework to develop and implement gender-transformative health promotion approaches in health promotion practice.

Key informants identified the knowledge translation challenge (and potential) in several ways:

> In our area, mainstream services struggle to understand the concept of gender and how it affects health and well-being. This framework could be used as a basis for training/capacity building for health promotion practitioners.

They also said:

> But we need to steer [practitioners] in some way, so they do get to say, you know, that there is actually a body of work on women and tobacco, or, you know, maternity care that isn't just about women as vectors, or ... whatever it is that we're trying to do in health promotion. Just so that it's encouraging and enabling. Otherwise, it could be quite daunting, I think.

Our consultative process was in alignment with established feminist principles of inclusion and of iterative processes that move from practice, to theory, to practice, and so on. To make the framework accessible to policy-makers, health care practitioners, researchers, communities, and women, we will again need to utilize mechanisms that support collective discussion and action on the framework, as well as practical tools for its application.

Building on Successful Engagement Methods from the Women's Movement

In the late 1960s and early 1970s, feminists pioneered facilitation processes that elicited evidence from women's lived experience to promote social change in the form of consciousness-raising (CR) groups (Poole, 2008; Shreve, 1989). The CR format for exchange, co-construction of knowledge, and activism involved women from all walks of life. The CR model usually involved a three-stage process of sharing, analysis, and action planning. The first step was to gather group members' experiences on a particular theme. Building from the sharing of each member's experience, the groups discussed the common elements in these experiences and how they related to the overall context of women's lives. CR was pivotal in crystallizing ideas, encouraging conscientization, inspiring action, and generating a social movement.

Keating (2005) describes the pedagogic and movement-building contributions of this initial CR process as providing a model for creating knowledge and theory in a participatory and collective manner, and proposes "coalitional consciousness building" as a contemporary CR model to engender awareness and solidarity across multiple lines of difference. Such a model of coalitional consciousness-building can bridge various forms of knowledge and wisdom arising from policy, practice, research, and direct experience of health issues. This model has relevance in examining the contexts of women's health, the multiple relations of oppressions and resistance at play (as outlined in the framework), and the possibilities for coalitional action on the experiences and knowledge that have been collectively shared and synthesized.

A currently operating example of coalitional consciousness-building is being employed by the Repairing the Holes in the Net research project,[1] which uses communities of practice (CoPs) as primary tools for stimulating gender-transformative improvements in the policy and service systems designed to address key facets of the determinants underlying women's homelessness and its attendant mental and physical health issues in northern Canada. In this project, CoPs in the three northern Canadian territories bring researchers, policy-makers, and frontline service providers together around a shared commitment to learn how to provide better outcomes for homeless women.

This approach draws participants into an iterative cycle of reflection, learning, planning, and action. Learning occurs as the knowledge and experience brought by those present is shared, as well as from literature and case studies from around the world and the new knowledge generated by the interviews conducted with service users and providers as part of the research study. CoP participants regularly reflect on the implications of what is learned for improving individual and collective practice as they discuss and formulate plans for the next steps for shifting policy and service delivery practice. As dialogue and planning are transformed into some form of action, undertaken collaboratively or by individuals within the context of their own agencies, intervention theories are tested and a new cycle of reflection, learning, and planning begins.

The communities of practice in the Repairing the Holes in the Net project, all of which are engaged in shifting systems that currently trap women in cycles of life crises, homelessness, and mental and physical health challenges, have consciously chosen to adopt a number of lenses for conceptualizing the challenges and emerging solutions. These include:

Gender: This was first aimed at enhancing gender sensitivity and developing gender-specific programs and approaches, but ultimately to stimulate gender-transformative innovations that challenge the current structures, attitudes, and practices that place women at such great risk for homelessness. These intolerable circumstances are described in *You Just Blink and It Can Happen: A Study of Women's Homelessness North of 60 Report* (Bopp et al., 2007) and have clear roots in societal attitudes and systems that marginalize, punish, and disadvantage women in so many ways.

Trauma: This lens is aimed at incorporating a deeper understanding of the impact of trauma on the lives of women who experience housing and mental health issues, and to incorporate it in policy and program initiatives at all levels and across sectors. These sites include primary health care, mental health, addictions, child and family protection, income support, policing and justice, and, if trauma-informed—that is, receptive to and safe for all—would create service environments that emphasize safety, choice, and agency for women.

Health promotion: This lens incorporates consideration of the broad range of determinants that contribute to women's homelessness and mental health challenges. These include (but are not limited to) poverty, domestic violence, addictions, a severe shortage of housing, weak social networks, and punitive and inadequate services.

Aboriginal cultural perspectives: This lens links efforts to address mental health issues to a larger political and social policy agenda of decolonization; introduces a focus on wellness rather than on addressing symptoms; offers services from a context-specific, strength-based, and trauma-informed perspective; and incorporates traditional medicines and cultural teachings.

The research findings from interviews and focus group sessions with service users and service providers in Whitehorse, Yellowknife, and Iqaluit, three main cities in Canada's North, are being compiled. These three territorial communities of practice are refining their action plans for a collaborative initiative aimed at shifting the service and policy environment related to addressing the mental health needs of homeless and at-risk women. Although it is far from clear where this path will lead, the participants in the Repairing the Holes in the Net initiative have built a collaborative culture and a focus on learning their way into improved health, social, and economic outcomes for the women of Canada's North.

It is approaches such as this—involving researchers, decision-makers, health providers, and women's health advocates—that are needed to effectively plan gender-transformative health promotion endeavours. A collaborative, multi-sectoral approach that embeds all these stakeholders in interactive and egalitarian contexts, respects different ways of knowing, and supports reciprocal learning will be transformative.

Getting Practical

Bringing Gender-Based Analysis and Action into a Health Promotion Planning Tool

To support implementation of gender-transformative health promotion, the research team envisaged a collective planning process that

- begins with engagement of multi-sectoral stakeholders;
- analyzes the diverse forms of evidence they bring to the table through a gender, sex, and diversity lens;
- reviews existing health promotion practice by critically examining gendered beliefs and discriminatory practices;
- identifies ways to improve women's health and change harmful gender norms, roles, and relations in the intervention; and
- leads to implementation of interventions that improve women's health and encourages equitable roles for women, as well as access to and control over resources.

Such gender-transformative health promotion efforts can be evaluated against the goals of promoting gender and health equity, and reported on in ways that lead to further engagement, collective analysis, and planning (see Figure 11.1).

Elements That Distinguish This Gender-Transformative Health Promotion Planning Tool

This tool acknowledges and values the various perspectives that health promotion practitioners and planners may have out of a concern for improving health outcomes for certain populations of women or for women in particular settings, or because they want to act on certain health issues that may be more prevalent, are changing in prevalence, be more serious, have gender-specific risk factors, or be uniquely experienced by girls and women (Poland, Krupa, & McCall, 2009). At the centre of the diagram are some core questions that may support bringing a gender lens and a gender-transformative lens to this work.

For example, health promoters may be considering interventions that address the needs of certain populations of girls and women, such as girls who are facing pressures to drink alcohol, and who are inundated with alcohol advertisements for coolers and "bikini-friendly" beers (Gammon, 2013) that promise health, low caloric content, and sexual prowess (Jernigan, Ostroff, Ross, & O'Hara, 2004; Kilbourne, 1999). Or health promoters may be considering interventions that address the multiple needs of Aboriginal women who are pregnant and who smoke—a recent Canadian study by Heaman and Chalmers (2005) found that 61.2 percent of pregnant Aboriginal women smoked compared to 26.2 percent of non-Aboriginal women. Aboriginal pregnant women who smoke are more likely to be young, single, low income, and less educated; use alcohol and illicit drugs; have inadequate prenatal care; suffer from physical abuse and violence; have low self-esteem, and lack social support.

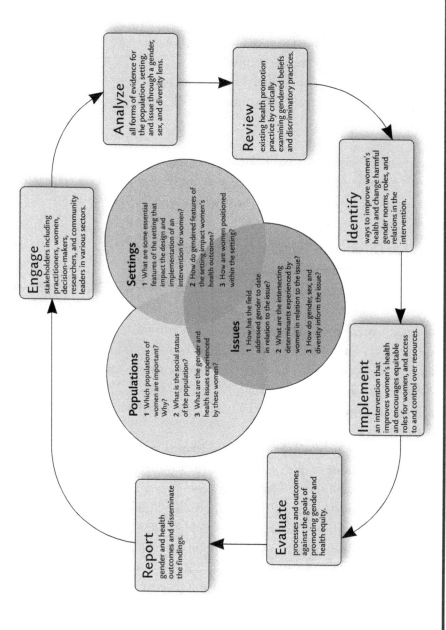

FIGURE 11.1: Creating Gender-Transformative Health Promotion Interventions for Women

Source: British Columbia Centre of Excellence for Women's Health.

Other examples of specific populations include younger women experiencing myocardial infarction or risk factors for cardiovascular disease (Chapter 7) or women planning to have children (Chapter 10). The planning tool poses specific questions related to populations (see the central circle in Figure 11.1), which facilitates intersectional analysis and supports a more complex approach to the analysis, review, and identification steps. These questions prompt a closer analysis of the "population" that highlights differential issues and needs among girls and women, and focuses health promotion planners on meaningful subtleties and inequities that matter. This approach leaves behind narrowly focused, gender-blind, and often paternalistic approaches that have often characterized health promotion efforts with such populations to date. These questions contribute to the development of more relevant and meaningful interventions and policies in health promotion for women.

Health promotion specialists, health system planners, and others interested in health promotion may sometimes be approaching gender-transformative health promotion from the location of a particular setting for enacting health promotion. For example, a setting offering assisted living care may be interested in encouraging older women with arthritis and osteoporosis to exercise; a hospital might offer mindfulness training for staff as they implement trauma-informed practice across the institution; a community centre might engage the local lesbian community in heart health awareness given their higher rate of obesity, smoking, and stress (Womenshealth.gov, 2011); or a prenatal program might start a walking program for new mothers. In this book, challenges related to gender-transformative approaches to health promotion in a range of settings such as workplaces (Chapter 9), supportive housing for women living in violent relationships (Chapter 8), and a women's hospital (Chapter 13) are considered. Questions from the tool designed to support reflection and action toward gender-transformative health promotion interventions by those working in such settings include the following:

- What are some essential features of the setting that impact the design and implementation of an intervention for women?
- How do the gendered features of the setting impact women's health outcomes?
- How are women positioned within the setting? (See the "Settings" circle in Figure 11.1.)

Such questions become particularly important to ask in settings such as the one described in Chapter 14 involving a male-dominated workplace in Australia engaged in promoting non-violence and gender equality. Asking these questions will focus health promotion designers and practitioners on the impact of gendered relations, roles, and the institutional expectations, specifically of women, regarding gender. Such questions will also highlight power differentials among women and between women and men in specific settings. All of these added inputs generate more information for tailoring health promotion more tightly and sensitively.

Health promotion specialists, health system planners, and others interested in health promotion may also be approaching gender-transformative health promotion from the perspective of work on a specific health issue that may be more prevalent in women, is increasing in prevalence, is more serious or unique to women, or has differing risk factors or associated risks for women. Conditions such as heart disease, diabetes, fibromyalgia, practices such as tobacco or alcohol use, or gendered conditions such as caregiving and/or overwork may all be issues through which gender-transformative health promotion may be achieved. For example, an innovative approach to heart health promotion (described in Chapter 7) was recently identified by women attending a clinic for pregnant women in Surrey, British Columbia, whose pregnancies are high risk due to substance use, exposure to violence, and poverty. They approached reducing their risk of heart problems through tobacco-reduction strategies that involved working in a paced, collaborative way tailored to individual women's needs (Urquhart, Jasuira, Poole, Greaves, & Nathoo, 2012). In doing so, they directly addressed the questions outlined in the "Issues" circle in Figure 11.1: What are the intersecting determinants experienced by women in relation to the issue? How do gender, sex, and diversity inform the issue? A key question is to assess the standard or typical approach to the issue and determine if it has addressed gender (or not). In Chapter 4, on tobacco, and Chapter 5, on alcohol use by women and girls, these kinds of questions form the foundation of analysis. The Surrey clinic approach went further and blended a complex analysis with women's input to expand the focus of substance-use interventions to include tobacco and then challenged traditional tobacco cessation-focused approaches to work from a harm-reduction stance. These actions point to the impact of the Review and Identify steps in the planning tool.

The Key Steps of Analyze, Review, and Identify

Analyze

Gender-transformative health promotion planning begins with engagement of multi-sectoral experts in girls' and women's health—women experiencing the health concerns being addressed, women's health advocates, practitioners, researchers, and decision-makers. This engagement supports the sharing of evidence and perspectives on evidence. This sharing is extended to the practice of sex-/gender-/ diversity-based analysis (SGDBA). Feminists and many global and national health organizations have practised and advocated for the use of SGDBA for decades, but it has yet to be adequately integrated in research and knowledge translation practice (Clow, Pederson, Haworth-Brockman, & Bernier, 2009). The Analysis step of the gender-transformative health promotion tool—as described in the previous section—becomes an avenue for expanding intersectional analysis and refining SGDBA skills.

Review

The proposed planning process both involves and goes beyond SGDBA. It also involves critical analysis of health promotion efforts to understand gendered assumptions and practices that fail to identify or address discriminatory barriers. In the case of the Repairing the Holes in the Net project on northern women's mental health and homelessness, this allowed for consideration of how to change barriers in income-support policies that do not allow women who are living in women's shelters to start jobs and receive income as they stabilize and make the transition from violent relationships and homelessness. Such policies, in addition to barriers such as housing shortages and the need for damage deposits, can result in another round of homelessness, lack of safety, and poor mental health for women in transition.

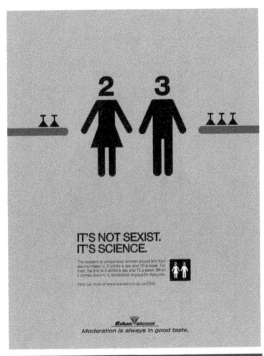

FIGURE 11.2: Poster Showing Sex-Specific Low-Risk Drinking Recommendations

Source: Éduc'alcool (http://educalcool.qc.ca/en).

Critical analysis of existing approaches may also address discriminatory practices such as those embedded in existing health promotion efforts related to alcohol, which appeal to gendered pressures to be thin by stressing the high caloric value of alcohol. Such approaches, beyond reinforcing unhealthy gender norms, can result in the "drunkorexia" phenomenon, whereby young women starve themselves and/or over-exercise during the day so that they may drink heavily in the evening (Beller, 2013). The posters shown here are designed to promote low-risk drinking. The stick figures with "2" and "3" as their heads (Figure 11.2) help-fully identify the differing low-risk drinking recommendations based on sex differences in the impact of alcohol on health. However, when designing these posters directed to young men and young women, the creators, unfortunately, reinforce gender stereotypes of men with interest in the workplace, and women with interest in dating relationships (Figure 11.3 and Figure 11.4).

Identify

The Identify step provokes collective creativity, aimed at identifying ways to improve women's health and change harmful gender norms, roles, and relations in an intervention. The poster from the Aboriginal Disability Network (Figure 11.5) illustrates gender-transformative health promotion and a conscious move from gender-blind/exploitative/accommodating approaches common to the field of prevention of alcohol use in pregnancy. It positions young men and young women sharing the responsibility for not drinking during pregnancy, a far cry from most pregnancy and alcohol material, which places the burden of responsibility squarely on women's shoulders, often with judgmental and demeaning messages. This gender-transformative health promotion message goes further to link the health of women during pregnancy with the health of their children and their cultural community.

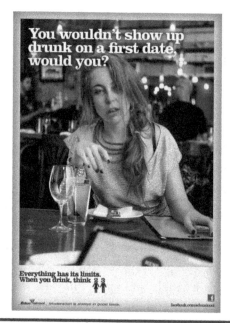

FIGURE 11.3: Éduc'alcool Student Campaign on Limiting Alcohol Consumption
Source: Éduc'alcool (http://educalcool.qc.ca/en).

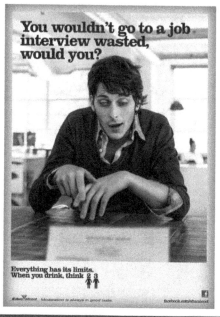

FIGURE 11.4: Éduc'alcool Student Campaign on Limiting Alcohol Consumption
Source: Éduc'alcool (http://educalcool.qc.ca/en).

Other organizations, such as the Calgary Fetal Alcohol Network, have employed the relational "friends-caring-for-friends" theme and have included the additional step of distributing booklets that give ideas for having collaborative conversations about alcohol with friends who are drinking during pregnancy. Again, this is a significant step forward from posters that commonly depict naked pregnant women, admonishing women to "take responsibility," to take note that "I'm here" (written on a woman's skin, presumably by the fetus), or that otherwise objectify, oversimplify, and demean women who consume alcohol during pregnancy. It invites an approach built not on isolating and shaming but rather on enhancing social support.

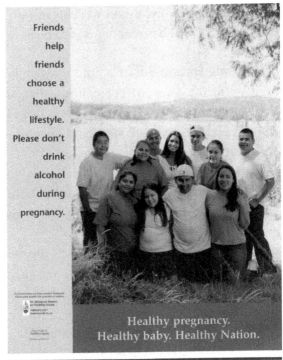

FIGURE 11.5: Friends Help Friends Poster
Source: BC Aboriginal Network on Disability Society.

Levels and Locations for Action

Our work on gender-transformative health promotion aims to promote awareness and action by individuals and groups, to change the way practitioners work in diverse settings, and to affect policy at micro, meso, and macro levels. For many, this work involves a perspective transformation as a key component of knowledge translation (McWilliam, 2007), in this case to enable health promoters to embrace gender-based analysis, intersectionality, the application of a critical lens to the field of health promotion, reflexive practice, and the linkage of health promotion and gender equity. For such multi-level, multi-sectoral, and transformative efforts, we need accessible forums for discussing the concepts of gender-transformative health promotion for women and for planning needed awareness-building efforts, practice interventions, policy changes, and research/ evaluation strategies.

There are existing examples of engaged, participatory work to achieve knowledge translation on gender-transformative health promotion—that is, work that supports this mutually respectful collective examination, questioning, and action on combining health promotion and gender-equity objectives.

Virtual and Face-to-Face Communities of Inquiry

Multi-sectoral communities of inquiry sponsored by the British Columbia Centre of Excellence for Women's Health have long provided the opportunity for co-learning, collective synthesis, and action planning on women's health. The following are key aspects of these communities of inquiry:

- Members participate as engaged professionals and paraprofessionals, not as representatives of agencies or governments.
- Membership is voluntary.
- These communities of inquiry are centred on learning together about complex issues by sharing multiple forms of evidence (research, practice wisdom, policy wisdom, experiential wisdom, and wisdom from traditional indigenous ways of knowing).
- They pay close attention to relationships, and are facilitated through a dialogic (Ackerly, 2007; Avis & Fisher, 2006; Baumgartner, 2001; Hunter, 2005) and appreciative (Ghaye et al., 2008; Marchi & Ciceri, 2011) approach.
- They are geared to stimulating change: individual, collective, organizational, and structural.
- They engage in and are linked to other forms of building awareness and stimulating action.

For example, in 2008 people working on the National Framework for Action to Reduce the Harms Associated with Alcohol and other Drugs and Substances in Canada were invited to participate in a virtual community as a mechanism for supporting learning about gender as it affects substance use—that is, for "gendering the National Framework" (Poole & Urquhart, 2009). Those who volunteered to participate included planners/decision-makers, direct service providers, educators, leaders from non-governmental organizations, policy analysts, researchers, and women's health advocates. The participation was pan-Canadian: people from 9 of 13 provincial and territorial jurisdictions participated, and 18 percent were from Canada's North (that is, at or above 53 degrees north latitude, excluding Edmonton) and 16 percent were from rural locations (living in communities with a population under 8,000 people). The community met over six months in six virtual one-hour sessions in which they learned about and discussed gender as it operates in the substance use field, and identified opportunities for gendered approaches to health promotion and prevention, treatment, and harm reduction involving girls and women. The community experience catalyzed many of its participants to take action on the links between violence and trauma and women's substance use, on enacting municipal policy as a strategy for preventing alcohol use during pregnancy, and on reducing harms such as homelessness as key to an intersectional approach to helping women with substance use and related social concerns. After the community sessions, the facilitator captured what was shared in the virtual community meetings (research, practice examples, web links, and questions raised) in discussion guides (see Gendering the National Framework series at www.bccewh.ca/publications), which have been used by others to spark further learning, synthesis, and action. In addition, a website was established as a repository for ongoing linkages to work in progress utilizing a gender lens on girls' and women's substance use in Canada (see www.coalescing-vc.org).

The community of inquiry/practice supporting the Gendering the National Framework project was short-term in length and entirely virtual in location. A related community of inquiry/practice on the topic on women's health promotion and prevention of alcohol use in pregnancy has been in operation for over four years, combining 11 monthly virtual meetings with one annual face-to-face meeting each year. It too includes researchers, clinical practitioners, policy analysts, representatives of community-based services, and women's health advocates who have had substance use problems and are mothers of children with fetal alcohol spectrum disorder. Their achievements in the 2012–2013 year are captured in the "word cloud" in Figure 11.6.

One product of this virtual community, designed to

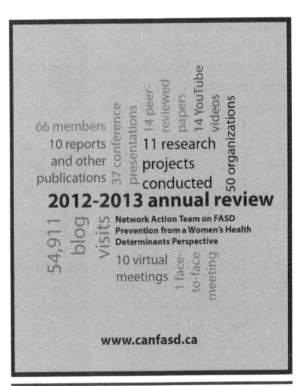

FIGURE 11.6: CanFASD Research Network, Network Action Team Annual Report Cover

Source: CanFASD Research Network, Network Action Team on FASD Prevention.

support awareness and action on the part of both its members and a wide international audience, is a highly popular blog.

Sharing Information and Commentary Utilizing a Blog Format

Blogs allow for just-in-time updates on research, policy changes, practice innovations, educational supports, and theory, coupled with short commentary to help the blog reader to contextualize the information and/or be inspired to act. As such they can be helpful mechanisms to facilitate gender-transformative health promotion. The blog associated with the virtual community of practice/inquiry on issues associated with prevention of alcohol use in pregnancy described above (http://fasdprevention.wordpress.com/) provides information; makes links between issues; promotes connections across distance (people in 166 countries access this blog); and inspires individual, local, regional, and national action. People interested in FASD prevention learn about everything from post-colonial theory to prenatal and postpartum clinical guidelines, to advances in screening for alcohol consumption using biomarkers, to integrating FASD prevention within municipal alcohol policy. One day blog readers might find information on an upcoming conference, the next on reaching college-age drinkers, the next on a gender-blind media campaign, and the next on developing holistic programs for women challenged by histories of violence and trauma. It exposes readers to the social, cultural, political, economic, environmental, and biological determinants as identified in the framework for gender-transformative health promotion for women; to issues and examples of health policy, research, and service delivery; and to analysis of interventions that attend not only to individual behaviour change but also to their achievement of health equity for women. As such, it can be an important adjunct to the learning fostered through deliberative dialogue in a virtual community of practice/inquiry, and an important potential tool for health promoters.

Online Linkages to Support Individual and Broad Health Outcomes

A key element of knowledge translation on gender-transformative health promotion is shifting the focus of education and action from individuals in a position to improve their health to ourselves as researchers, educators, practitioners, and policy-makers who are in a position to support both individual and broader change. For us to think large—to connect our research, policy, and practice work to achieve improved health outcomes for women, as well as increasing gender equity overall— requires multiple, ongoing, and non-threatening opportunities for connecting and for reflective practice. With new technologies we are finding new ways to achieve this. We are hosting online discussions of complex health and social issues such as trauma-informed practice (Poole et al., 2010); we are collectively synthesizing and sharing what we know about holistic care for pregnant women based on the experience of one-stop clinics in multiple cities (Bryans et al., 2012); and we are creating and posting video clips that explicate complex health outcomes from multiple expert perspectives (BCCEWH, 2012; Network Action Team, 2013). In working together online we are achieving the analytic, review, and identification steps of the planning tool. And we are able to share the results of this work in a relational way, thus enhancing what can be learned from published articles and reports. It is critical to have such mechanisms for meaningful engagement, as individuals or as groups, with the principles and concepts underlying the framework: to critically consider how gendered structures and polices affect health, and how we can identify and implement gender-transformative health promotion.

Conclusion: Provoking Action

Working on gender-transformative health promotion for women has been inspired in part by the women's consciousness-raising movement of the 1970s, which demonstrated how sharing experiences, collective analysis, and action planning can bring attention to important women's health concerns and prompt iterative cycles of action based on evolving understandings of inequities and how to overcome them. It has also been inspired by the opportunities presented by new technologies and virtual and digital innovations. Both the framework and the planning tool invite multi-sectoral engagement, instill a gender- and diversity-based analysis, inspire a collective review of current health promotion practices, and generate ideas for how to improve health and change harmful gender norms, roles, and relations as we implement health promotion in varied settings with diverse populations of women. The processes also require a simultaneous addressing of a range of issues and determinants of women's health. We have numerous and growing examples of engaged, participatory work (online and off) to achieve knowledge translation on women's health promotion through these processes of collective examination, questioning, and action, which combine both health promotion and gender-equity objectives. With these foundations and mechanisms, enacting gender-transformative health promotion need not feel daunting. These foundations both invite and provoke our action.

NOTE

1 Repairing the Holes in the Net is an applied health services study funded by the Canadian Institutes for Health Research (CIHR) in partnership with the Mental Health Commission of Canada (MHCC) under a Partnerships for Health System Improvement (PHSI) Program. It is

being conducted by the British Columbia Centre of Excellence for Women's Health in partnership with the Yukon Status of Women Council and the Council of Yukon First Nations Health Department, the YWCA Yellowknife and the Centre for Northern Families, the Qulliit Nunavut Status of Women Council, and the Four Worlds Centre for Development Learning. Its aim is to improve the mental health of northern women who have unstable housing or who are homeless through the development of research-based models for more effective health services delivery and policy in Canada's three northern territories.

REFERENCES

Ackerly, B. (2007). "How does change happen?" Deliberation and difficulty. *Hypatia, 22*(4), 46–63.

Avis, J., & Fisher, R. (2006). Reflections on communities of practice, on-line learning, and transformation: Teachers, lecturers, and trainers. *Research in Post-Compulsory Education, 11*(2), 141–151.

Baumgartner, L. M. (2001). An update on transformational learning. In S. B. Merriam (Ed.), *The new update on adult learning theory* (pp. 15–24). San Francisco: Jossey-Bass.

BCCEWH. (2012). *Expecting to quit, finding what works for you—digital narratives about change from women who are current or recent smokers.* Retrieved from www.expectingtoquit.ca/resources/

Beller, S. (2013, April 1). *"Drunkorexia" is double trouble.* Retrieved from www.thefix.com/content/drunkorexia-double-trouble91481

Bopp, J., van Bruggen, R., Elliott, S., Fuller, L., Hache, M., Hrenchuk, C., ... & McNaughton, G. (2007). *You just blink and it can happen: A study of women's homelessness north of 60.* Yellowknife: Four Worlds Centre for Development Learning, Qulliit Nunavut Status of Women Council, YWCA of Yellowknife, Yellowknife Women's Society, Yukon Status of Women's Council.

Bryans, M., Dechief, L., Hardeman, S., Marcellus, L., Nathoo, T., Poag, E., & ... Taylor, M. (2012). *Supporting pregnant and parenting women who use substances: What communities are doing to help.* Vancouver: British Columbia Centre of Excellence for Women's Health, CanFASD Research Network. Retrieved from www.canfasd.ca/files/What_Communities_Are_Doing_to_Help_February_7_2013.pdf

Clow, B., Pederson, A., Haworth-Brockman, M., & Bernier, J. (2009). *Rising to the challenge: Sex and gender-based analysis for health planning, policy, and research in Canada.* Halifax: Atlantic Centre of Excellence for Women's Health.

Gammon, A. (2013). 15 bikini-friendly beers: The best low-cal brews to still feel (and look) amazing in your two-piece. *Shape Magazine.* Retrieved from www.shape.com/healthy-eating/healthy-drinks/15-bikini-friendly-beers

Ghaye, T., Melander-Wikman, A., Kisare, M., Chambers, P., Bergmark, U., Kostenius, C., & Lillyman, S. (2008). Participatory and appreciative action and reflection (PAAR)—democratizing reflective practices. *Reflective Practice, 9*(4), 361–397.

Heaman, M., & Chalmers, K. (2005). Prevalence and correlates of smoking during pregnancy: A comparison of Aboriginal and non-Aboriginal women in Manitoba. *Birth, 32*(4), 299–305.

Hunter, S. (2005). Negotiating professional and social voices in research principles and practice. *Journal of Social Work Practice, 19*(2), 149–162. doi:10.1080/02650530500144709

Jernigan, D. H., Ostroff, J., Ross, C., & O'Hara, J. (2004). Sex differences in adolescent exposure to alcohol advertising in magazines. *Archives of Pediatric Adolescent Medicine, 158*(7), 629–634.

Keating, C. (2005). Building coalitional consciousness. *NWSA Journal, 17*(2), 86–103.

Kilbourne, J. (1999). *Deadly persuasion: Why women and girls must fight the addictive power of advertising*. New York: Simon & Schuster.

Marchi, S., & Ciceri, E. (2011). Login and logout: Practices of resistance and presence in virtual environments as a kind of reflective learning activity. *Reflective Practice, 12*(2), 209–223. doi:10.1080/14623943.2011.561533

McWilliam, C. L. (2007). Continuing education at the cutting edge: Promoting transformative knowledge translation. *Journal of Continuing Education in the Health Professions, 27*(2), 72–79.

Network Action Team. (2013, February 28). *Shining a light on Canada's multi-layered approach to FASD*. Video clips from a special evening session at the 5th International Conference on Fetal Alcohol Spectrum Disorder, Vancouver, BC. Retrieved from www.youtube.com/watch?v=roNcobFMlWw&list=PLCuxEw01QE5kYyBBgpp-DMae95ZQ8C8Wj

Poland, B., Krupa, G., & McCall, D. (2009). Settings for health promotion: An analytic framework to guide intervention design and implementation. *Health Promotion Practice, 10*(4), 505–516. doi:10.1177/1524839909341025

Poole, N. (2008). How can consciousness raising principles inform modern knowledge translation practices in women's health? *Canadian Journal of Nursing Research, 40*(2), 77–93.

Poole, N., Brown, V., Byrans, M., Capyk, S., Dechief, L., Hache, A., & Mason, R. (2010, November 18). *What do we mean by trauma-informed care?* Retrieved from www.coalescing-vc.org/virtualLearning/section1/trauma-informed-care/webcasts.htm

Poole, N., & Urquhart, C. (2009). Trauma-informed approaches in addictions treatment. *Gendering the National Framework Series: Vol. 1.* Vancouver: British Columbia Centre of Excellence for Women's Health.

Shreve, A. (1989). *Women together, women alone: The legacy of the consciousness-raising movement*. New York: Viking Press.

Urquhart, C., Jasuira, F., Poole, N., Greaves, L., & Nathoo, T. (2012). *Liberation! Helping women quit smoking: A brief tobacco intervention guide*. Vancouver: British Columbia Centre of Excellence for Women's Health.

Womenshealth.gov. (2011). *Lesbian and bisexual health fact sheet*. Retrieved from http://womenshealth.gov/publications/our-publications/fact-sheet/lesbian-bisexual-health.cfm#c

12

Creating Lasting Change: Advocacy for Gender-Transformative Health Promotion

Petra Begnell and Rose Durey

Introduction

The women's movement is characterized by advocacy that has improved and transformed women's status and health outcomes—from the creation of women's health services, to access to contraception and safe, legal abortion, to changes in the way women are represented in the media. Yet for a number of reasons, advocacy has become the poor cousin to other more accepted health promotion interventions. But gender-transformative health promotion, which strives to improve both the health and status of women, could and should use an array of tools and strategies to achieve this goal. Advocacy is a powerful tool for gender-transformative health promotion, which, despite its ability to bring about significant, long-lasting change, is often misunderstood and underutilized by the health promotion and women's health sectors. This chapter explores the role of advocacy in gender-transformative health promotion, challenges misconceptions about advocacy, and highlights its potential as an instrument for lasting change to improve women's health. Advocacy to reduce the objectification of women in Australia is used as an example of effective gender-transformative health promotion.

Advocacy Is Central to Health Promotion

Advocacy influences outcomes and achieves change (Cohen, de la Vega, & Watson, 2001), and can be used to redefine the structures, norms, attitudes, and behaviours that support inequity. Advocacy has been defined by the World Health Organization as "a combination of individual and social actions designed to gain political commitment, policy support, social acceptance and systems support for a particular health goal or program" (World Health Organization, 1998, p. 5). It is a legitimate and necessary health promotion activity and one of three core strategies described in the Ottawa Charter for Health Promotion—enable, mediate, and advocate (World Health Organization, 1986). The Ottawa Charter recommends the application of these three strategies to the following action areas:

- strengthen community action
- develop personal skills
- create supportive environments
- reorient health services
- build healthy public policy

Advocacy spans the breadth of health promotion activity defined by the action areas above—from working downstream with individuals and communities (often referred to as "individual advocacy") to working at an upstream level (often referred to as "systemic" or "structural advocacy"), which targets public policy and societal structures (Carlisle, 2000). Individual advocacy can be a good place to start—much of what health promotion practitioners do is essentially advocating for individuals and empowering them to improve their health. This can be achieved through health promotion activities such as behaviour-change programs, interventions to build community capacity, or running community groups. However, health promotion practitioners must also act on the determinants of health and ill health to make lasting change—this is where upstream health promotion and systemic advocacy come to the fore. Systemic advocacy can be more efficient, effective, and long-lasting, and "acknowledges that barriers to health can lie beyond the control of individuals and that structural factors need to be addressed if gender roles are to be transformed and health inequalities are to be reduced" (Carlisle, 2000, p. 370). By influencing public policy and resource allocation within political, economic, and social systems and institutions (Cohen, de la Vega, & Watson, 2001), health promotion has the potential to be gender-transformative.

Barriers to Advocacy

Barriers to advocacy come from a range of sources—employers, funding bodies, those with power and influence, and even health promotion practitioners themselves. Advocacy, by its very nature, is about challenging the status quo, confronting injustice, and changing traditional attitudes, so it is often met with resistance. However, without advocacy as a tool for gender-transformative health promotion, achievements may be limited, as it is advocacy that will bring about lasting change to the systems, policies, practices, and attitudes that contribute to gender inequality.

Real barriers to the uptake of advocacy as a strategy in health promotion remain, and these may also apply to gender-transformative health promotion.

Advocating for changes to policy, legislation, or regulation requires significant effort and takes time. Despite this, the changes achieved are more likely than individual advocacy to bring long-term and sustainable benefits (Boender et al., 2004; United Nations Educational, Scientific and Cultural Organization, 2010). Overall, changes to systems, and to the conditions in which people live, can be less expensive and more efficient than health promotion efforts aimed directly at individuals (Chokshi & Farley, 2012).

Advocacy, especially systemic advocacy, is often not regarded as part of the work of health promotion practitioners and organizations. It can be seen as too political, disconnected from health promotion work "at the coalface," or too difficult to demonstrate outcomes for—all of which can also make it difficult to secure funding. Organizations face an additional challenge in advocating for changes to government policy when it relates to the very government that provides their funding. In addition to all this, there are limits to health promotion practitioners' ability to engage

 ## BOX 12.1: **CHARITIES AND ADVOCACY**

In Australia, there has been debate about the legitimacy of advocacy by charitable organizations. In 2006, Aid/Watch,[1] an Australian watchdog organization focused on aid, trade, and debt, had its charitable tax status revoked by the Commissioner of Taxation because its activities were deemed to be "too political" and was therefore not considered to be a charity. Charitable status is important for many not-for-profit organizations in Australia because of the tax concessions that it bestows. The case went to Australia's highest court, which upheld Aid/Watch's charitable tax status. The court (*Aid/Watch Incorporated v. Commissioner of Taxation* [2010]) noted that "the generation by lawful means of public debate ... is a purpose beneficial to the community" (para. 47), and that "in Australia there is no general doctrine which excludes from charitable purposes 'political objects'" (para. 48). This decision meant that advocacy and the public critique of government policy were deemed a significant part of the work of charitable organizations, which include many health promotion organizations. It provided health promotion practitioners in Australia with the endorsement to advocate within their sphere of influence to achieve changes that will benefit the populations they are working with.

In other parts of the world, however, barriers such as this may still exist. Therefore, systemic advocacy may need to begin with advocacy about the very need for advocacy. This case could also be referred to as a precedent in this type of advocacy, which occurs internally in organizations.

in advocacy activities, which relate to both the project-based nature of funding for health promotion work, as well as to the limited coverage of advocacy as a part of health promotion and public health practice in university courses.

The term "advocacy" itself may be a hindrance as it can conjure up daunting thoughts of rallies and marches, intensive media campaigns, meetings with legislators, and the potential for backlash. Yet advocacy can encompass a whole range of activities that have the purpose of contributing to change, some of which are set out in this chapter. Framing and reclaiming advocacy as a means of improving health outcomes is vital to ensure change.

Advocacy Is Necessary for Gender-Transformative Health Promotion

Health promotion needs to reshape the context in which individual decisions are made (Dworkin, Dunbar, Krishnan, Hatcher, & Sawires, 2011), and to do this,

---

BOX 12.2: **STEPS IN DEVELOPING GENDER-TRANSFORMATIVE HEALTH PROMOTION**

Practitioners using a gender-transformative approach to health promotion should:

- *Encourage critical awareness of gender roles and norms (Boender et al., 2004):* This is the foundation of gender-transformative health promotion and should form part of any advocacy activities. Advocate for policy and legislative change that supports equitable social systems (Health Rights Advocacy Forum, 2012). An example of this is affirmative action to ensure women are represented in political leadership positions.
- *Ensure that policy and practice challenges the imbalance of power, the distribution of resources, and the allocation of duties between women and men (Boender et al., 2004; Health Rights Advocacy Forum, 2012):* This could include advocating for changes to support parents to more equitably share care for children, through flexible working arrangements or parental leave.
- *Promote the position of women across policy, programs, and advocacy (Boender et al., 2004; Health Rights Advocacy Forum, 2012):* Including and consulting with women in program and policy design, and ensuring their involvement in advocacy campaigns, are critical to embedding change.
- *Work with men to improve gender equality and health, leading to better health outcomes for both women and men (Dworkin et al., 2011):* Men are an integral part in the reshaping of traditional gender norms, structures, and attitudes. They must be part of the change process.

advocacy is needed. Advocacy's legitimate and important place in health promotion practice (Chapman, 2004; Pettersson, 2011) extends to the improvement of women's health and status through gender-transformative health promotion. It is therefore imperative to include advocacy activities in gender-transformative health promotion. Advocacy can

- interrogate the different gender norms and roles that affect women and men;
- address the causes of gender inequality;
- create conditions that increase shared power, control of resources, and decision making between women and men; and
- promote gender equality.

If health promotion is to be gender-transformative, it must target the societal systems and structures that lie at the root of gender inequality, which have a profound influence on women's health.

What Does Advocacy for Gender-Transformative Health Promotion Look Like?

Conceptualizing advocacy as a tool for gender-transformative health promotion across the spectrum of health promotion activities enables practitioners to recognize that much of their work could be considered advocacy. Advocacy is about action for change, and so advocacy for gender-transformative health promotion can encompass a range of activities including

- bringing together evidence on a topic;
- writing a paper;
- sharing ideas and resources with other like-minded organizations and individuals;
- scanning the environment to understand what others are doing about an issue and where the opportunities or gaps are through the media, policy development, professional and interest groups, or informal networks;
- conducting workshops for practitioners about how to challenge norms and change practice;
- writing a letter to a decision-maker;
- building a social media campaign to raise awareness and encourage supporters to take action;
- creating, circulating, and/or signing a petition;
- using social media;

- writing a submission to a government inquiry;
- writing a letter to the editor to highlight concerns or correct misinformation;
- developing a media campaign; and
- meeting with the elected official with responsibility for the health or women's or other related portfolio.

Simple actions like these can contribute to a shift in understanding regarding gender norms, roles, and structures, and simple actions can be gender-transformative. Having a goal in mind and setting out to capitalize on the work that is already being done to purposefully and strategically achieve change broadens health promotion activity into advocacy activity.

As with any health promotion intervention, good planning can make all the difference to achieving the desired outcomes, and this extends to advocacy. Despite organizations having defined agendas, priorities, key performance indicators, and targets to meet, re-examining health promotion work with a gender-transformative lens and an advocacy lens is a worthwhile activity. Doing this can highlight the ways in which existing work can contribute to gender-transformative health promotion.

Advocacy for Gender-Transformative Health Promotion in Action

The example below applies the gender-transformative health promotion framework and planning tool to advocacy to challenge the objectification of women in media and advertising. While this example is Australian, the application of this approach is relevant in many other countries.

Analyze All Forms of Evidence for the Population Setting and Issue through a Gender, Sex, and Diversity Lens

Women's Health Victoria is a not-for-profit organization focused on improving the health of women in Victoria, a state of Australia. The impact of the objectification of women on their health, as well as its effect on the community, has been a long-standing concern of the organization, and evidence was gathered and analyzed about objectification and its impact on women's health. Objectification occurs when "a woman's sexual parts or functions are separated out from her person, reduced to status of mere instruments, or else regarded as if they were capable of representing her. To be dealt with in this way is to have one's entire being identified with the body" (Bartky, cited in Moradi & Huan, 2008, p. 377). While many factors affect women's body image, the media is repeatedly identified as a significant contributor to the predominant image of the ideal female body (Lawrie, Sullivan, Davies, &

Hill, 2006). The media provide women with constant messages that the perfect body is thin and beautiful: images presented in the media are typically of women who are unnaturally slim and who have often undergone cosmetic surgery. The images themselves are often digitally enhanced, and are both unreal and unrealistic.

Objectification has a number of significant personal and social consequences. The American Psychological Association Task Force on the Sexualization of Girls (2007) notes that objectification affects:

- girls' health and well-being, including cognitive and physical functioning, body dissatisfaction and appearance anxiety, mental and physical health, sexuality, and attitudes and beliefs.
- boys, men, and adult women. For example, exposure to narrow ideals of female sexual attractiveness may make it difficult for some men to fully enjoy intimacy with a female partner. Adult women may suffer by trying to conform to a younger standard of ideal female beauty.
- society, including through sexism, sex bias, and sexist attitudes. "Across several studies, women and men exposed to sexually objectifying images of women from mainstream media ... were found to be significantly more accepting of rape myths ... sexual harassment, sex role stereotypes, interpersonal violence, and adversarial sexual beliefs about relationships than were those in control conditions" (American Psychological Association Task Force on the Sexualization of Girls, 2007, pp. 30–31). Exposure to sexualized content has also been shown to affect how women behave and how men treat and respond to real women in subsequent interactions. These studies have found that after men are exposed to sexualized content, their behaviour toward women is more sexualized, and they treat women like sexual objects.

This analysis of evidence gathered by Women's Health Victoria was collated into a gender impact assessment on women and body image (Main, 2009).

Review Existing Health Promotion Practice by Critically Examining Gendered Beliefs and Discriminatory Practices

The work that Women's Health Victoria had carried out at the analysis stage showed clearly the gendered beliefs and discriminatory practices in the portrayal of women in media and advertising.

Women's Health Victoria also learned about other interventions that had been carried out in relation to objectification. This included work by other women's organizations across the world, such as presentations by the National Organization for Women in the United States to draw attention to the widespread nature of objectification, and efforts to regulate the media industry, such as through the development of a Voluntary Industry Code of Conduct on Body Image (Australian Government, 2009). Complaints to media and advertising regulators were also reviewed. However, it was discovered that the self-regulation of Australia's advertisers had been ineffective in preventing the objectification of women, primarily because objectification was not identified as a separate grounds for consideration in the Australian Association of National Advertisers Code of Ethics (the Code). As it stood, the Code did not identify discrimination and vilification as distinct from objectification, which is particularly relevant to women's experiences. This meant that gendered beliefs and discriminatory practices relating to the portrayal of women in the media and advertising could continue unabated.

Making complaints against individual advertisements was felt not to be the most effective or efficient use of Women's Health Victoria's time, nor did it represent upstream health promotion. The advocacy of Women's Health Victoria moved on from the discussion of problems to the exploration of solutions that aimed to achieve positive and lasting change.

Identify Ways to Improve Women's Health and Change Harmful Gender Norms, Roles, and Relations in the Intervention

In order to identify ways to improve women's health and change harmful gender norms, roles, and relations, Women's Health Victoria began a structured environmental scanning process of news, research, policy, programs, and services to identify trends, gaps, and opportunities in relation to challenging and confronting the objectification of women. One way of addressing objectification was to target media and advertising institutions that perpetuate the objectification of women.

A process of reform around media and advertising presented an ideal opportunity for advocacy on this issue. During 2010 and 2011, advocacy opportunities included the following:

- the Australian Association of National Advertisers reviewed their Code of Ethics (Australian Association of National Advertisers, 2010)
- the federal government announced a Senate Inquiry into the National Film and Literature Classification Scheme (Senate Legal and Constitutional Affairs Committee, 2011)
- the Australian Law Reform Commission undertook a review of the National Classification Scheme (Australian Law Reform Commission, 2011)

All of these inquiries included body image, the objectification of women, or the sexualization of girls in their terms of reference. This provided Women's Health Victoria with the opportunity to advocate for changes to advertising and media in Australia that would make them more gender-equitable.

Implement an Intervention That Improves Women's Health and Encourages Equitable Roles for Women, and Access to and Control over Resources

Women's Health Victoria made submissions (2010, 2011a, 2011b) to each of these inquiries, recommending that objectification should be included in the National Film and Literature Classification Scheme and in the Advertisers Code of Ethics. How other countries had responded to this issue was researched, and model clauses were provided as examples in the submissions. Women's Health Victoria was also invited to present verbal evidence that built on the information and recommendations provided in the written submissions.

During this time, Women's Health Victoria also engaged the media through the distribution of media releases and letters to the editor that were then published in Australia. This media engagement aimed to draw attention to the pervasiveness of the objectification of women, its health impacts, and the potential for change.

Engage Stakeholders, Including Practitioners, Women, Decision-Makers, Researchers, and Community Leaders in Various Sectors

Women's Health Victoria's advocacy on this issue also involved sharing information with other women's health services, so that they could use their own influence as pressure-makers. A fact sheet was developed on how to make a complaint about advertisements and music videos and was distributed through networks so that others could also challenge the harmful portrayal of women in advertising and the media. Women's Health Victoria's submissions were also shared among wider networks of women's organizations so that others could draw from and use the analysis and recommendations to advocate in their own spheres.

Evaluate Processes and Outcomes against the Goals of Promoting Gender and Health Equity

Evaluation of advocacy can differ from the evaluation of other health promotion programs, but it is important to record outcomes in order to demonstrate the impact of the advocacy. Following up on inquiries, tracking the development of government recommendations and their implementation, monitoring policy developments, and reviewing media reports are all important ways to measure the outcomes of structural advocacy.

The outcomes of the advocacy of Women's Health Victoria on the objectification of women represented an important achievement for the status of Australian women. For example, the Senate Committee Inquiry into Film and Literature Classification recommended that the classification scheme should be expanded to encompass concerns about the objectification of women (Senate Legal and Constitutional Affairs References Committee, 2011). In addition, in 2011, the Australian Association of National Advertisers released their revised Code of Ethics, which states for the first time that "advertising or marketing communications should not employ sexual appeal in a manner which is exploitative and degrading of any individual or group of people" (2012, para. 2.2). This allows the Advertising Standards Board to consider objectification when making decisions, and this has begun to happen (Canning, 2012; News Limited Network, 2013). A growing number of media reports highlighting rulings using this clause are also important measures, as what is reported in the media contributes to changing attitudes.

These outcomes represent an important step toward transforming the structures and systems that perpetuate gender inequity, improving women's health, and redefining the way in which women are viewed in society. While it is only a small step on a longer journey toward gender equity in the advertising and media world, it nonetheless represents significant progress in this area.

In the evaluation of gender-transformative health promotion, it is also worth considering how women and men adjust to and use redefined gender norms through evaluation. Further research is needed to find out "how women and men actually wrestle with and use new notions of masculinity and femininity in their relationships and communities" (Dworkin et al., 2011, p. 999).

Report Gender and Health Outcomes and Disseminate the Findings

The more advocacy is reported among the women's health and health promotion sectors, the more mainstream the practice will become. Women's Health Victoria has shared learnings and outcomes in a range of ways, including articles, workshops, media releases, and letters to the editor. Knowledge and outcomes have also been shared informally through networks. All of these represent important means by which advocacy to reduce the objectification of women and its associated health impacts have been disseminated.

Conclusion

This chapter has explored the key elements of advocacy for gender-transformative health promotion using the example of Women's Health Victoria's advocacy on the objectification of women. This example demonstrated the range of activity that contributes to advocacy, and how gender-transformative health promotion can improve health and achieve gender equality. By challenging the objectification of women, traditional gender norms and roles are interrogated, such as the inappropriate value that society places on women's appearance.

Advocacy is an important tool in health promotion efforts to transform gender roles, norms, and structures. It can lever change at a systemic and structural level, thus enabling lasting change to occur and potentially reaching a great number of people. Advocacy can also take place at the individual and community level. Many health promotion practitioners will find that their work already encompasses advocacy activities to address gender inequality at these levels.

Fundamentally, gender-transformative health promotion aims to create conditions that increase shared power, control of resources, and decision making between women and men. Changing the way women are represented in the media and advertising makes this aim more achievable. Without advocacy, this could not happen. Harnessing the work already being done, building on it, and using it as a lever to bring about positive change in women's health and status will move health promotion practice toward the outcomes needed for lasting change.

NOTE

1   Retrieved from http://aidwatch.org.au/

REFERENCES

Aid/Watch Incorporated v. Commissioner of Taxation [2010]. HCA 42. Retrieved from www. austlii.edu.au/au/cases/cth/HCA/2010/42.html

American Psychological Association Task Force on the Sexualization of Girls. (2007). *Report of the APA Task Force on the sexualization of girls.* Retrieved from www.apa.org/ pi/women/programs/girls/report.aspx

Australian Association of National Advertisers. (2010). *Code of Ethics review.* Retrieved from www.aana.com.au/pages/code-of-ethics-review-2010.html

Australian Association of National Advertisers. (2012). *Australian Association of National Advertisers Code of Ethics.* Retrieved from www.aana.com.au/pages/codes.html

Australian Government. (2009). *Voluntary industry code of conduct on body image.* Canberra: Australian Government. Retrieved from www.youth.gov.au/sites/Youth/bodyImage/ codeofconduct

Australian Law Reform Commission. (2011). *National classification scheme review.* Retrieved from www.alrc.gov.au/publications/national-classification-scheme-review-ip-40

Boender, C., Santana, D., Santillan, D., Hardee, K., Greene, M. E., & Schuler, S. (2004). *The "So what?" report: A look at whether integrating a gender focus into programs makes a difference to outcomes.* Washington, DC: Interagency Gender Working Group Task Force. Retrieved from www.prb.org/igwg_media/thesowhatreport.pdf

Canning, S. (2012, July 17). ASB bans shorn woman ad. *The Australian.* Retrieved from www.theaustralian.com.au/media/asb-bans-woman-shearing-ad/story-e6frg996-1226428259109

Carlisle, S. (2000). Health promotion, advocacy, and health inequalities: A conceptual framework. *Health Promotion International, 15*(4), 369–376.

Chapman, S. (2004). Advocacy for public health: A primer. *Journal of Epidemiological Community Health, 58*(5), 361–365.

Chokshi, D. A., & Farley, T. A. (2012). The cost-effectiveness of environmental approaches to disease prevention. *New England Journal of Medicine, 367*(4), 295–297.

Cohen, D., de la Vega, R., & Watson, G. (2001) *Advocacy for social justice: A global action and reflection guide.* Bloomfield: Kumarian Press Inc.

Dworkin, S. L., Dunbar, M. S., Krishnan, S., Hatcher, A. M., & Sawires, S. (2011). Uncovering tensions and capitalizing on synergies in HIV/AIDS and antiviolence programs. *American Journal of Public Health, 101*(6), 995–1003.

Health Rights Advocacy Forum. (2012). *Gender sensitive and gender transformative responses to HIV and AIDS.* Nairobi: Health Rights Advocacy Forum.

Lawrie, Z., Sullivan, E. A., Davies, P. S. W., & Hill, R. J. (2006). Media influence on the body image of children and adolescents. *Eating Disorders, 14*(5), 355–364.

Main, A. (2009). *Women and body image gender impact assessment.* Melbourne: Women's Health Victoria. Retrieved from http://whv.org.au/publications-resources/publications-resources-by-topic/post/women-and-body-image-gender-impact-assessment/

Moradi, B., & Huan, Y. P. (2008). Objectification theory and psychology of women: A decade of advances and future directions. *Psychology of Women Quarterly, 32*(4), 377–398.

National Organization for Women. *The ABCs and Ds of commercial images of women.* Retrieved from http://loveyourbody.nowfoundation.org/presentations/SexStereotypesBeauty/index.html

News Limited Network. (2013, April 15). Advertising watchdog upholds complaints against Wicked Campers over "offensive" van slogans. *The Australian.* Retrieved from www.news.com.au/travel/travel-updates/advertising-watchdog-upholds-complaints-against-wicked-campers-over-offensive-camper-van-slogans/story-e6frfq80-1226621001186

Pettersson, B. (2011). Some bitter-sweet reflections on the Ottawa Charter commemoration cake: A personal discourse from an Ottawa rocker. *Health Promotion International, 26*(S2), 173–179.

Senate Legal and Constitutional Affairs Committee. (2011). *Inquiry into the Australian film and literature classification scheme.* Retrieved from www.aph.gov.au/Parliamentary_Business/Committees/Senate_Committees?url=legcon_ctte/completed_inquiries/2010-13/classification_board/index.htm

Senate Legal and Constitutional Affairs References Committee. (2011). *Review of the national classification scheme: Achieving the right balance.* Canberra: Commonwealth of Australia. Retrieved from www.aph.gov.au/Parliamentary_Business/Committees/Senate_Committees?url=legcon_ctte/completed_inquiries/2010-13/classification_board/report/index.htm

United Nations Educational, Scientific and Cultural Organization. (2010). *Short guide to the essential characteristics of effective HIV prevention.* Paris: UNESCO. Retrieved from http://portal.unesco.org/en/ev.php-URL_ID=48359&URL_DO=DO_TOPIC&URL_SECTION=201.html

Women's Health Victoria. (2010). *Submission to the Australian Association of National Advertisers' review of code of ethics.* Melbourne: Women's Health Victoria. Retrieved from http://whv.org.au/publications-resources/publications-resources-by-topic/post/australian-association-of-national-advertisers-code-of-ethics/

Women's Health Victoria. (2011a). *Submission to the national classification scheme review.* Melbourne: Women's Health Victoria. Retrieved from http://whv.org.au/publications-resources/publications-resources-by-topic/post/national-classification-scheme-review/

Women's Health Victoria. (2011b). *Submission to the inquiry into the Australian film and literature classification scheme.* Melbourne: Women's Health Victoria. Retrieved from http://whv.org.au/publications-resources/publications-resources-by-topic/post/australian-film-and-literature-classification-scheme/

World Health Organization. (1986, November). *Ottawa Charter for health promotion.* Retrieved from www.who.int/healthpromotion/conferences/previous/ottawa/en/

World Health Organization. (1998). *Health promotion glossary.* Geneva: Author. Retrieved from www.who.int/healthpromotion/about/HPG/en/

13 Promoting Women's Hospitals as a Site for Change

Lorraine Greaves and Elizabeth Whynot

This chapter examines the potential for health promotion in a key setting: the women's hospital. Women's hospitals, especially independent ones, are scarce but critically important institutions for not only providing women's health care, but also generating improved health for women through health promotion. However, they are subject to numerous pressures that make this task a challenge. In this chapter Lorraine Greaves describes some of these overarching challenges, and Elizabeth Whynot reflects on her experiences with the goals of health promotion while president of the British Columbia Women's Hospital & Health Centre.

Introduction

Lorraine Greaves

Women's hospitals have historically been established to address key women's health issues such as maternity care, care for indigent women, or as sites for employing women physicians when women doctors were barred or unwelcome in mainstream hospitals.

In Canada, Women's College Hospital in Toronto and British Columbia Women's Hospital & Health Centre in Vancouver stand out as leaders in providing women's health care. Women's College Hospital has a long history of providing care for women in Toronto, having been established in 1883 as a women's medical college and in 1913 as a women's hospital. More recently it has had a rocky history in defending its existence during constant health reform amid the growing complexities of the health care system in Ontario and elsewhere in Canada. Nonetheless, despite many threats to its mandate and very existence, including losing its ability to provide birthing care for women, it has survived and has recently been redeveloped into a short-stay ambulatory care centre addressing a wide range of women's health needs.

In contrast, BC Women's Hospital in Vancouver is relatively new, established out of a transformed Grace Hospital in 1994. It has a thriving maternity service that serves all of British Columbia for high-risk cases and the local area in Vancouver for low-risk birth, and is one of the largest providers of maternity care in Canada. In Australia, The Royal Women's Hospital in Melbourne is 157 years old, and has also been recently redeveloped. It provides a local low-risk and a regional high-risk maternity service, along with a growing range of other women's health services. Some of these newer services reflect emergent community needs, such as a de-in-fibulations clinic for women who have experienced genital mutilation, and require considerable commitment and thought on the part of the hospital to provide sensitive and consistent care.

Women's hospitals, whether they are new or established, or whether they provide full hospital care or not, struggle with a range of issues. They are often marginalized from mainstream hospitals, which reflect male-dominated and medicalized models of care that emerged during the last century and eclipsed many women-centred services such as midwifery, birth attendance, and caring for indigent women. They often struggle to maintain their scope and have to defend their focus on women or even the necessity for the fields of women's health, women's health care, and women's health research. They often struggle with amalgamation forces in constant health reform situations, and put major political and strategic effort into holding on to central services such as birthing and maternity care, often without the support of on-site general surgery or a full range of other medical services for women, such as treating women's reproductive cancers.

Even when women's hospitals are politically supported and well funded, expand-ing services is difficult, and they are often pressed into partnership and shared service arrangements with bigger and better-funded hospitals. Women's hospitals also struggle with fundraising, and often have weaker charitable foundations and donor systems than mainstream hospitals. As a result, critical but often invisible infrastructural supports for strong research functions and innovative evaluation and policy development are underfunded. Further, expanding innovative non-maternity women's health services—such as sexual assault, domestic violence, mental health and addictions programs, among many others—is often done on a shoestring.

Women's hospitals have often created special approaches to health care, such as women-centred care frameworks, adhering to a social model of health, or working in close partnership with women's community-based services to co-create pro-gramming and outreach. They have tried to be highly responsive to women's health needs, and typically lead broad consultative processes to document and collect women's opinions on their health needs as part of their planning processes. Indeed, all three of the women's hospitals mentioned earlier have carried out large consultative processes with broad populations of women in their recent histories. These distinguishing features reflect the influences and processes of the women's movements of the past century—developing birth-control services, changing abortion laws, calling for more women doctors, inserting elements into a patriarchal agenda for health such as domestic violence awareness and prevention, or generating more understanding of women's mental health and addiction issues. Much of this agenda has involved engaging women, communities, and community organizations in agenda-setting, research, and program development.

These sorts of issues demand an understanding of community settings, the social determinants of health, and cultural and linguistic diversities, and require more comprehensive non-medical approaches to women's health and health care. Inevitably when following these models, women's health promotion becomes a critically important issue. How does a hospital move beyond the provision of care for women who are ill to create health in women, prevent illness, generate improved attitudes and access to care, and work more closely and respectfully with women and communities on a wider range of issues?

Women's hospitals have had to struggle with their scope, role, and mandate in order to delve into many of these issues, and have had to do so in the context of underfunding, complicated health reform, inconsistent political support, the constant need for reinforcing the role and history of the women's hospital, and rising economic pressures in complex health care delivery systems. But they have, when they survive, been beacons in the landscape of health service development. Addressing these tasks presents challenges for leaders working within women's health. How do they generate strong partnerships with women's groups, be on the frontiers of change for women's health, and concurrently maintain legitimacy with the system? How do they maintain and protect a strong voice and authority for women's health services and women's hospitals? How do they protect financing and independent governance when simple efficiency models push for amalgamations? How do they grow a flourishing women's health research system based on advanced thinking on sex and gender when universities and disciplinary practices do not support or teach these approaches?

These challenges are being met by the leading women's hospitals in Canada and Australia. They all have an enhanced version of the social model of health, respecting the impact of the social determinants. They are all grappling with community needs in their locales, often shifting quickly as populations change and diversify. They all struggle with funding for research and health promotion, and need more help, financing, and direction in these areas. Critical and time-sensitive care decisions take daily priority, eclipsing these overarching concerns. It is in this context and vortex that Elizabeth Whynot addresses the place of health promotion in a women's hospital, and the struggles that she encountered in making headway in this area.

Reflecting on the Role of the Hospital in Women's Health Promotion

Elizabeth Whynot

"Complex adaptive systems are characterized by a high degree of adaptive capacity, giving them resilience in the face of perturbation" (Wikipedia, n.d.). "So they definitely change; they just don't change into something else" (Whynot, 2010). I included these sentences a few years ago as part of a talk I was invited to provide on the subject of leadership in health care. The invitation came at a good time for me as I had recently retired after eight years as president of the largest maternity hospital in Canada, the British Columbia Women's Hospital & Health Centre (BC Women's), an intense experience that I really needed to think about.

Over 40 years my professional life has been divided more or less equally among clinical practice, community or public health, and acute care administration. Before joining BC Women's in 1998, I provided primary care in clinics for disenfranchised and marginal populations, as well as in private practice, and had worked two stints in medical (public) health officer roles, including eight years in Vancouver's Downtown Eastside (DTES), which is often referred to as the poorest postal code in Canada. Since leaving BC Women's in 2008, I have rejoined a clinical practice in Vancouver's inner city and now participate as a director on the board of the new First Nations Health Authority.

In the early 1970s, I had been a marching, picketing, protesting feminist and women's health advocate, a pro-choice activist, a member of the Vancouver Women's Health Collective, and an early member of the Rape Relief Board. In the early 1980s, I worked with Dr. Carol Herbert, another family physician, to set up the women-centred Vancouver Sexual Assault Service. But for about 10 years before I worked at BC Women's, my work had focused on community health activities that were, for the most part, "gender-neutral" and driven by the DTES's prevailing health emergencies, including uncontrolled epidemics of HIV, hepatitis C, and drug overdose deaths. All of these affected women, of course, but there was almost no gendered approach in our responses.

So when I joined BC Women's in 1998, I felt like I was coming home after quite a long absence. Over time I came to realize I was also entering a complicated administrative environment that I knew nothing about, including a women's health community that had advanced in its understanding and strategies to address women's health issues, increasingly incorporating its analyses into mainstream health planning and services such as those that BC Women's was offering.

Despite having only been established in 1994, by 1998 BC Women's was already a well-recognized institution in British Columbia, combining a very large maternity and neonatal program with a broad spectrum of women's health services. Some of these were new and some were inherited from other agencies, and included the sexual assault service, abortion services (CARE Program), osteoporosis, breast health, Aboriginal health, reproductive mental health, and many others. Dr. Penny Ballem, BC Women's first leader, effectively drove forward an agenda to develop BC Women's as a provincial women's health resource, facilitating the first British Columbia Women's Health consultation in 1995 (Ballem, 1995) and establishing the groundwork for a unique applied research endeavour, the British Columbia Centre of Excellence for Women's Health (BCCEWH), established in 1996 with federal funds.

This emergence of BC Women's as a provincial leader occurred over a period when the concepts of both women's health and health promotion were emerging and being increasingly refined. Working from the premise that women's health included the social, political, and economic context as well as biology (United Nations, 1995) meant that BC Women's vision had to move beyond provision of women's health services to engage in systemic advocacy about all factors affecting women's health, political or otherwise—health promotion, in other words. Health promotion is a broad concept, defined in the Ottawa Charter as a set of strategies covering a range of interventions, from the individual to the population level, to improve "well-being" and the proportion of healthy individuals within society as a whole (World Health Organization, 1986). The potential scope for any health institution's participation in the project of health promotion is very wide.

Like all publicly funded health institutions in Canada, BC Women's ultimately gets its mandate from the provincial government, and is part of a complex system whereby government implements its policies and allocates its resources. A redesign of the health system in British Columbia began in the early 1990s, the same time that BC Women's began its life as a comprehensive women's health organization. In the 20 years that BC Women's has existed, the government has worked to fundamentally change the way it manages health care resources, finally settling (for now) on a system of health authorities, five regional and one provincial. For the last 12 years, BC Women's has been administered as part of the Provincial Health Services Authority (PHSA).

Hence, the BC Women's I came to work in was not then and still is not a truly independent entity, but one medium-sized agency in a much larger system, albeit charged with a unique provincial focus on women's health and some helpful partnerships with both government policy-makers and community-based women's advocates.

In our system of public administration, policy, mandate, and funding are derived from "above," but interpretation and broadening of policy and mandate is developed at the institutional level. Leadership and vision are very important in this process because the clearer the vision, the stronger the ability to advocate from the "bottom up" for more relevant and supportive government policy. As leaders of large, government-funded institutions, senior hospital administrators can exercise important influence on policy, especially from a platform of community-based political support and/or compelling evidence for action or change.

The relationships among government, health care institutions, and health authorities are complex, made even more so by whatever may be the current political context and the mixed interests of various stakeholders such as patients, community groups, target populations, other health agencies and authorities, health unions, professional groups, researchers, communications departments, and universities. In order to consider the role of a hospital like BC Women's in women's health promotion and what it has been and what we might wish it to be, we must first acknowledge the institution's geographical, structural, social, and political location. A hospital/health centre is a complex system within a larger complex adaptive system. Let's refer to this larger system from here on as the CAS. With this structure in mind, we can better understand the hospital's difficulty in developing a clear expression of its direction in supporting the health of women, in promoting health, and/or in changing the health system's relationship with women and girls.

Currently the government's language and policy direction in relation to health authorities is dominated by the need to justify the very large expenditures that go to support the acute care system, and to demonstrate accountability. Therefore, the strategic vision, and ultimately the activities, of the hospital incorporate language and values that reflect the mandate from the larger CAS, such as better value, sustainability, and improved service design. Dedication to other values—such as promoting the broadly defined health of women, the health of the women's population in general, or that of specifically marginalized populations—must somehow be expressed and acted upon within the dominant values and direction of the CAS, which are generally laid down by government and, in the case of BC Women's, the Provincial Health Services Authority.

Health Promotion in a Women's Hospital

Leaving aside for the moment the question of the impact of gender analysis and its implications for both planning and action, I would like to explore where "health" and "health promotion" fit in a hospital setting. Health and health promotion are usually defined in gender-neutral terms: Health is "a state of complete physical, mental and social well-being and not merely the absence of disease or infirmity," enabling individuals to realize their aspirations (World Health Organization, 1946, p. 1).

Health promotion is the process of enabling people at the individual and population level to increase control over and to improve their health, to reach a state of complete physical, mental, and social well-being (World Health Organization, 1986).

These concepts are taken to be applicable to both individuals and populations, and to include some acknowledgement of the impact of external environmental, societal, and political factors. The health of the individual is seen to be dependent not only on her genetic inheritance (biology) but also on the context in which her life is lived. Unfortunately, when health and health promotion are discussed, it is often unclear whether the state of well-being to which we aspire and the actions to enable achievement of that state are referring to the individual or to the population.

"Enabling people to increase control over and improve their health" is a process that can be enacted at a number of levels, depending on where we assume the locus of control to be, or where we think we can be most effective, or where we think the fundamental problem lies. Our actions could focus on individuals, a community/population of individuals, or government decision-makers or policy-makers. What we choose to do will be determined by our understanding of the evidence, by our own beliefs about how people and institutions change, by our own location in the greater system, and by what power we may have to effect positive change at whatever level.

In general, hospitals, as the most expensive component of our health care system, are in the business of restoring physical and mental health by responding to and mitigating the illnesses or injuries threatening the well-being and independence of individuals. With some notable exceptions (maternity hospitals), these institutions minister to people only because they are, will be, or have been sick.

Hospitals are very much worlds of their own, often existing apart from the community at large except as they interact one on one with individuals and their families and/or are beholden/accountable to government or health authorities for their operating funding and mandate. The acuity and complexity of the work, complicated more and more by the advances of technology, are so engrossing for those who work there that they are usually quite happy to leave the questions of population health and health promotion to other, in their view more appropriate, sectors. When hospitals get involved in health promotion activities, it is usually in the context of broadening the dissemination of the demonstrably positive effects of lifestyle changes or medications to reduce the incidence and impacts of illnesses on individuals who might eventually need and use expensive hospital resources, or better managing the "high fliers," those whose lives of physical and social vulnerability lead to frequent visits or stays in hospitals, where they use up a lot of resources.

Hospitals' health promotion activities, then, are more likely to focus on achieving positive changes for the individuals who come to the door—such as reducing their risk of heart attack or stroke, or connecting them to a service system that can address health determinants such as housing and poverty—and then get them out the door. This is a very targeted approach, starting from specific medical concerns such as cardiac illness, and working backwards or upstream of the illness to reduce the impact at the acute care site by improving the health of the individual. In Canada, hospitals usually do not engage as institutions in broader, more social, or political advocacy.

Hospitals also provide a place of work and significant income for large numbers of people, including support staff and professionals who spend their entire careers in these environments. At BC Women's, there are about 2,000 staff, most of whom are women. Increasingly, government, the health authority, and hospital leadership are acknowledging the importance of the health of their workforce, which is by far the highest expenditure in the health system. Developing health promotion strategies for staff to address such issues as depression, influenza risk, and cardiovascular disease within hospitals has now become a priority in most settings. However, health promotion responsibility for staff is usually assigned to the human resources department and includes development and dissemination of educational materials and resource links for staff to support their individual knowledge and capacity to reduce risk or seek assistance. Health promotion activities that might address more social or environmental determinants of staff well-being (such as on-site child care, self-determined schedules, or work-life balance) are much more difficult within a system with such structural issues as collective agreements, autonomous professional groups, and resource restraints.

Systemic Challenges in Improving Women's Health

> Women's health involves women's emotional, social and physical well-being and is determined by the social, political and economic context of their lives, as well as by biology. This broad definition of women's health recognizes the validity of women's life experiences and women's own beliefs about and experiences of health. Every woman should be provided with the opportunity to achieve, sustain and maintain health, as defined by the woman herself, to her full potential. (Phillips, 1995, pp. 507–508)

Since its inception in 1994, BC Women's leadership has taken on a much broader health promotion agenda than most other hospitals. The hospital's development over the 1990s coincided with the emergence of new definitions of women's health and new approaches to public health, including the articulation of the importance of health promotion as a strategy. The governments of the day, both provincial and federal, were supportive of population health initiatives addressing a range of health determinants and accepted that gender was one of them. In British Columbia, the government regarded and promoted BC Women's as a resource providing provincial leadership and expertise in all areas of women's health, and its early leadership strengthened this perception through innovative actions such as convening a provincial women's health forum and wide consultation, developing the British Columbia Centre of Excellence for Women's Health, and advocating publicly for reproductive choice.

Nevertheless, as a publicly funded hospital within this complex adaptive system where it must line up its activities to be consistent with government and health authority directions, its extended mandate and activities had to be seen to rest firmly on government priorities and specific clinical service responsibilities, a requirement that has only increased over the last 10 or 12 years. So, for example, by 2003, in *Advancing the Health of Girls and Women*, the provincial women's health strategy, BC Women's is described as

> the lead agency ... with the mandate to address the broad range of health issues for women in BC. [D]evoted primarily to the health of women of all ages and backgrounds, BC Women's provides a broad range of specialized health services and is the largest single provider of maternity services in Canada. It coordinates and evaluates specialized health services, disease prevention and health promotion activities, and works with other health authorities in BC to support equitable and cost effective health care for girls and women. (BC Women's Hospital & Health Centre & British Columbia Centre of Excellence for Women's Health, 2004, p. 9)

In this description, the hospital is "devoted to health of women," but it enacts this value largely through its clinical services.

In its 2012–2013 strategic plan update (BC Women's Hospital & Centre, 2012), the description of priority and focus is much the same: "Improving quality outcomes and providing better value for patients; Contributing to a sustainable health care system in BC; and Deliver[ing] the best care for women, girls and newborn babies" (p. 1). The provincial leadership role to advocate for women's health is still discernible within the overall context of government and health authority priorities, but the language has changed. Thus the hospital's stated aims are to include a broader understanding of women's health in the way it provides care "beyond traditional medical interventions," and "lead the women's population health agenda," "serving as a catalyst to identify key issues and contribute to ... policies ... aimed at improving the health of BC's population, especially girls and women" (ibid.).

So, here is BC Women's, one of only a few institutions in Canada with a mandate (in its very name, even) to address women's health issues, struggling nevertheless to articulate this calling as part of a much larger, compelling, politically sensitive system (complex and possibly adaptive) of health services. In the project of improving women's health, this institution has had a lot going for it, including consistent female leadership; a preponderance of women staff (like most hospitals); strong feminist analyses of some issues and the people to apply them; at least intermittent government support for a broader role; and some very strong researchers across the spectrum of health policy, health system, and clinical research. But it is challenged in claiming the ground of women's health by its position in the larger system whose prevailing and compelling direction is emphatically not gendered.

A recent letter from a senior health authority administrator in response to a community-generated letter advocating for continuation of a specific service demonstrates this challenge well: "[The Health Authority] spends health care dollars on health care services but cannot support non-clinical items." Health promotion is not a clinical activity. This is the classic health system paradox—all our money goes into restoring health, that is, treating the sick, and woe unto the health care provider who tries to optimize health.

The Meaning of Health Promotion for a Women's Hospital

In the context of health promotion, gender transformation would require examining the role of gender as it affects a woman's ability to respond to health information and effect changes in her own health behaviour. However, most (health researchers) still focus on how the behaviours of the "recipients" of health promotion practices are affected by social constraints. This work fails to consider how those who can change social conditions, such as health promotion programmers, health practitioners, and local policy-makers, might impact meso- or community-level issues, thereby mediating between individual women and broader structural influences (Women's Health Victoria, 2012).

In spite of the structural and political challenges over the years, I believe BC Women's has been at least partly successful in many activities that can be categorized as health promotion. These endeavours have been facilitated by the previously described strategic partnerships with community, researchers (British Columbia Centre of Excellence for Women's Health), and government. Three BC Women's initiatives (among many others) can provide some insight into how this particular hospital has engaged in health promotion: *Advancing the Health of*

Girls and Women, Sheway/Fir Square, and the Woman Abuse Response Program.

Advancing the Health of Girls and Women is a Women's Health Strategy for British Columbia published in 2004 (BC Women's Hospital & Health Centre & British Columbia Centre of Excellence for Women's Health, 2004). BC Women's was a partner in its production with the BCCEWH and these agencies together led a broad consultation with community women across British Columbia, health providers and health authorities, government, and researchers over many months to gather the information for the plan. Key sources included updates on data in the 1995 Provincial Health Officer's report on women's health (Ministry of Health & Ministry Responsible for Seniors, 1996), community-based focus groups and women's health analyses, and plans developed by regional health authorities. The stated purpose of the report was to "improve the health of girls and women throughout BC." The partners set the platform for this in the report by providing substantial background on women's health in general and specifically in British Columbia (history, definitions, indicators, analysis) and extrapolating a number of recommendations to strengthen the system's ability to monitor women's health and to focus on some priority health issues such as access to a sustainable maternity care system and improved support for women with mental health and addictions problems. The plan was disseminated through various venues, including a presentation to the executives of all BC health authorities who, we hoped, would mandate activity within their structures.

As one of the leaders in the development of *Advancing the Health of Girls and Women*, BC Women's explicitly assumed a health promotion role. With the support of the British Columbia Centre of Excellence for Women's Health, it produced a robust document that is still very relevant. There were a couple of important gains made as a result of the development and articulation of the strategy. First, there was a very broad engagement in the discussion of what girls' and women's health is and should be, and it enhanced the reputation of BC Women's as a source of expertise on all women's health issues. Second, the recommendations provided priorities that coincided with anticipated directions of the Ministry of Health. For example, maternity care access was selected from a myriad of other issues specifically because the government was indicating an interest in this area, which set the stage for the development of the BC Maternity Care Enhancement Strategy (BC Ministry of Health, 2004). On the other hand, there was relatively little uptake on other priorities, especially at the regional health authority level, where other problems, usually involving acute care hospitals, were top of mind. And when *Advancing the Health of Girls and Women* was complete, it included discussion of women's poverty and homelessness, issues that were so sensitive for the provincial government of the day that it withdrew as an official partner in releasing the report even though the Ministry of Health had provided the early funding. Arm's-length institutions such as hospitals can sometimes perform a helpful function for the larger system by voicing issues that are politically difficult or impossible for those closer to its centre.

Sheway and Fir Square are a linked set of clinical support services for pregnant women who have alcohol and/or other substance use problems that can potentially affect their own health and the health of their fetus or infant. Sheway is a community-based program that provides multidisciplinary support and advocacy, and Fir Square is a dedicated preconception and postpartum clinical care unit located in a ward of BC Women's. The hospital is a partner in the community-based service, providing core funding as well as the services of a special family practice maternity care team. Women attending the community program are provided with support in obtaining information on nutrition, housing, personal safety, social support, harm reduction, and addictions treatment in addition to prenatal and postnatal care. While in Fir Square, women are provided with similar supports as well as in-patient medical and nursing care.

On the face of it, this support continuum is a clinical program, not a health promotion activity per se, yet this program's success rests on the degree to which participating women can claim their own health. Women in Sheway/Fir Square are provided with care based on a harm-reduction paradigm, which on an individual basis implies providing a woman with the tools to ensure her own safety and her own agency in becoming healthier. Of course, not all participants are able to succeed in reclaiming their health and in so doing that of their children and families, but a large proportion do, and retention in the Sheway program itself approaches 100 percent, an unheard of number in addiction treatment programs generally.

The role of the hospital in this case has been to work in partnership with women and their team to support them as they need to be supported, which has often meant advocating for them within the larger systems of social supports and child protection. The hospital's role has also been to support champions of a new understanding of how communities view women who drink alcohol or use illicit drugs during pregnancy, to change how the problem is defined, to change the standard of care that is offered to them, to change the rules, and to educate other communities and providers. This is a type of gendered health promotion that aims to transform assumptions about these heath issues and therefore the way in which women are perceived and supported in taking control of their health.

BC Women's Woman Abuse Response Program provides a third example of the hospital's involvement in health promotion. The goal of this program is to enhance safety for women within health care settings, especially those who may be experiencing relationship abuse. Many health care initiatives to address the issue of interpersonal violence focus only on identifying women at risk through enhanced screening, with the criteria of success being the proportion of women screened by health providers and the proportion of women thereby identified as victims. This approach is similar to most clinical initiatives in the health care system—that is, to identify and respond on an individual level—but it is simplistic and ineffective in improving women's health or even increasing women's safety.

The BC Women's Woman Abuse program is built on an analysis of the context of women's lives and what is required to increase safety and a woman's empowerment within that context. The program has been responsible for the development and dissemination of extensive training materials to enhance health (and community) system competence in ensuring safety and safe responses for women experiencing abuse that do not compound harm. Within the hospital setting, the aim is to develop a context in which women both understand that it is safe to disclose and ask for assistance, and where they will receive support appropriate to their individual circumstances. The training aims to contextualize the in-hospital response to relationship violence within the social and political realities of violence in the community. The program educates workers about gender-based violence and develops practical ways in which health sector staff can both support women to make the decisions to enhance their safety and provide linkages and resources to help with that process.

As stated in the framework that guides the program,

> the Woman Abuse Response program at BC Women's is educating health professionals to shift practice rather than place responsibility on women to disclose abuse. The guiding principles are adapted from the anti-violence field, acknowledging the centrality of women's safety and the need to mitigate the intersecting discriminations of gender based violence, social circumstance and culture and race. The program recognized that staff may bring their own experiences of abuse to their work, and this experience can be helpful in creating strategies for responding appropriately to abuse in the lives of their patients. (Cory & Dechief, 2007, p. 36)

The Woman Abuse Response Program is a demonstration of implementing gendered health promotion within the hospital setting. Such work is not easily accomplished within this setting because of the acuity of the work and the challenges posed by providing the time and space needed for staff education. Because any hospital stay represents a tiny proportion of a woman's life, it is argued (as it is in other acute settings about cardiac disease, for example) that health promotion advocacy is better applied at the community level. But again this raises the question of the scope of the hospital's role in the community, and specifically whether the hospital has a greater community role.

I think the answer is yes. The BC Women's Woman Abuse Response Program has been widely influential across the province partly by virtue of its location within BC Women's, which has strengthened its credibility among other ministries and agencies that have significant impact on women's safety, including the Ministry of Justice and the Ministry for Children and Families. The program leaders, with support of hospital leadership, have worked with such external agencies to develop higher quality, more gender-informed training and responses within their respective systems, as well as offering training and facilitation for other hospitals in partnership with communities.

We can try to push a system in some way, but it is moving by itself and has its own momentum, so then we can try to grab a corner and pull it off course, at least a little. We might or might not have any impact on its speed or direction. In any case, I would say it's very hard to tell what our impact is on the large CAS but whatever we may wish, we are stuck within it. But the system is also stuck with us, and its overall direction, its meaning, is undoubtedly influenced by our active participation in it.

The BC Women's Hospital & Health Centre is a medium-sized agency in a large, ponderous, complex, moving health care system. With its unique mandate, however, as a women-centred agency, I believe it has a responsibility to engage not only with the individuals who come to it for clinical expertise and support but also with the system as a whole. The hospital can and has done this in several different ways, depending on the expertise and resources available, whether developing provincial momentum to improve women's health, working with women to reduce their risk in a clinical program, or changing staff and community perspective on a pervasive women's health issue, as the three examples illustrate.

If the hospital leadership and staff maintain their commitment to improving the health of girls and women, then the hospital must necessarily embrace gendered health promotion at whatever level it finds itself working with individuals or the greater system. In this way, it may be possible to gradually transform how women's health is perceived and supported in our complex world from a key vantage point within that system.

REFERENCES

Ballem, P. (1995). *The challenges ahead for women's health: BC Women's community consultation report.* Vancouver: BC Women's Hospital and Health Centre Society.

BC Ministry of Health. (2004). *Supporting local collaborative models for sustainable maternity care in British Columbia: Recommendations from the Maternity Care Enhancement Project.* Victoria: British Columbia Ministry of Health.

BC Women's Hospital & Health Centre. (2012). *Strategic plans and publications.* Retrieved from www.bcwomens.ca/AboutUs/BCWomens/StrategicPlan.htm

BC Women's Hospital & Health Centre & British Columbia Centre of Excellence for Women's Health. (2004). *A women's health strategy for British Columbia: Advancing the health of girls and women.* Vancouver: BC Women's Hospital and Health Centre & British Columbia Centre of Excellence for Women's Health.

Cory, J., & Dechief, L. (2007). *SHE framework: Safety and health enhancement for women experiencing abuse: A tool kit for health providers and planners.* Vancouver: BC Women's Hospital and Health Centre & BC Institute Against Family Violence.

Ministry of Health & Ministry Responsible for Seniors. (1996). *A report on the health of British Columbians: Provincial health officer's annual report feature report: Women's health.* Victoria: Author.

Phillips, S. (1995). The social context of women's health: Goals and objectives for medical education. *Canadian Medical Association Journal, 152*(4), 507–511.

United Nations. 1995. Fourth World Conference on Women: Action for Equality Development and Peace, Beijing, China, September 4–15.

Whynot, E. (2010, January 8). *Both sides now: Realities and illusions in health care leadership.* Paper presented at the 3rd Annual Anne Crichton Memorial Seminar, Vancouver, BC.

Wikipedia. (n. d.). *Complex adaptive system.* Retrieved from http://en.wikipedia.org/wiki/Complex_adaptive_system

Women's Health Victoria. (2012). Gender transformative policy and practice. Retrieved from http://whv.org.au/static/files/assets/e98b657e/Gender-transformative-policy-and-practice.pdf

World Health Organization. (1946). *Constitution of the World Health Organization.* Geneva: Author.

World Health Organization. (1986). *Ottawa Charter for health promotion.* Ottawa: Author.

14 Taking a Stand: A Gender-Transformative Approach to Preventing Violence against Women

Rose Durey

Introduction

Violence against women is a damaging and pervasive issue that cuts across all sectors of society. It impacts the health and well-being of women, families, and communities, as well as the economy. But it is preventable. The determinants of violence against women are strongly linked to gender inequality and it is these determinants that must be challenged in the primary prevention of violence against women. This chapter explores the strong parallels between the primary prevention of violence against women and gender-transformative health promotion. Both address gender inequality as a determinant by confronting and reshaping traditional gender roles, norms, and structures.

This chapter explores a violence prevention program implemented in a male-dominated workplace. From 2007 to 2012, Women's Health Victoria, an Australian women's health promotion organization, partnered with Linfox, a male-dominated transport and logistics company, to prevent violence against women. This chapter explores the development of the program called Take a Stand Against Domestic Violence: It's Everyone's Business (Take a Stand) that emerged from this work, and the impact the program had at Linfox. It also discusses the elements that make Take a Stand gender-transformative, and the importance of taking a gender-transformative approach to the prevention of violence against women.

Preventing Violence Against Women/ Gender-Transformative Health Promotion

The United Nations Declaration on the Elimination of Violence Against Women defines violence against women as "[a]ny act of gender-based violence that results in, or is likely to result in, physical, sexual or psychological harm or suffering to women, including threats of such acts, coercion or arbitrary deprivation of liberty, whether occurring in public or in private life" (United Nations, 1993, Article 1). Violence against women affects individuals, families, communities, and society as a whole. In Australia, one in three women over the age of 15 have experienced physical assault (Australian Bureau of Statistics, 2006), and over half of all women in Australia have experienced at least one incident of physical and/or sexual violence in their lifetime (Australian Bureau of Statistics, 2006; Mouzos & Makkai, 2004). Violence against women is the leading contributor to death, disability, and illness in Victorian women ages 15 to 44 (VicHealth, 2004). Most violence against women occurs in the home and is perpetrated by a male known to the victim, predominantly an intimate partner (Australian Bureau of Statistics, 2006). It has significant and often devastating consequences for victims, including death, homelessness, and poor social, mental, and physical health outcomes (Marcus & Braaf, 2007; National Council to Reduce Violence Against Women and Their Children, 2009; World Health Organization & Liverpool John Moores University, 2009). Violence against women also impacts the economy. In 2009, the cost of violence against women and their children to the Australian economy was estimated to be $13.6 billion (National Council to Reduce Violence Against Women and Their Children, 2009).

The primary prevention of violence against women aims to prevent it before it occurs. It does this by addressing the causes of violence against women rather than the more visible "symptoms" (World Health Organization, 2002, 2010; VicHealth, 2007b). It differs from secondary prevention, which targets at-risk populations, and tertiary prevention, which aims to prevent future incidents of violence by responding to past victims or perpetrators (VicHealth, 2011).

These underlying causes or determinants of violence against women are strongly linked to gender inequality (United Nations, 1993). They include

- unequal power relations between women and men;
- adherence to rigid gender stereotypes; and
- broader cultures of violence (Barrett Meyering, 2011; VicHealth, 2007b).

By addressing these causes, change is possible. That change is the transformation of traditional gender roles, norms, and structures, and in this way the primary prevention of violence against women aligns strongly with gender-transformative health promotion. Gender-transformative approaches

actively strive to examine, question, and change rigid gender norms and imbalance of power as a means of reaching health as well as gender equity objectives.

> Gender transformative approaches encourage critical awareness among men and women of gender roles and norms; promote the position of women; challenge the distribution of resources and allocation of duties between men and women; and/or address the power relationships between women and others in the community, such as service providers or traditional leaders. (Rottach, Schuler, & Hardee, 2009, p. 8)

Like the primary prevention of violence against women, gender transformative health promotion aims to redefine harmful gender norms, challenge gender stereotypes and develops and strengthens equitable gender roles and relationships (Boender et al., 2004; Greene & Levack, 2010).

Violence-supportive attitudes and behaviours form part of a culture in which traditional notions of gender are prevalent. A key study into community attitudes to violence against women in Australia found that the strongest and most consistent predictor of holding violence-supportive attitudes was being male, and having weak support for gender equality (VicHealth, 2007a; VicHealth, 2010). Violence-supportive attitudes and behaviours

- trivialize violence and its impacts;
- attribute blame to the victim of violence;
- deny that violence occurred or that certain behaviours are violence;
- deny that public agencies or the community have a responsibility to prevent violence or to hold violent people to account; and/or
- justify or excuse violence.

Jokes, remarks, aggressive or demeaning behaviour, or displaying offensive materials could all support violence (VicHealth, 2007a). This resonated with Women's Health Victoria and underscored the need to design a program that challenged violence-supportive attitudes and behaviours among men and promoted non-violent norms. Men as well as women must be meaningfully engaged in interventions to promote gender equality and prevent violence against women (World Health Organization & Liverpool John Moores University, 2009).

In exploring ways in which men could be engaged to prevent violence against women, workplaces were identified as a key setting. Not only are workplaces directly impacted by instances of domestic violence, they also play a role in influencing the behaviour of individuals and groups. They can reinforce or challenge normative beliefs and can also model equitable and respectful gender relations (Connell, 2003; Cunradi,

Ames, & Moore, 2008; VicHealth, 2007b). Workplaces therefore are a site in which non-violent norms can be promoted. This is an emerging area of practice (VicHealth, 2011). Workplaces also offer an opportunity to reach individuals who would not otherwise come into contact with health promotion interventions. In addition, workplaces are also a site in which organizational systems and structures can be adapted to promote gender equity. The following section describes the workplace-based program that was designed by Women's Health Victoria to prevent violence against women.

Designing and Implementing "Take a Stand"

In 2007, Women's Health Victoria was funded by the Victorian Health Promotion Foundation (VicHealth) to prevent violence against women by strengthening the organizational capacity of a male-dominated workplace to promote gender equality and non-violent norms. Women's Health Victoria worked with Linfox, a privately owned company with over 16,000 employees worldwide, to test the design and implementation of Take a Stand, a primary prevention workplace program. The project focused on employees located in Victoria, a state of Australia, and was evaluated with the support of VicHealth. Take a Stand is a comprehensive workplace program that addresses the prevention of violence against women at a range of levels within the workplace. It is premised on the understanding that the health and safety of employees at home affects their health and safety at work. It takes a whole-company approach, addressing all systems, staff, and levels of a company (Versola-Russo & Russo, 2009). The program promotes non-violent social norms and challenges violence-supportive attitudes and behaviours. It also ensures that employees who are experiencing intimate partner violence are supported. Take a Stand recognizes that—whether through the victim, perpetrator, or wider community—the workplace is impacted by violence.

Some key principles regarding men's involvement in violence prevention were considered in the design and implementation of Take a Stand. Pease (2008) notes that these include the need to

- ensure that men's violence prevention was linked to the promotion of gender equality;
- ensure that a feminist analysis remained the central underpinning of the work;
- refocus primary prevention of men's violence to system interventions;
- work with non-violent men whose silence perpetuates other men's violence;
- locate men in their specific context;

- interrogate masculinity; and
- ensure that men's violence-prevention work is accountable to women.

These principles guided the development of Take a Stand. The heart of the program is about changing the attitudes and behaviours that sustain violence. This is achieved through awareness-raising, corporate leadership, workplace policy, training, and promotion of violence-prevention messages throughout the workplace. Women's Health Victoria worked with Linfox to implement these elements, aligning them with the company's goals, values, and existing initiatives.

Take a Stand uses a bystander approach to violence prevention. The bystander approach is a means by which individuals are equipped to take a stand against violence against women in the context of their working and personal lives. It also has the potential for broader community and societal change. A bystander is not a victim or perpetrator, but a friend, colleague, or family member who takes action to "[i]dentify, speak out about or seek to engage others in responding to: specific incidents of violence; and/or behaviours, attitudes, practices or policies that contribute to violence" (VicHealth, 2011, p. 8).

The bystander approach sends a message that violence against women is everyone's business, and that everyone has a positive role in eliminating it. It provides the mechanism to challenge violence-supportive attitudes and behaviours. The approach has been used successfully in programs across the United States (Katz, 2006; Dyson & Flood, 2007), and underpins the Australian Football League's (2007) Respect and Responsibility program.

By focusing on positive messages, Take a Stand reinforces healthy, respectful behaviours and centres on what people in the workplace can do to make a difference. This is important because an approach in which all men are regarded as potential perpetrators would alienate most men from the outset (Katz, 2006). Blame does not create attitudinal, behavioural, or organizational change (Funk, 2006). Instead, it individualizes violence against women so that it is understood as a result of individual men's dysfunctional behaviour (Katz, 2006). This ignores the fact that violence against women is a part of a pervasive system of gender inequality (ibid.). By increasing receptiveness to violence prevention using the bystander approach, broader community change is envisaged (Banyard, Plante, & Moynihan, 2004). The approach

- encourages men and women to speak out against violence-supportive attitudes and behaviours;
- provides practical tools for challenging violence-supportive attitudes and behaviours;

- recognizes the long-term benefits of a preventative approach; and
- regards men as partners in prevention and not perpetrators.

This approach was vital in gaining support for the project among managers and employees. A program in which men felt targeted, or one that was more confrontational, would not have gained traction in a male-dominated company. The bystander approach was therefore key to the adoption of the program and the receptiveness of employees in training.

In challenging sexist behaviour, the bystander approach also provided a link to gender inequality as a determinant of violence against women. This connection, so crucial to the primary prevention of violence against women, is often difficult to grasp. At Linfox, this was achieved by discussing sexist behaviour in training activities, by addressing sexism in the Take a Stand principles, and by including respectful relationships between women and men in a prevention of domestic violence policy. Take a Stand demonstrated the potential for workplaces to transform understandings of gender given that workplaces have the power to reinforce or disrupt conventional notions of masculinity (Ely & Meyerson, 2010). Through adapting practices, policies, and norms, "organizations can equip men to undo gender by giving them the motivation, a model, and a margin of safety to deviate from conventional masculine scripts" (ibid., p. 27). This is what Take a Stand sought to achieve.

Evaluation of Take a Stand

This section explores the extent to which messages about how to challenge violence-supportive attitudes and behaviours were heard and adopted by staff at Linfox. These messages, together with practical tools to implement them, were conveyed through training.

In total, 515 employees participated in the training, across 11 work sites in Victoria. Results showed that

- 87 percent of participants felt that the training helped them gain a better understanding of domestic violence;
- 87 percent of participants felt that the training helped them understand how things people say or do can support domestic violence; and
- 89 percent of participants felt that they were very likely or quite likely to speak out against domestic violence as a result of the training.

Comments from participants included the following:

- "Made me think twice about my behaviour and response to situations."
- "There are people that know people that do it [perpetrate domestic violence] and they might learn something from this and as a friend can say something. I've said to a friend 'Why are you talking to your wife like that?'"

Managers were also positive about the impact of the training on their work sites: "The blokes get a new view on things and start thinking more about their actions."

Findings also showed that participants felt they were more likely to challenge violence-supportive attitudes and behaviours as a result of the training, and understood how sexism occurs on a continuum of violence against women. The training may also continue to promote organizational culture change within individual work sites as staff come to discuss domestic violence more openly, and are more cognizant of how what they say or do can contribute to a culture in which violence against women is prevalent. Almost all participants felt that the training should be provided more widely. The majority of focus group participants, who were consulted six months after the training, felt that the training had changed the way they thought about violence against women and what they could do about it.

Although Women's Health Victoria's work at Linfox is now complete, the Take a Stand program continues. Women's Health Victoria is currently working to implement the program in a number of other workplaces in Victoria. Women's Health Victoria is also committed to sharing learnings with other organizations interested in working with business to prevent violence against women.

Conclusion

Take a Stand is a unique, whole-company program aimed at the primary prevention of violence against women. It uses the workplace as a setting to engage men in the prevention of violence against women and, in doing so, challenges traditional notions of gender. This is what makes the program gender-transformative—it endeavours to confront attitudes and behaviours that support violence against women, change them, and promote gender equity. The alignment between the primary prevention of violence against women and gender-transformative health promotion is clear. Both are about transforming gender roles, norms, and structures. And ultimately, if violence against women is to be prevented, it is these that must be transformed.

REFERENCES

Australian Bureau of Statistics. (2006). *Personal safety survey 4906.0*. Canberra: Australian Bureau of Statistics. Retrieved from www.abs.gov.au/ausstats/abs@.nsf/mf/4906.0

Australian Football League. (2007). *Respect and Responsibility: Creating a safe and inclusive environment for women at all levels of Australian Football and in the broader community.* Melbourne: Australian Football League. Retrieved from www.afl.com.au/staticfile/AFL%20Tenant/AFL/Files/Practical_Education.pdf

Banyard, V., Plante, E., & Moynihan, M. (2004). Bystander education: Bringing a broader community perspective to sexual violence prevention. *Journal of Community Psychology, 32*(1), 61–79.

Barrett Meyering, I. (2011). *Thematic review 1: What factors shape community attitudes to domestic violence?* Sydney: Australian Domestic and Family Violence Clearinghouse. Retrieved from www.adfvc.unsw.edu.au/PDF%20files/Thematic%20Review_1.pdf

Boender, C., Santana, D., Santillan, D., Hardee, K., Greene, M. E., & Schuler, S. (2004). *The "So what?" report: A look at whether integrating a gender focus into programs makes a difference to outcomes.* Washington, DC: Interagency Gender Working Group Task Force. Retrieved from www.prb.org/igwg_media/thesowhatreport.pdf

Connell, R. W. (2003). *The role of men and boys in achieving gender equality.* Brasilia: UN Division for the Advancement of Women: Expert Group Meeting. Retrieved from www.un.org/womenwatch/daw/egm/men-boys2003/documents.html

Cunradi, C., Ames, G., & Moore, R. (2008). Prevalence and correlates of intimate partner violence among a sample of construction industry workers. *Journal of Family Violence, 23*, 101–112.

Dyson, S., & Flood, M. (2007). *Building cultures of respect and non-violence: A review of literature concerning adult learning and violence prevention programs with men—Respect and Responsibility Program.* Melbourne: VicHealth. Retrieved from www.vichealth.vic.gov.au/en/Publications/Freedom-from-violence/Building-Cultures-of-Respect-and-Non-Violence.aspx

Ely, R., & Meyerson, D. (2010). An organizational approach to undoing gender: The unlikely case of offshore oil platforms. *Research in Organizational Behaviour, 30*, 3–34.

Funk, R. E. (2006). *Reaching men: Strategies for preventing sexist attitudes, behaviors, and violence.* Indianapolis: JIST Life.

Greene, M. E., & Levack A. (2010). *Synchronizing gender strategies: A cooperative model for improving reproductive health and transforming gender relations.* Interagency Gender Working Group. Washington: Population Reference Bureau. Retrieved from www.engenderhealth.org/files/pubs/gender/Synchronizing_Gender_Strategies.pdf

Katz, J. (2006). *The macho paradox: Why some men hurt women and how all men can help.* Naperville, IL: Sourcebooks Inc.

Marcus, G., & Braaf, R. (2007). *Domestic and family violence studies, surveys, and statistics: Pointers to policy and practice.* Sydney: Australian Family and Domestic Violence Clearinghouse. Retrieved from www.austdvclearinghouse.unsw.edu.au/PDF%20files/Stakeholderpaper_1.pdf

Mouzos, J., & Makkai, T. (2004). *Women's experiences of male violence: Findings from the Australian component of the International Violence Against Women Survey (IVAWS).* Canberra: Australian

Institute of Criminology. Retrieved from www.aic.gov.au/publications/current%20series/rpp/41-60/rpp56.aspx

National Council to Reduce Violence Against Women and Their Children. (2009). *Background paper to Time for Action: The National Council's plan for Australia to reduce violence against women and their children, 2009–2021.* Canberra: Australian Department of Families, Housing, Community Services, and Indigenous Affairs. Retrieved from www.fahcsia.gov.au/our-responsibilities/women/publications-articles/reducing-violence/national-plan-to-reduce-violence-against-women-and-their-children/background-paper-to-time-for-action-the-national-councils-plan-for-australia-to-reduce-violence-against-women-and-their

Pease, B. (2008). *Engaging men in men's violence prevention: Exploring the tensions, dilemmas, and possibilities.* Sydney: Australian Domestic and Family Violence Clearinghouse. Retrieved from www.austdvclearinghouse.unsw.edu.au/issues_Papers.htm

Rottach, E., Schuler, S. R., & Hardee, K. (2009). *Gender perspectives improve reproductive health outcomes: New evidence.* Interagency Gender Working Group. Retrieved from www.igwg.org/igwg_media/genderperspectives.pdf

United Nations. (1993). *Declaration on the elimination of violence against women.* Geneva: Author. Retrieved from www.un.org/documents/ga/res/48/a48r104.htm

Versola-Russo, J., & Russo, F. (2009). When domestic violence turns into workplace violence: Organizational impact and response. *Journal of Police Crisis Negotiations, 9*(2), 141–148.

VicHealth. (2004). *The health costs of violence: Measuring the burden of disease caused by intimate partner violence.* Melbourne: VicHealth. Retrieved from www.vichealth.vic.gov.au/en/Publications/Freedom-from-violence/The-Health-Costs-of-Violence.aspx

VicHealth. (2007a). *Preventing violence before it occurs: A framework and background paper to guide the primary prevention of violence against women in Victoria.* Melbourne: VicHealth. Retrieved from www.vichealth.vic.gov.au/Publications/Freedom-from-violence/Preventing-violence-before-it-occurs.aspx

VicHealth. (2007b). *Two steps forward, one step back: Community attitudes towards women.* Melbourne: VicHealth.

VicHealth. (2010). *National survey on community attitudes to violence against women 2009.* Melbourne: VicHealth. Retrieved from www.vichealth.vic.gov.au/en/Publications/Freedom-from-violence/National-Community-Attitudes-towards-Violence-Against-Women-Survey-2009.aspx

VicHealth. (2011). *Review of bystander approaches in support of preventing violence against women.* Melbourne: VicHealth. Retrieved from www.vichealth.vic.gov.au/Publications/Freedom-from-violence/Review-of-bystander-approaches-in-support-of-preventing-violence-against-women.aspx

World Health Organization. (2002). *World report on violence and health.* Geneva: Author. Retrieved from www.who.int/violence_injury_prevention/violence/world_report/en/index.html

World Health Organization. (2010). *Preventing intimate partner and sexual violence against women: Taking action and generating evidence.* Geneva: Author. Retrieved from www.who.int/violence_injury_prevention/violence/activities/intimate/en/index.html

World Health Organization & Liverpool John Moores University. (2009). *Violence prevention: The evidence—promoting gender equality to prevent violence against women.* Geneva: Author. Retrieved from www.who.int/violence_injury_prevention/violence/4th_milestones_meeting/publications/en/index.html

15 Catalyzing Gender-Transformative Health Promotion

Lorraine Greaves

Introduction

Going forward, there are many challenges at many levels in enabling communities, agencies, and governments to develop gender-transformative health promotion. Charlene Cook (2009), who works in social work practice and teaches at the University of Toronto, recently reflected on the state of women's health theorizing, observing that many forces are rapidly changing—biomedical advances, demand for bioethical responses, and globalization of health—and she keenly observes that although there is increased knowledge of the social determinants of health, there is also an increasing political resistance. She reasserts a call for an "epistemological understanding to women's health that is reflexive, progressive and actionable" (Cook, 2009, p. 151–152). Such an understanding would also be a boon to generating better health promotion for women. At the moment, however, we face an uphill struggle in generating understanding and enthusiasm for gender-transformative health promotion. Not only has the health promotion movement been largely silent on gender in the past 40 years, there has been virtually no ground tilled on the ideas of gender transformation. But the need is clearly there: currently, the links between health and gender and equity loom large across the globe, whatever the income level or development stage of a country, and a range of actions are essential to address these links.

The gender-transformative health promotion framework and tool we have developed represent praxis in health promotion. We have taken current gender theory, blended it with a social determinants approach, and focused our attention on how to make action and change happen in health promotion for women. The idea and goal of turning health promotion into a gender-transformative activity is inherently feminist and radical in the sense of going to the root of the problems of

250

women's health and women's inequity and inequality. But the challenges inherent in accomplishing gender transformation are cultural, economic, political, and intellectual. This task requires strategy, imagination, creativity, courage, and passion, as well as a critical evidence base. It also requires work on several levels, including personal, institutional, social, political, and economic.

Sites for Understanding Gender

Although gender is often simplistically understood (and sometimes conflated with "sex"), the concept of gender itself is very complex and constantly subject to changing meanings, depending on time, place, and culture. Gender is a product of culture and can be transformed through action, advocacy, evidence, experience, and the generation and diffusion of new ideas. There are many levels at which gender is expressed and experienced. Understanding these myriad manifestations of gender is essential in order to accurately and effectively create gender-transformative health promotion. These include gender relations, gender identity, and institutional gender, to name some (Johnson, Greaves, & Repta, 2007). These sites or categories of understanding gender also define for us the opportunities and sites for change.

For example, gender relations affect individual, couple, and family interactions, and define relationships between women and men, women and household members, and women and their work colleagues. Gender relations are very contingent on ascribed or achieved power, both stemming from and reinforcing stereotypes, sexism, patriarchal attitudes, gender role socialization, and varied gender-related cultural assumptions. These relations are culture-bound and affect a wide range of experiences for women, such as gender roles, the allocation of power in households, the ability to influence household and relationship dynamics, levels of interpersonal violence, women's reproductive choices, and their freedom of movement and decision-making powers. These elements of the impact of gender relations are often ignored by health promoters, who may be singly interested in strictly health-related results and measures that pertain to health. In addition, these kinds of social processes may seem hard to affect and beyond the scope of health promotion or health care. However, it is possible to measure these sorts of indicators and link them to interventions in health or economic or social life (CARE International, 2012; Ibrahim & Alkire, 2007).

Gender identity is another level of experiencing and understanding gender. While often seen as an individual experience of one's notions of femininity and masculinity, sexual orientation, and sexual identity, it also determines how others respond. However, this too resists a uniform definition and understanding as gender identity is movable and different from place to place and over time, reflecting social

and cultural assumptions and stereotypes that affect individual and group definitions of self and identity, experiences of the body and body image, experiences and
opportunities for sexuality, and sexual and self-expression. In the main, though,
gender identity ascribes dominant culture-bound expectations of being male or
female, and inherently indicates the preferred ways of being. For those who do not
fit the prevailing norms of gender identity, it is difficult to fit in and may lead to
stigmatization, discrimination, or marginalization.

Institutional gender, on the other hand, is all around us, expressed through our
social systems and institutions such as law, education, religion, media, and politics.
These are large systems and can be formidable as they govern us through rules,
regulations, and opportunities for participation in public institutions, education,
labour force, and public life. These operate on all levels—local, regional, national,
and international—and we are all affected by them to some extent. These have often
been predicated and built upon social assumptions about biologically based traits,
and have been particularly inequitable and, in some cases, restrictive, for girls and
women. But these elements of life also respond to advocacy, revolution, and public
social movements. The history of the women's, gay rights, suffrage, and abolitionist
movements illustrates the non-static nature of law, rules, and regulation, and the
pliability of social assumptions about biologically based traits. These histories give
us a basis and inspiration for continued change, and outline the opportunities for
constructing channels or opportunities for women to achieve economic or social
status and to improve their health. They also point to the constrictions and blockages
in attempting to do so. Restrictions (or freedoms) in engaging in public life affect
the opportunity for health and may produce resulting inequities in health.

Gender-Transformative Praxis

Given that these elements and experiences of gender can often appear so ingrained
and formidable, it is essential to approach the task of gender-transformative health
promotion with a strategy and a sound evidence base. The planning tool (outlined
in Chapter 11), along with the overriding framework (described in Chapter 1) offer
some basic approaches to this task. In addition, the examples in Part 2 illustrate a
range of struggles and successes in addressing gender and ultimately gender-transformative health promotion on a wide variety of health issues. Some lessons can be
derived from these cases, including the importance of generating accurate evidence
of the impact of gender on various health issues, but also the importance of generating and accessing a range of types of evidence, and using it to make cases for change.

The cases described in this book also indicate that some areas of health promotion
are more evolved than others, as some issues are just emerging onto the agenda in a

gendered manner, such as workplace mental health, whereas others report on decades of attempts to integrate and transform gendered understandings of the issues, such as in the field of tobacco use. Other cases, such as preconception care, illustrate how a sex-linked issue—reproduction—is also highly gendered, and is therefore a useful training case for those researchers and practitioners who think sex-specific issues such as pregnancy are women's issues, and do not necessarily need a gender analysis.

Part 3 indicates how important it is to do effective and creative knowledge transfer and exchange, how to engage women and health practitioners in conscious-ness-raising using technology and other means, and how advocacy is a critical tool for health promotion, despite sometimes hostile or unreceptive political climates. Part 3 also delves into some difficult structural issues affecting how hospitals, whose mandate is delivering care to people with illnesses and conditions, can engage with health promotion principles and policy, and how in the interests of changing negative gender norms, men must become actively involved.

But what concrete measures can be taken to include the required strategic thinking, creativity, imagination, and courage in the task of generating more gender-transformative health promotion? We must actively link the outputs of women's economic, social, and political status to their health and that of their com-munities and families. These are outputs in the framework diagram (Figure 1.1) for a reason. They are the ultimate goals and measuring rods for the effectiveness of gender-transformative women's health promotion. Luckily, evidence is building on these links. Keleher and Franklin (2008) report on a wide review of studies and projects that attempt to change norms about women regarding education, vio-lence, female genital cutting (mutilation), and in male attitudes. While consistent evaluations and randomized control trials are rare, descriptive research indicates that it is clear that increasing education for girls, for example, not only results in better health for girls, women, and their children, but also better economic growth at the individual and country levels (Keleher & Franklin, 2008). Microeconomic anti-poverty projects have similar impact, but have the added benefit of increasing respect for women and developing leadership skills (CARE International, 2012). Keleher and Franklin (2008) report a less clear picture on changing men's attitudes of dominance and control, and indicate that in all of these areas, changing norms is difficult work, and needs to be supported at multiple levels within supportive policy and human and women's rights frameworks. Some work in the field of reproductive health, maternity, and HIV/AIDS shows that gender equality and men's attitudes and behaviour toward women can be influenced by health promotion efforts (Feldman-Jacobs, Yeakey, & Avni, 2011). Many of these elements of changing norms are interrelated—for example, when women's economic independence increases, so does the respect they receive and, as a consequence, practices such as female malnutrition and violence against women may decrease.

Overcoming Formidable Challenges

We must be blatant and very specific about the goals of women's health promotion in generating specific improvements in women's well-being, utilizing specific indicators such as freedom of movement and household decision-making power, political and labour force participation, and community engagement. Developing these sorts of specific indicators is an ongoing task, but often relies on the concepts of agency and empowerment. These efforts are gaining ground in efforts to understand how multi-level indicators such as household decision-making, autonomy, political empowerment, and access to credit can be used to measure, across a range of surveys, their impact on health, education, equity, or access to governance and leadership roles (Ibrahim & Alkire, 2007).

We must also be clear and creative about the principles and practices of participation, using new technologies to engage with women in both old and new ways—generating circles of consciousness-raising, information-sharing, social support, organizing and action in communities, politics, and research. Despite technological innovations not imagined 40 years ago, age-old principles of engagement, co-learning, respect, and action remain critically important elements of empowerment, especially for women and girls, who still experience basic structural inequalities such as limited access to education, land, food, or money.

Accountability cannot be overlooked. There are mechanisms, both formal and informal, for holding people, families, communities, countries, and international bodies to account for the impact of their actions, attitudes, policies, and legal decisions. These mechanisms can be used to expose and shame, punish and educate, set examples and chart new rules. Murthy (2008) suggests that there are several elements to accountability: answerability, enforcement, and responsiveness, among others. Murthy (2008) applies these concepts to gender and health by noting that women's health issues are often seen as controversial or of low priority. While these assessments reflect politics, religious, or cultural attitudes, there are mechanisms in use in several countries to insert rights to engagement, participation, information, access to services, patient's rights charters, report cards, and preservation of human rights (Murthy, 2008). While governments are often pressured for accountability, there is also opportunity for pressuring for accountability at multi-levels and in multi-sectors, including private donors and NGOs, and to include gender-based accountability mechanisms into these approaches. This area is ripe for gender-transformative accountability measures.

Overriding all of these measures, though, sexism and misogyny must be consistently confronted. They persist despite (or because of) gains in women's status in some countries. Even in a country like Australia, when a woman, Julia Gillard, was the prime minister until 2013, she remained the butt of constant sexist and disparaging attacks. These attacks were so marked and consistent that national organizations were publishing reports about it (Crooks, 2012), international media reported on it (*The New York Times*, for example), and the then prime minister herself addressed it in a long and strongly worded speech on October 10, 2012, in the House of Parliament (www.welvic.org.au/issues/sexism/). Reacting to such blatant attacks of sexism, especially against women leaders, is a constant preoccupation in contemporary Australia, with groups springing up to confront it publically (www. seeitsayitstopit.com, for example). Reacting to and naming such attitudes is important as changing the climate for women can be dependent upon such simple and broad-based actions. The same principle underpins the project described in Chapter 14 on the importance of addressing bystander attitudes about men's violence against women in male-dominated workplaces: changing the climate so that such misogyny and sexism do not go unremarked.

Equally formidable, yet less visible, are global forces such as globalization, capitalism, and various legislative and regulatory vacuums that create unequal and unhealthy conditions for women. Examples such as exploited beedi rollers and garment workers, human trafficking in women and girls, state-sanctioned tolerance and lack of responses to violence against women, or female genital mutilation are just a few examples of forces that create ill health in gendered ways. These forms of inequity require global action and advocacy, and there are encouraging signs (see, for example, the resistance to female genital mutilation, the Girl Effect, at www.girleffect.org/news/2013/03/ending-female-genital-mutilation-dr-isatou-tourays-fight-against-fgm/; and Hands Off!, http://nowscape.com/islam/FGM-Africa1.htm; and Human Rights Watch, www.hrw.org/topic/womens-rights/trafficking-women-and-girls, the resistance to human trafficking of and violence against girls and women).

Inspiring Rights- and Principle-Based Starting Points

Several waves of intellectual change offer support for addressing these multi-level barriers, and for creating gender-transformative health promotion. There is growing theory, practice, and awareness of women's health and health promotion as a distinct enterprise, and supportive research deriving more and more sex- and gender-related evidence to support change. There is growing interest in the conversation about the social determinants of health and their effects on inequity and women's health, despite the huge challenges they represent. Feminism and other social justice movements continue to offer homes for generating new health promotion practice, building on the waves of social change generated by women's and other social movements over the past centuries. There are international documents and, in some cases, instruments or treaties that form a bedrock for country-based action and advocacy, offering support for activists around the world. Examples of these include the Convention on the Elimination of All Forms of Discrimination Against Women (United Nations, 1979), the World Health Organization gender policy (World Health Organization, 2002), and human rights instruments. International public health treaties such as the WHO-Framework Convention on Tobacco Control (WHO-FCTC) (World Health Organization, 2003) and the global alcohol strategy (World Health Organization, 2010) address specific issues such as tobacco use and alcohol use respectively, offering a framework for action and improved regulation. These documents offer opportunities for change in line with their expressed goals and conforming with their articles or sections. Organizations such as the Framework Convention Alliance, which is aimed at monitoring the FCTC progress, are also avenues for action and advocacy. In the case of the WHO-FCTC, over 170 countries have ratified the treaty and are bound to uphold its components, offering more than 170 potential sites for national advocacy and international pressure. Due to activism and the Kobe Declaration (World Health Organization, 1999), there is a strong gender statement in the preamble: "Alarmed by the increase in smoking and other forms of tobacco consumption by women and young girls worldwide and keeping in mind the need for full participation of women at all levels of policy-making and implementation and the need for gender-specific tobacco control strategies...." This statement, which precedes the articles of the WHO-FCTC, offers a guide for action and results as the monitoring of the FCTC is carried out. Despite this, the application of a gender lens in tobacco control, let alone a gender-transformative lens, requires constant vigilance (Amos, Greaves, Nichter, & Bloch, 2012).

Even when there is willingness to integrate gender and to engage with the complexities of gender in its many moving forms and meanings, and potentially to engage with gender-transformative ideas, however, there is a need for ongoing education, training, and creative sharing of ideas. Even when parties express good-will and a desire to change negative gender norms, they are often dependent upon ideas from the women's health movement. Hence, the biggest barrier and limit to gender-transformative health promotion may be our own imaginations.

A place to start is to engage with the principles identified in Chapter 1 that underpin the framework for gender-transformative health promotion. The integration of various principles into health promotion—such as capacity-building and engagement on elements of women-centredness, harm-reduction, and trauma-informed approaches—is key. Other principles—such as being equity-oriented, culturally safe, action-oriented, and strengths-based—all contribute to the receptivity and relevance of the health promotion initiative, policy, or program. And above all, making sure that initiatives are evidence-based is critical. Funders, sponsors, and donors can use their accountability to insist on evidence-based initiatives and proposals, while widening the notion of what constitutes "evidence" to include all kinds of data, released in a variety of formats, not strictly limited to highly controlled studies published in academic journals.

All of these aspects, as we have seen, are critically important for women, are very gendered, and are among the principles we used to move the framework development forward. Inherent in the project of creating gender-transformative health promotion, then, is more understanding and training on the utility of these principles and approaches. For example, the notion of women-centredness often includes respect for and understanding the social determinants of health; attention to inequity and social justice; and commitment to sex- and gender-specific research, program, and policy development. There are many health promotion projects aimed at women that do not include much consideration of these. For example, traditional behaviour-change approaches to tobacco reduction during pregnancy have often been devoid of sensitivity to inequities and social justice concerns such as poverty or violence, thereby losing their potential effectiveness in a sea of irrelevance or low priority. Using the same example of tobacco control, there has been little respectful attention paid to harm reduction in messaging to women and girls in health promotion campaigns regarding tobacco use, whether during pregnancy or not. More often, there has been reluctance to engage meaningfully with harm reduction in tobacco control, perhaps as it was seen to undermine the message that any tobacco use is unsafe. This omission, though, contributes to a lack of realism and relevance for many women (and others) who may be struggling with inequity, stigma, and mental health and addiction issues, complicating their responses to mainstream health promotion messages regarding tobacco use.

Finally, and more recently, the concept of trauma-informed approaches is gaining more ground, especially in mental health and addictions services (Poole & Greaves, 2012). This assumes that many individuals and some subpopulations are likely holding trauma from past and current experiences, such as violence, sexual assault, torture, disaster, or war. Addressing the possibility of this requires a broad trauma-informed framework that does not require personal disclosure but rather creates services, messages, and health promotion approaches that do not re-traumatize, coerce, or command, but alternatively engage in more sensitive ways. Health promotion for women is a particularly fertile arena for trauma-informed approaches, given the highly gendered nature of much trauma and violence. Following our example, how does this apply to tobacco control? Reducing the authoritative and coercive nature of tobacco reduction messages and tobacco-free health promotion would involve a more strengths-based approach, generating support and receptivity for tobacco reduction, prevention, or cessation based on individuals' current attributes and desires for change. It would also generate a more gender-sensitive and context-sensitive set of messages about tobacco use, and not assume that all women have equal resources, personal and economic, to apply to tobacco reduction or cessation. It would be less directive and more supportive and acknowledge the adaptive and coping-related functions of tobacco use for women, especially those with violence and trauma experiences (Urquhart, Jasiura, Poole, Nathoo, & Greaves, 2012). Similarly, when in personal contact, motivational interviewing by a health provider specifically builds upon such strengths and ideas for change, generating support for change within the individual or group.

Another starting point is media literacy. Examining mainstream health promotion from a critical standpoint is essential to generating gender-transformative health promotion. This is possible only if training in critical thinking and media literacy is part of training and education for all. Unless such training is incorporated into health promotion training, as well as into public education, especially for young people, there will be no reaction to the ongoing reinforcement of negative gender norms that is the crux of much standard health promotion. For example, if the notion of appealing to girls and women via their vanity, as opposed to their health, persists unremarked upon and without negative feedback from audiences, such approaches will reinforce such gendered stereotypes and notions and feed a vicious circle. But critiquing is not enough. There is a need for creativity in generating gender-transformative health promotion as well. And many interested and willing parties will look to the women's health movement for inspiration. We will need to partner with creative and progressive advertising agencies and social marketers, conversant in all digital media to up-end typical health promotion treatment of gender, women, and girls. This will allow for more inventive and creative approaches to be floated, as part of the changing of the normative culture.

Articulating the links between economic development and the reduction of gender inequity offers another key opportunity for making the argument for gender-transformative health promotion. What economic improvements can be accomplished through doing gender-transformative health promotion? As discussed in the Introduction, the empowerment of women and girls liberates energy and intellect from half of the population to be applied to economic activity and development. This is a formidable augmentation in any country, whether high, middle, or low income. Such a release enables entire families and communities to change their economic outlook. The empowerment of women also potentially engages a broader proportion of the population in governance, although not without considerable backlash in some settings. Engagement of women in health promotion design will escalate and spread into collective engagement in community life, politics, and spinoff leadership efforts. The integration of health promotion initiatives into a political cycle involving advocacy, activism, policy change, and engagement lead to more participation in public life. Being able to measure these effects in increasingly specific ways is critical to understanding the effects on multiple levels, from individual empowerment and agency to broad-based political and legal changes. Changes in women's health and status for the better lifts all as they invariably improve infant, child, and family health as well.

The challenge of generating a sea change in health promotion practice, research, and policy to introduce gender transformation is a tall order and a big issue. It may even be a wicked problem, reflecting multiple aspects and interrelated issues and a feeling of intractability. The record of making progress on similar big issues, such as improving the social determinants of health or generating inter-sectoral and inter-ministerial "health in all policies" initiatives, is discouraging. These types of challenges are meant to raise the bar on thinking about health and health equity, as well as on the recommended solutions. But generating changes on social determinants, for example, often feels formidable and requires engagement with broader issues such as housing or poverty, which can seem intractable and beyond the scope of singular health promotion specialists. "Health in all policies" has been touted in several countries as a solution to such big problems by suggesting that policies be designed in all areas of government with a view to their impact on health and health equity outcomes (Kickbusch & Buckett, 2010; Leppo, Ollila, Pena, Wismar, & Cook, 2013), but this approach has been slow to get off the ground. The reasons for this are many—from short-sighted politicians unwilling to look beyond their mandates, to ministry-bound thinking, to lack of economic resources, leadership, and lack of training and tools for doing so (Greaves & Bialystok, 2011). But overall, changing deep-seated issues such as gendered and often sexist and inequitable social and economic conditions is often considered an insurmountable challenge.

Conclusion: Creating a Sea Change

Nonetheless, we have cause to be optimistic. This book and the notion of gender-transformative health promotion offer a path forward for improving women's health and status in tandem. We hope that there is within it the inspiration to reach higher and to pursue more lofty goals than mainstream health promotion currently does. We hope that the framework and planning tool serve as a map for change, and inspire all who are engaged in health promotion initiatives, programming, and policy to reach for transformations.

There have been many positive legal and social changes for women and girls over the past century on a range of multi-level issues; global movements for change are engaging women; there is renewed disgust and reaction to global violence against women; and increased sharing of women's knowledge through new technologies and digital media. They can all give us cause for hope. Even sparks of creativity and hope dot the field of health promotion, such as the I Stand campaign, which resists weight bigotry for girls (see Figure 15.1 and more images at http://istandagainstweightbullying.tumblr.com/). This controversial campaign was derived in response to the State of Georgia's Strong4Life campaign (www.strong4life.com), which used images of an overweight girl (among others) with the tag line "WARNING: It's hard to be a little girl if you're not" to address one of the most mainstream issues in contemporary health promotion: obesity. The I Stand campaign neatly articulates a clear, realistic, and relevant response that simultaneously respects and celebrates strong girls and presents a real-life image to counter linear and punitive interpretations of weight-control messaging. The counter-advertising stirred controversy, but persisted in making the point that shaming young girls (and others) who were overweight was inhumane and counterproductive. Such organizations as About-Face, a website devoted to equipping girls with media literacy skills, articulate the response and why the Strong4Life campaign was ill conceived. See www.about-face.org/georgias-strong4life-campaign-relies-heavily-on-fat-shaming/#.UdN8l-Co5vA for the full story.

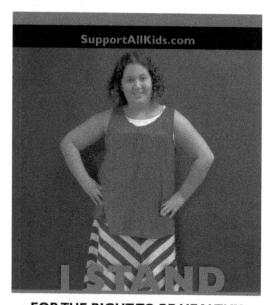

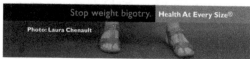

FIGURE 15.1: I Stand against Weight Bullying Campaign Poster

Source: I Stand against Weight Bullying (http://istandagainstweightbullying.tumblr.com).

Our contribution in this book has been to design a concrete tool and an overarching framework that, if enacted, will assist in designing health promotion that will further such efforts and assist in improving girls' and women's health and status at the same time. Creating a sea change in the valuation of women and girls is one starting point, and involves the recognition that health promotion issues are perhaps a wider and longer list than typically assumed. In addition, as the engagement of women, communities, and government increase, this will go a long way to generating more realistic and respectful gendered health promotion, thereby transforming itself.

REFERENCES

Amos, A., Greaves, L., Nichter, M., & Bloch, M. (2012). Women and tobacco: A call for including gender in tobacco control research, policy, and practice. *Tobacco Control, 21*(2), 236–243.

CARE International. (2012). *Reaching new heights. The case for measuring women's empowerment*. Retrieved from www.care-international.org/uploaddocument/news/publications/reports%20and%20issue%20briefs/english/international%20womens%20day_women%20empowerment_care%20report%202012.pdf

Cook, C. (2009). Women's health theorizing: A call for epistemic action. *Critical Public Health, 19*(2), 143–154.

Crooks, M. A. (2012). *Switch in time: Restoring respect for Australian politics*. Victoria, Australia: Victorian Women's Trust.

Feldman-Jacobs, C., Yeakey, M., & Avni, M. (2011). A summary report of new evidence that gender perspectives improve reproductive health outcomes: U.S. Agency for International Development and Interagency Gender Working Group. Washington, DC: Population Reference Bureau.

Greaves, L., & Bialystok, L. (2011). Health in all policies: All talk and little action? *Canadian Journal of Public Health, 102*(6), 407–409.

Ibrahim, S. A., & Alkire, S. (2007). *Agency and empowerment: A proposal for internationally comparable indicators*. Oxford: Oxford Poverty and Human Development Initiative (OPHI) Working Paper Series.

Johnson, J. L., Greaves, L., & Repta, R. (2007). *Better science with sex and gender: A primer for health research*. Vancouver: Women's Health Research Network.

Keleher, H., & Franklin, L. (2008). Changing gendered norms about women and girls at the level of household and community: A review of the evidence. *Journal for Research, Policy, and Practice, 3*(S1), 42–57.

Kickbusch, I., & Buckett, K. (2010). *Implementing health in all policies*. Geneva: Government of South Australia & World Health Organization.

Leppo, K., Ollila, E., Pena, S., Wismar, M., & Cook, S. (Eds.). (2013). *Health in all policies: Seizing opportunities, implementing policies* (Vol. 2013). Helsinki: Ministry of Social Affairs and Health, Finland.

Murthy, R. S. (2008). Strengthening accountability to citizens on gender and health. *Global Public Health, 3*(S1), 104–120.

Poole, N., & Greaves, L. (2012). *Becoming trauma informed.* Toronto: Centre for Addiction and Mental Health.

United Nations. (1979). *Convention on the elimination of all forms of discrimination against women.* Retrieved from www.un.org/womenwatch/daw/cedaw/cedaw.htm

Urquhart, C., Jasiura, F., Poole, N., Nathoo, T., & Greaves, L. (2012). *Liberation! Helping women quit smoking: A brief tobacco-intervention guide.* Vancouver: British Columbia Centre of Excellence for Women's Health.

World Health Organization. (1999). *Kobe declaration.* Retrieved from www.who.int/tobacco/framework/conferences/k_declaration/en/

World Health Organization. (2002). *Integrating gender perspectives in the work of WHO.* Geneva: Author.

World Health Organization. (2003). *WHO-Framework convention on tobacco control.* Geneva: Author.

World Health Organization. (2010). *Global strategy to reduce the harmful use of alcohol.* Geneva: Author.

Afterword

Helen Keleher

Over the years, health promotion as a field of research and practice has clearly struggled to demonstrate intended impacts and levels of effectiveness. Too often the results of health promotion initiatives have shown less than expected results. While we struggle to convince funding bodies to understand the long-term work that health promotion requires, this book also clearly shows that a lack of focus on gender and health undermines both effort and investment in health promotion, and that transformative approaches are critically necessary.

Globally, the field of health promotion has been patchy in its understanding of how to make a difference in women's health outcomes. Women around the world have fewer financial resources, less wealth and property, and higher burdens in the dual economies of paid and unpaid work. As well, women ensure the reproduction, well-being, and survival of others across the lifespan from youth to old age. As a result, there are significant groups of women whose health is compromised by their life experiences. The editors and the contributing authors of this book have clearly made the case that when health promotion is gender-neutral, it is missing key elements necessary for effectiveness.

While other frameworks have been put forward to assist health promoters and policy-makers to apply an equity lens over their work, one key premise of this book is that an equity lens alone is not sufficient. The authors clearly demonstrate that goals to achieve gender-equity outcomes from health promotion are necessary, and that dominant approaches to health promotion tend to be derived from male-centred norms that fail women and do little, if anything, to increase gender equity. Indeed, health promotion that lacks gender-equity strategies is likely to increase gender inequities for women. So despite the proliferation of charters, guidelines, policies,

263

and strategies developed since the Ottawa Charter in 1986, the lack of focus on gender equity is a vital missing link that must be fixed if health promotion work is to reach its potential for improving women's health.

The discussion and analysis, examples, case studies, and theoretical advances put forward in this book are relevant not only to developed countries—they apply to any country, globally. The framework for gender-transformative health promotion is applicable universally to different cultures and diverse places. Certainly, the concepts of the gender lens and gender equity are not new, nor is the rationale for a focus on women, and yet health promotion and indeed the broader fields of public health are not thought of as fields where breakthroughs in gender thinking and practice have been achieved. That said, neither health promotion nor public health has had the benefit of such a coherent and cogent approach as this book offers. Those at all levels of development and decision making involved in policy and practice guidelines, as well as academics involved in theory and practice, should read this book and reflect on what the authors are saying about how to increase the effectiveness of their work by using gender approaches to health promotion.

This book has the potential to transform health promotion. The framework for gender-transformative health promotion is a breakthrough for health promotion and provides a solid anchor for the book. Many topics are covered—tobacco, alcohol, housing, violence, preconception care, mental health promotion, workplace health, advocacy, and women's hospitals—and are all blended with a focus on the social determinants of women's health. Through these case studies and examples, the authors set out to show how we can reconceptualize health promotion for women to make health promotion more effective, and they have achieved just that. Chapter after chapter illustrates the benefits of working from a position that seeks to improve gender equity along with women's health, illustrating how such a reframing of thinking and actions makes a difference in health promotion practice, theory, and policy.

The authors have not ignored the very real challenges of the widespread and deeply rooted resistance to notions of gender equity for women. Rather, they have carefully thought through the feasibility and future of the framework and gender-transformative health promotion amid the politics of gender and women's health. The rationale they provide will be useful to all of us who face the often relentless opposition to a focus on women and to the concept of gender equity for women. They remind us that the task of gender transformation requires creativity, a gender-informed imagination, courage, patience, and resilience, but, most importantly, a critical evidence base. They also remind us that men can be directly involved in addressing women's health, and gender-transformative approaches to men's health would benefit all. All of these approaches are necessary to effect change.

There are many lessons learned and shared in this book to which we can and will return, over and over, as we navigate the challenging change processes that will bring gender-transformative health promotion into everyday practice. I look forward to seeing new units of study in health promotion courses based on this work that are focused on gender-transformative health promotion. Both women and men will benefit from the learning that such courses offer, with the support of this book for guidance to theory and practice and to inform learning. Everyone working in health promotion (and public health) has the responsibility to understand gender power relations and their relevance for their work, as well as a clear responsibility to understand the social factors and conditions of living in determining health and illness outcomes. Once these are acknowledged, the next step is to find solutions to gender-neutral health promotion by using the framework and planning tool in this book to transform practice and outcomes.

I was first invited two years ago to participate in a Melbourne consultation examining the preliminary elements of the framework, and to discuss issues in its application. Since then, I have been struck by the detailed development and consultation processes that underpin it and its important relevance to our work in the field, the academy, and in communities. Most of all, I am struck by how important this book could be to the health and welfare of women and girls worldwide. I have keenly awaited the publication of the book, and reading it has been an uplifting experience. Some books become good friends because they are so interesting, useful, inspiring, and original, and this is one of them. Thank you to all involved in its creation.

Helen Keleher is director of population health at the Frankston-Mornington Peninsula Medicare Local, where she is developing both population health knowledge and an applied research program. She is professor (adjunct) with the School of Public Health and Preventive Medicare, Monash University, and has published widely in health promotion, primary health care, and health equity. She was national convenor of the Australian Women's Health Network from 1999 to 2005 and a member of the Women and Gender Equity Knowledge Network of the WHO Commission on Social Determinants of Health from 2006 to 2008. She is a board member of the South East Melbourne Medicare Local, and immediate past president of the Public Health Association of Australia.

Contributor Biographies

Paola Ardiles, MHSc, is an immigrant woman and mother of two. She obtained her master's degree in health promotion from the University of Toronto in 2006. Paola has since served as a knowledge-broker by linking research, policy, and practice in mental health promotion, health equity, health literacy, cultural competency, immigrant and refugee health, women's mental health, workplace health, and social inclusion. She participates in capacity-building work and research on ethno-cultural and social determinants of postpartum depression. Paola is an adviser to the PhiWomen research team and also a knowledge-user on a provincial research program investigating health equity in British Columbia. In 2012, CMHA-BC awarded Paola with the Dr. Nancy Hall Public Policy Leadership Award of Distinction for her local, provincial, and national work to advance mental health. Today, she is the founder and leader of Bridge 4 Health, a dynamic collective platform to foster interdisciplinary collaboration and citizen engagement to promote health and well-being for all.

Jill Atkey, MA, is director of research and education at BC Non-Profit Housing Association. She has been involved in community-based research and community development in the non-profit sector for 15 years in British Columbia and Alberta. She has co-written numerous reports on housing, income security, and poverty-reduction policies and programs. Recent projects include the development of 25-year projections of rental housing demand and core housing need for British Columbia and 28 regional districts. She recently worked with a team to develop a tool kit to raise awareness of the barriers to housing for women leaving violence, which includes a short film and facilitator's guide. She is the co-leader on a project exploring housing barriers for immigrant and refugee women leaving violence. Jill has an MA from the School of Community and Regional Planning at the University of British Columbia.

Petra Begnell is program and strategic development manager for Women's Health Victoria. She has a background in nursing, education, and health promotion. Her current focus is the prevention of violence against women. Career highlights include leading Women's Health Victoria's involvement in the successful advocacy campaign that removed abortion from the Crimes Act in Victoria, creating a suite of workshops for health professionals that build skills around gender-sensitive practice, and developing an Australian first program that uses the workplace as a setting to engage men in preventing violence against women.

Lauren Bialystok, PhD, has worked in women's health as a policy analyst, researcher, and peer educator. She has held positions at the Ministry of Health and Long-Term Care (Ontario), Planned Parenthood of Toronto, and as a researcher at the British Columbia Centre of Excellence for Women's Health. She is trained in philosophy and brings feminist and ethical theory to her study of women's health issues. Lauren is an assistant professor in the Department of Humanities, Social Science, and Social Justice Education at the Ontario Institute for Studies in Education, University of Toronto.

Judie Bopp, MA, PhD, is a co-founder of the Four Worlds Centre for Development Learning. She holds a master's degree in multicultural education and a doctorate in organizational development, and has provided training, technical support, and evaluation services related to program development and organizational change to many groups, ranging from the ministries of national governments to small non-governmental organizations and professional bodies in Asia, the South Pacific, Africa, Eastern Europe, the Caribbean, and indigenous North America. Judie's publications include a basic text on community development entitled *Recreating the World: A Practical Guide to Building Sustainable Communities, Aboriginal Domestic Violence in Canada,* and *Mapping the Healing Journey.* She has worked in Canada's North since 2006 on issues related to women's homelessness and mental health. She is also currently working with village leaders in northern Pakistan to build sustainable solutions to their economic and social development challenges.

Sophie Dupéré, PhD, is assistant professor in the Faculty of Nursing at Université Laval. She has been involved in community health/health promotion in Canada and internationally for the last 15 years, working as a nurse, consultant, researcher, and activist. She is the co-editor of three books, one of which was the third edition of *Health Promotion in Canada*, and has written a number of articles on poverty, social health inequalities, gender and women's health, and participatory approaches.

Rose Durey, LLB, MA, is a senior policy officer in the Screening and Cancer Prevention Unit at the Department of Health in Victoria, Australia. She previously worked as policy and health promotion manager at Women's Health Victoria, where she coordinated *Working Together Against Violence*, a VicHealth-funded project aimed at the primary prevention of violence against women. Prior to joining Women's Health Victoria, Rose worked in policy and research at an adoption and fostering organization in the United Kingdom. Rose has a law degree from the University of Western Australia and a master of social science (policy and human services) from RMIT University in Melbourne.

Mei Lan Fang, MPH, holds a master of public health degree from Simon Fraser University. Her capstone project was entitled, "Coping with Bereavement: Exploring Psychological Well-being, Religious Practices, Beliefs, and Support Needs of Manchester's Chinese Population." She is a research trainee at the Centre for the Study of Gender, Social Inequities, and Mental Health, focusing on health needs and social justice initiatives for immigrant and refugee populations.

Wendy Frisby, PhD, is a professor in the School of Kinesiology and the former chair of women's and gender studies at the University of British Columbia. She has received several grants and a number of awards for her community-based health promotion research with immigrant women and women living on low incomes. Dr. Frisby and her collaborators use a feminist participatory action research approach to examine the role of community physical activity in reducing social isolation. In 2011, the Canadian Association for the Advancement of Women and Sport listed her as one of the most influential women in Canada.

Julieta Gerbrandt, MSc, holds a master of science degree in human nutrition from the University of British Columbia. Her graduate work focused on human nutrition and food security of people living with disabilities. Her experience includes working as a research assistant in the Institute of Health Promotion Research as well as in the Nursing and Health Behaviour Research Unit at the University of British Columbia. She was a project coordinator for the British Columbia Centre of Excellence for Women's Health, where she focused on research relating to promoting health in women.

Kathy GermAnn, PhD, is an independent researcher, writer, and consultant in health and human services and an adjunct assistant professor at the Centre for Health Promotion Studies at the University of Alberta's School of Public Health. Informed by over 30 years of practice in the health system, a PhD in organizational analysis, and a master's degree in health promotion, her key areas of interest include mental health promotion, particularly the organizational determinants of working and well-being; organizational capacity for health promotion and community development; and the complex, emergent dynamics of organizational change, inter-organizational collaboration, and system-level change in the public sector.

Lorraine Greaves, PhD, is a medical sociologist, senior investigator at the British Columbia Centre of Excellence for Women's Health and its former executive director from 1997 to 2009. She has worked in academic, government, education, and NGO settings. Dr. Greaves is an international expert in tobacco use, women and gender, and also does research on addictions, violence, and trauma. She is the lead mentor of IMPART, a Canadian Institutes for Health Research-funded training program in gender, women, addiction, and mental health issues. She has published numerous books on subjects such as: social research methods, the inclusion of sex and gender in health research, women's smoking, women's substance use in Canada, and trauma-informed health systems. Dr. Greaves also carries out a knowledge translation program aimed at integrating gender and diversity analyses into health knowledge, programs, interventions, policies, and organizational development. Among her awards are the Laura Jamieson Prize, the YWCA Woman of Distinction Award, and an honorary doctorate from the University of Ottawa.

Natalie Hemsing, MA, is a research associate at the British Columbia Centre of Excellence for Women's Health. She has an extensive background in primary and secondary research on sex- and gender-based analysis; smoking prevention, cessation, and tobacco policy among diverse populations; and systematic reviews and knowledge syntheses. She has been involved in research projects on smoking reduction and cessation among pregnant women and their partners; the impact of second-hand smoke policies; smoking cessation in substance use and trauma treatment settings; tobacco use among Aboriginal girls; women's respiratory and heart health; and domestic violence.

Karin H. Humphries, PhD, holds the UBC-Heart and Stroke Foundation Professor in Women's Cardiovascular Health and is an associate professor in the Faculty of Medicine at the University of British Columbia. She has a doctorate in epidemiology and a background in biochemistry, kinesiology, and experimental pathology. Her areas of special interest are in cardiovascular epidemiology with a focus on outcomes following coronary interventions. Dr. Humphries is a co-investigator on three national teams: two looking at cardiovascular outcomes, the Canadian Cardiovascular Outcomes Research Team (CCORT), Gender and Sex Differences in Cardiovascular Disease (GENESIS); and one with the British Columbia Centre of Excellence for Women's Health, which built a health promotion framework for women's health promotion. Her primary research focus is sex differences in the diagnosis, treatment, and outcomes of patients with coronary disease. Dr. Humphries is conducting studies on the sex differences in health-related quality of life in young adults who have suffered a myocardial infarction and an institutional ethnographic approach to understanding inequities in health-related experiences among mid-life men and women following an acute myocardial infarction.

Mona Izadnegahdar, PhD, completed her doctorate in epidemiology at the University of British Columbia, School of Population and Public Health, and her master's degree in epidemiology at the University of Calgary, Department of Community Health Sciences, Faculty of Medicine. Her main research interests include cardiovascular epidemiology, quality of life, access to care, and in particular understanding the contributing factors to the poor outcomes and health status of younger adults following a heart attack. Her doctoral thesis examined sex differences in outcomes of younger adults following a heart attack, and was supported by the Canadian Institutes of Health Research Frederick Banting and Charles Best Doctoral Award and the Canadian Cardiovascular Outcomes Research Team (CCORT). Over the last 10 years, she has developed expertise in the area of cardiovascular research, working at the Centre for Health Evaluation and Outcomes Sciences, the Providence Health Research Institute and Cardiac Services BC, and currently as an epidemiologist at the British Columbia Centre for Improved Cardiovascular Health (ICVHealth).

Donna S. Lee, MA, holds a master of arts degree (kinesiology) and a bachelor of arts degree (sociology), both from the University of British Columbia. Her research interests include immigrant women's health and well-being, intersectionality, and interculturalism. She is a former municipal recreation programmer and coordinator of a provincial health promotion initiative to increase access to physical activity for adults living on low income. She plans to pursue a PhD, which will build on her research interests and explore the use of visual methods in community-based research.

Farah Mawani is a PhD candidate at the Dalla Lana School of Public Health, University of Toronto, and a visiting scholar at Massey College. She has experience in global research, policy, teaching, writing, and advocacy in social determinants of mental health inequalities. She currently focuses on the negative impact of workplace environments, discrimination, and human rights abuses on mental health inequalities. She also focuses on the positive and transformative capacity of peer support to reduce mental health inequalities. She has experience in national roles, including as senior policy and research analyst, mental health strategy, at the Mental Health Commission of Canada; Multicultural Mental Health Resource Centre Steering Committee member; Mental Health Reform and Policy research team, Centre for the Study of Gender, Social Inequities, and Mental Health; and national coordinator for numerous national health research projects. She is a founding member of the Centre for Social Innovation—Regent Park in Toronto.

Ann Pederson, MSc, is director of population health promotion at British Columbia Women's Hospital & Health Centre, and was previously at the British Columbia Centre of Excellence for Women's Health for over 15 years. She has co-edited three books on health promotion in Canada, and is engaged in several projects related to healthy living and women. In particular, she is involved in research on efforts to support women's involvement in physical activity and chronic disease prevention, and is completing a study using an equity lens to examine the introduction of the smoking ban on parks and beaches in Vancouver. She has created numerous guides, curricula, and training packages on gender-inclusive health planning and the use of sex-, gender-, and diversity-based analysis in the health field. Ann is also a member of the board of the Canadian Public Health Association.

Pamela Ponic, PhD, was a post-doctoral research trainee on the Promoting Health in Women Emerging Team. She uses feminist participatory research and knowledge translation to understand and address the social determinants of women's health and health promotion. Her primary post-doctoral work was a Photovoice project on the barriers to housing for women fleeing violence, from which an advocacy report and digital storytelling tool kit was produced. She worked with a team of researchers at the British Columbia Centre of Excellence in Women's Health to explore how trauma-informed approaches to physical activity can improve opportunities for marginalized women.

Nancy Poole, MA, is director of research and knowledge translation at the British Columbia Centre of Excellence for Women's Health in Vancouver. She has over 20 years of experience in research, policy, and practice relating to health promotion, prevention, treatment, and harm reduction for women with alcohol, tobacco, and other substance use problems. She is well known for her leadership in fetal alcohol spectrum disorder prevention, trauma-informed systems, and women-centred responses to substance use. She was the 2009 Healthway Health Promotion visiting research fellow sponsored by Curtin University and the Government of Western Australia. Nancy is also known in Canada for leadership in piloting online participatory methods for knowledge generation and exchange on women's health, including virtual networks and online communities of inquiry.

Colleen Reid, PhD, teaches in the Faculty of Child, Family and Community Studies at Douglas College. She earned her PhD from the University of British Columbia in 2002 and completed a post-doctoral fellowship from Simon Fraser University in 2007. Colleen's areas of interest include gender and women's health, intersectionality, health promotion and community development, the determinants of health, and community-based research.

Gerald Thomas, PhD, received his doctorate in political science from Colorado State University in 1998 and has worked in Canada in addictions research and policy since 2001. He served on the secretariat of the group that created Canada's first National Alcohol Strategy in 2007, and has collaborated with researchers from the British Columbia Centre of Excellence for Woman's Health on a number of projects involving women and alcohol. Dr. Thomas is a senior research and policy analyst with the Canadian Centre on Substance Abuse and a collaborating scientist with the Centre of Addictions Research of British Columbia.

Elizabeth Whynot, MD, led British Columbia Women's Hospital & Health Centre for eight years, retiring as president in 2008. While at BC Women's, she was responsible for patient services for a variety of provincial initiatives to improve the health of women. As a member of the Provincial Health Services Authority Executive Committee, Liz was responsible for the development of its HIV/AIDS and Aboriginal health strategies. BC Women's was awarded the 2007 Arthur Kroeger Public Affairs Award for Management. Liz is a board member of the First Nations Health Authority, and works part-time as a locum physician at inner city clinics in Vancouver.

Lynne Young, RN, PhD, is professor at the University of Victoria's School of Nursing. She completed a PhD in nursing with a focus on health promotion and women's health. Her work focuses on developing knowledge for nursing and nursing education. She is co-editor of an award-winning book on health promotion and co-editor of a book on student-centred teaching. She is a member of a Canadian Institutes for Health Research-funded research team developing knowledge for health promotion for women and co-site leader for the Victoria site of the Canadian Longitudinal Study on Aging.

Index

Copyright Acknowledgements